NATURAL ALTERNATIVES

to Over-the-Counter and Prescription Drugs

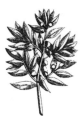

Michael T. Murray, N.D.

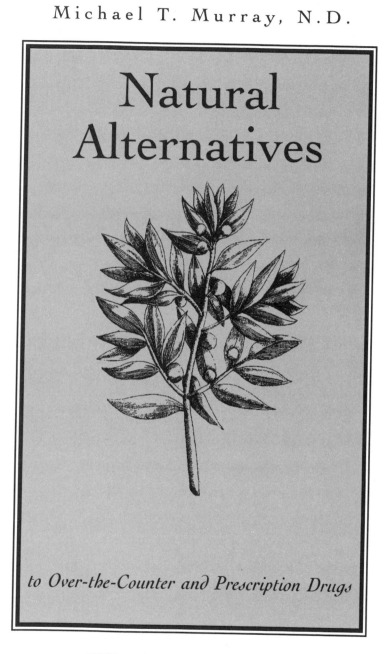

Natural Alternatives

to Over-the-Counter and Prescription Drugs

William Morrow and Company, Inc.
New York

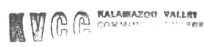

IMPORTANT: PLEASE READ

The information in this book is intended to increase your knowledge about natural remedies and by no means is intended to diagnose or treat an individual's health problems or ailments. The information given is not medical advice nor is it presented as a course of personalized treatment. There may be risks involved in connection with some of the natural remedies suggested in this book, just as there may be risks involved in connection with prescription drugs. Therefore, before starting any type of natural remedy or medical treatment, or before discontinuing any course of medical treatment you may now be undergoing, you should consult your own health-care practitioner.

Copyright © 1994 by Michael T. Murray and Trillium Health Products

It is the policy of William Morrow and Company, Inc., and its imprints and affiliates, recognizing the importance of preserving what has been written, to print the books we publish on acid-free paper, and we exert our best efforts to that end.

Library of Congress Cataloging-in-Publication Data

Murray, Michael T.
    Natural alternatives to over-the-counter and prescription drugs /
    Michael T. Murray.
        p.   cm.
    Includes bibliographical references and index.
    ISBN 0-688-12358-9
    1. Naturopathy. I. Title.
RZ440.M87   1994
615.5'35—dc20   93-14152
                                                       CIP

Printed in the United States of America

First Edition

1 2 3 4 5 6 7 8 9 10

BOOK DESIGN BY PATRICE FODERO

To Dr. Ralph Weiss,
my inspiration to become a naturopathic physician,
and
Dr. Joseph Pizzorno,
for his incredible accomplishments
on behalf of naturopathic medicine

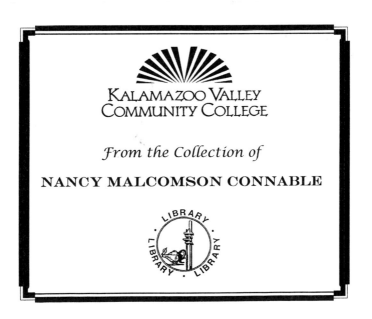

PREFACE

My journey into the area of natural medicine began like that of so many others who seek an answer to their health problems. Frustrated by conventional medicine, at the urging of my father I went to see a naturopathic physician, a doctor of natural medicine, Dr. Ralph Weiss. It was an experience that changed my life forever.

Eighteen months before seeing Dr. Weiss, my leg had been operated on for a long-standing knee injury. I was a freshman at the University of Oregon at the time of the operation. After the four-hour operation, my orthopedic surgeon stated that I would be very fortunate if I were ever able to walk without a limp. He recommended that I take up golf and swimming for exercise. Jogging, basketball, and similar activities were out of the question. After having my leg in a cast for three months, I began doing everything in my power to rehabilitate the knee. I wanted to have a full and physically active life that included basketball, racquet sports, and jogging, but after a year and a half, I was still unable to place any significant stress on my knee. My left leg was still only about 50 percent as strong as my right leg. I could walk without a noticeable limp, but I wasn't happy with my situation. I finally gave in to my father's request to see Dr. Weiss.

I was very skeptical about naturopathic medicine at first. Sure, I knew Dr. Weiss had helped people I knew, including family members, but I did not believe that he would be able to help me. After all, I had been to one of the top knee specialists in the world. My doubts about Dr. Weiss were quickly eliminated the moment we met. I could tell he was a different kind of doctor. He was concerned about my knee, but he was also interested in my diet and life-style. He explained things to me about my body in terms that I could understand. He spoke with great confidence about how the body possesses a tremendous ability to heal itself. In a long-standing condition like mine, it was necessary to remove obstacles that were preventing my knee from healing properly.

He explained to me the basic principles of acupuncture. He told me that there are energy channels known as meridians, which flow through the body, and how scientists now know these energy patterns exist. He felt that perhaps my knee was not responding because there was a blockage of energy flow. This information all sounded a bit strange, but somehow, it made sense to me. The principles behind acupuncture struck a chord deep within me and resonated with truth.

Dr. Weiss then proceeded to give me an electro-acupuncture treatment; that is to say, he used an electrical device to stimulate acupuncture points around my knee corresponding to the meridians he felt were blocked. In a matter of minutes, my weak leg became about 80 to 90 percent as strong as my healthy leg. I could literally feel my leg come alive again. I was totally amazed. As far as I was concerned, it was a miracle. That evening, I played basketball without pain for the first time in many years.

I decided I had to learn more about naturopathic medicine. I changed my major to premed so that I could meet the admission requirements of the four-year doctor of naturopathic medicine program at the Bastyr College of Natural Health Sciences in Seattle, Washington.

My first class at Bastyr was Naturopathic Philosophy. Dr. Joe Pizzorno, president of Bastyr College, led a discussion concerning the scientific validity of naturopathic medicine. The discussion inspired me, and I remember saying, "If naturopathy is based on truth, then it should be able to be explained in current scientific thought." Dr. Pizzorno was quick to point out that while there was substantial information on the effects of diet and life-style routinely prescribed by naturopaths, some of the more esoteric healing methods used by naturopaths have not been fully investigated from a scientific perspective. He explained that it would probably be many years in the future before science had evolved to a level of sophistication necessary to understand some of these techniques. He encouraged me to seek out scientific explanations for the therapies that could be expressed in current terminology associated with nutrition and herbal medicine.

My interest in naturopathic medicine having been galvanized, I have since dedicated my life to collecting and disseminating information that supports the use of natural medicines from a scientific perspective.

This book is designed to inform readers about the many natural alternatives to the drugs they are taking. My belief is that the natural approach will provide a safer, more effective, and permanent means of restoring health.

May you live in good health.

—Michael T. Murray, N.D.

FOREWORD

The health-care system in the United States is in a state of crisis. We are bankrupting our economy by spending nearly a trillion dollars a year on medical care—and the types of treatments we are offered are often inappropriate, ineffective, and unnecessarily dangerous.

Over the years, I have heard horror stories from hundreds of patients who have been injured or harmed by "usual and customary" medical treatments. The number of patients who have failed to find relief from the conventional drug-and-surgery approach is even greater.

Health-care reform is now on the minds of millions of Americans, and rightly so: The current system does not work. Practitioners of nutritional and natural medicine have known for a long time that, to be successful and cost-effective, the health-care system must emphasize proper diet, exercise, stress reduction, and appropriate use of nutritional supplements, plant extracts, and other naturally occurring substances.

Several years ago, while giving a presentation to a group of naturopathic physicians, I asked if anyone in the audience frequently heard that natural medicine had helped patients after conventional medicine failed. Nearly everyone in the room raised their hands. The response did not surprise me. Although I was trained as a conventional M.D., it had not taken me long to discover that natural medicine was safer, less expensive, and often more effective that the medicines I had been taught to prescribe.

Most conventional doctors continue to resist what they call "alternative medicine." Of course, what is labeled "alternative" sometimes has more to do with who controls the media and the medical disciplinary boards than what is in the best interests of the patient. The medical establishment maintains that nutritional therapy, botanical (herbal) medicine, and other alternative treatments are "unproven," and should therefore not be accepted into the medical mainstream. However, that argument ignores two important facts.

First, the practice of medicine is an art rather than a science. Most of the treatments that doctors prescribe every day are no more "proven" than are the alternative methods they criticize. Accepting unproven and dangerous treatments, while rejecting safer and less expensive natural alternatives, is a bizarre double standard.

Second, those who decry the lack of scientific data supporting alternative medicine have not been keeping up with the medical literature. During the past ten years, hundreds of scientific papers have been published that document the safety and effectiveness of dietary modifications, nutritional supplements, herbs, exercise, acupuncture, and other alternative treatments. These reports have appeared in mainstream medical journals.

For almost twenty years, Jonathan Wright, M.D., and I have been collecting scientific papers related to the field of natural medicine. The Wright/Gaby research files now contain more than twenty-two thousand articles from medical journals. Since 1984, most of the responsibility for this ongoing collection has been assumed by Dr. Michael Murray. Dr. Wright and I are fortunate to be associated with a man whose encyclopedic knowledge of the current natural-medicine literature is matched by his capacity to search tirelessly through thousands of titles each week, looking for new advances.

When I met Michael Murray in 1984, he was a brilliant and highly motivated naturopathic medical student. Since that time, he has become recognized as one of America's leading authorities on natural medicine, with a particular expertise in herbal medicine. In this book, Dr. Murray describes effective natural remedies for many common medical conditions.

It is noteworthy that most of the substances mentioned in this book can be purchased in a health-food store or supermarket—without a prescription. However, self-care should never be a substitute for proper diagnosis and follow-up by a trained professional. While many doctors are so closed-minded that their patients are afraid to tell them they are using alternative treatments, a growing number are becoming interested in natural medicine. I have observed that doctors who try incorporating natural medicine into their practice almost always continue to do so. There is, of course, something appealing about increasing your success rate while dramatically reducing the incidence of side effects.

Special interests that profit from the status quo are threatened by even the thought of a system that emphasizes self-care and relies mainly on inexpensive, nonpatentable medicines. Those special-interest groups spend billions of dollars each year to market the type of medical care from which they profit. A portion of that money is used to disseminate propaganda against natural alternatives.

Because of the efforts of Dr. Murray and others, the medical profession is slowly becoming aware that there are legitimate alternatives to drugs and surgery. As the research and data supporting natural medicine continue to increase, and as the limitations and dangers of conventional medicine become more widely appreciated, natural medicine will emerge as the only reasonable alternative.

—Alan R. Gaby, M.D.

Alan R. Gaby, M.D., is a member of the advisory panel of the National Institutes of Health Office of Alternative Medicine.

ACKNOWLEDGMENTS

Most of all, I would like to acknowledge my wife, Gina. Her love, support, and patience are the major blessings in my life. Also, I want to give a very heartfelt thanks to my parents, Cliff and Patty Murray, and my parents-in-law, Robert and Kathy Bunton, for their incredible love, support, and true friendship.

There are numerous other people to whom I owe my deepest appreciation: Terry Lemerond and everyone at Enzymatic Therapy for all of their support over the years; Dr. Alan Gaby for his friendship and for writing the foreword to this book; Dr. Walter Cannion and everyone at The Northwest Healing Arts Center; students and faculty at Bastyr College who have given me encouragement and support; and my editors, Will Schwalbe and Zachary Schisgal and copy editor Robbie Capp for their contributions to this book.

I must also acknowledge the researchers, physicians, and scientists who over the years have striven to better understand the use of natural medicines. The evolution in understanding occurring in medicine is largely a result of long, hard hours of study and research by individuals who never experience the public spotlight. Without their work, this book would not exist, and medical progress would halt.

And finally, I would like to thank you, the reader, for granting me the opportunity to share with you *Natural Alternatives to Over-the-Counter and Prescription Drugs*.

CONTENTS

Section Three — Staying Healthy

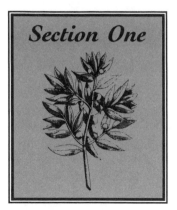

Section One

The Current State of Health in America:

The Need for Natural Medicine

Health-care reform is a topic of considerable interest today. There are numerous problems with the current system: Millions of Americans have no health insurance; medical costs are skyrocketing; many surgical procedures are performed unnecessarily; and there is growing concern over the safety of many prescription drugs.

The first section of this book is devoted to examining the relationship between the drug companies and medical doctors, the system they are a part of, and some solutions to the problems in the health-care industry today. Modern medical care is changing. As we enter into the information age, the relationship between doctors and patients is moving toward a partnership in healing. Patients are better informed now, allowing them to participate fully in their health-care decisions. Unfortunately, in many cases neither the doctor nor the patient is aware of natural alternatives that exist. It is not the doctor's fault, as he or she has probably never been exposed to the philosophy and science behind natural medicine.

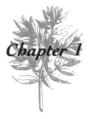

Chapter 1

MAKING MEDICINE

OR MAKING MONEY?

The United States spends more money on health care than any country in the world. For 1994, the projection is that the total will exceed one trillion dollars. Despite this tremendous financial commitment, are Americans getting their money's worth? If so, why is the United States ranked sixteenth in terms of life expectancy and why are there more people in nursing homes in this country than anywhere else in the world? Where is all this money spent on health care going? Are drug companies and doctors more concerned about making money than making people healthy?

Since the 1950s, the drug industry has been the most profitable industry in America. In December 1959, the last year of the Eisenhower administration, the Senate Subcommittee on Antitrust and Monopoly heralded a year-long investigation of the drug industry with the declaration that the public was not only being overcharged for drugs, but was being ripped off by more than $250 million a year for useless and sometimes harmful medicines.[1] The drug industry was harshly criticized for its unrestricted promotional, marketing, and pricing practices.

Have things changed in the last thirty-five years? Yes, they have gotten much better for the drug companies at the public's expense. During the past thirty-five years, drug costs have skyrocketed at a rate four times that of inflation. In 1960, the drug industry was the most profitable industry in America, with a profit margin of 10.6 percent of sales. By 1992, this had increased to 13 percent.

In 1980, the average prescription cost was $6.52. In 1992, the cost of the same prescription was $22.50. Since 1980, prescription drug costs have risen nearly three times higher than the consumer price index. Projections are that drug costs will continue to rise at a rate of nearly 10 percent per year for the next few years. Some drugs will see rises even steeper. Not surprisingly, the drugs most likely to rise in cost are those in highest demand among aging baby-boomers. For example, Premarin, a drug used primarily in women around the time of menopause, is being prescribed more. In 1985, the price of one hundred tablets of Premarin was $13.34; in 1991, the price had increased by nearly 2.5 times that amount to $33.09.

Lack of Profit Control and Competition Keep Drug Costs High

Drug costs are higher in the United States than anywhere else in the world. Most major industrial nations employ profit-control measures that limit how much a drug company can charge for a drug.[2] Because most drug companies market the same drug throughout the world, they rely on American sales for the bulk of their profits.

In the United States, drug companies can increase their prices without fear, because there is very little competition. In fact, there is more cooperation than competitiveness among drug companies to keep prices high. There are also several built-in barriers to competition in the current system. When a drug company develops a drug, it is granted a patent that can last up to twenty-two years with extensions. The drug company that developed the drug has exclusive marketing rights.

When the patent expires, other drug companies are then allowed to market the same drug. However, instead of lowering the price of the "brand name" drug to compete with "generic" brands, the drug company will usually raise the price. The drug company can increase the price of the drug without the fear of losing the loyalty of doctors largely because they spend billions of dollars each year paying for that loyalty. About twenty-six cents of every dollar spent on a drug goes toward promotion and marketing. This cost translates into about thirteen thousand dollars per doctor per year that the drug company spends in an attempt to get the doctor to prescribe its drug. Although drug companies often cite increased research and development costs as a reason for rising drug costs, the truth of the matter is that they spend much more money on marketing than on research and development. Less than sixteen cents of every dollar spent on a drug goes to research and development.

Drug Companies Control Medical Education

Most physicians receive very little formal education in the area of pharmacology—the study of drug actions and effects. Medical students are taught general principles of pharmacology, but the bulk of their understanding is derived from hospital training with practicing physicians. So, from whom do these practicing physicians learn about pharmacology? From the drug companies, of course.

There are 45,000 drug-company sales representatives (often referred to as detail persons) who provide the majority of drug information to the 550,000 prescribing physicians. Yet less than 5 percent of these sales representatives have had formal training in pharmacology.

Drug companies also sponsor most of the continuing-education courses that physicians are required to attend to keep their licenses. The drug companies will not only cover the costs of the educational program, they may also "sponsor" the physician by offering to cover all travel expenses or, at the very least, pay for meals.

Drug companies have also infiltrated medical schools and journals. What all this comes down to is that because the drug companies control medical education, doctors learn only about the use of prescription drugs in healing. This system feeds a medical process that is predicated on treating disease with drugs. The current system is not based on helping people achieve health through prevention of disease.

What Determines Which Drug a Doctor Will Prescribe

Most physicians do not make decisions about which drug to use on the basis of scientific research or cost. They base their decision almost entirely on which drug is the most popular choice of their colleagues.[3] What determines popularity? The effectiveness of the drug company's marketing and advertising efforts. In essence, doctors are often bribed or lied to so that they will prescribe certain medications.

The bribing aspect is well known. In 1990, the American College of Physicians authored a position paper to set guidelines in an attempt to address the long-standing practice of drug companies influencing doctors' decisions by giving them extravagant "gifts" or stipends.[4] According to this paper, the giving of "gifts" by the drug company is now firmly established as part of drug promotion and continuing medical education (CME). These "gifts" range from the trivial to all-expense-paid trips for two to resort settings for special CME programs. Elegant dinners, recreational outings, and tickets to celebrity performances or sporting events reside somewhere in the middle. So, what was the primary guideline set by the American College of Physicians?

"Gifts, hospitality, or subsidies offered to physicians by the pharmaceutical industry ought not to be accepted if acceptance might influence or appear to others to influence clinical judgment. A useful criterion in determining acceptable activities and relationships is: Would you be willing to have these arrangements generally known?"[4]

The American Medical Association (AMA) has also set guidelines for physicians' relationships with drug companies. The AMA's guidelines, like those of the American College of Physicians, allow for gifts of modest value and for financial support for educational functions.[5]

If the drug company didn't expect the gift to influence the doctor's decision, why would it give the gift? According to a 1992 article published in *The New England Journal of Medicine* written by Douglas Waud, M.D., the term *gift* should read *bribe*.[6] A gift implies that no strings are attached. Dr. Waud criticized the American College of Physicians' and AMA's guidelines because they seem to recommend that physicians "stick to bribes that are small enough to be swept under the rug if someone asks."

Although most physicians are well aware of how drug companies seek to gain their loyalty through these methods, very few are aware of how effective the companies are in lying to them about the virtues of a particular drug. In 1981, the Food and Drug Administration (FDA) established that "advertisements must present true statements relating to side effects, contraindications, and effectiveness" and that advertisements not meeting this requirement would be considered false and misleading. Despite these explicit standards, misleading advertising abounds in medical journals. An expert panel recently judged that over 92 percent of all advertisements in a leading medical journal failed to comply with the FDA guidelines, and concluded that 34 percent of all advertisements contained misleading or erroneous information.[7] While doctors like to believe that they make drug decisions based upon medical knowledge, the fact of the matter is, studies have shown that advertising influences doctors' decisions much more than scientific evidence.[4,8]

The cost of the drug is not a major consideration to physicians in determining which drug to prescribe. In many cases, it simply does not matter to them or to the patient because insurance companies are footing the bill. But perhaps the biggest reason cost is not a factor in choosing which drug to prescribe is the fact that most doctors do not have a clue to how much drugs cost.[3]

Do Doctors Make Too Much Money?

Few would argue that America has some of the best, most dedicated, and most honest doctors in the world, doctors who put in long hours of work and study to make a genuine difference in the lives they touch. Yet, are doctors worth the amount of money they earn? Doctors make considerably more money in the United States than anywhere else in the world.[9] The average income for a medical doctor is nearly $150,000 per year. Specialists such as radiologists and heart surgeons have an average income of more than $250,000 per year.[9,10]

Are doctors worthy of this high compensation? According to the four prominent principles of economic justice (Aristotle's Income Principle, the Free Market Principle, the Utilitarian Income Principle, and Rawls' Difference Principle), the answer is a resounding *no*.[10] Although most physicians have endured over ten years of intense education and training, and work long, hard, stress-filled hours, there is absolutely no justification for the high salaries.

One of the best ways to reduce skyrocketing medical costs is to focus on preventing illness. There is an increasing demand for medical doctors specializing in preventive medicine. However, despite this demand, there is a severe shortage of doctors specializing in this field. This shortage is surprising. Why isn't the supply meeting the demand?

One very big reason medical doctors do not practice preventive medicine is obvious: money. The average yearly income for a member of the American College of Preventive Medicine, a group of preventive medical doctors, is ninety thousand dollars.[11] Granted, ninety thousand dollars is a good income. Yet it is considerably less than the average income for other medical specialists.

Which is more valuable to society: a physician who can prevent disease through educating patients on healthful living, or a physician who performs a surgery that could have been entirely prevented by healthful diet and life-style? Benjamin Franklin is credited with saying, "An ounce of prevention is worth a pound of cure." In regard to health, few people would argue with this principle. However, in our current medical system, the treatment is the focus, and it is the treatment that rewards doctors with their fees.

Final Comments

Doctors are beginning to see how they have been pawns of the drug companies. The influence of the pharmaceutical industry on medical practice was clearly stated in a recent editorial entitled "The Addiction to Drug Companies" that appeared in the medical journal *Biological Psychiatry*.[12] It stated:

> The overall influence of the industry is to emphasize drug treatment at the expense of other modalities: psychotherapy, social ap-

proaches, nutritional, herbal, and natural remedies, rehabilitation, general hygienic measures, nonpatentable drugs, or other alternative approaches. It focuses attention on disorders that are treatable by drugs, and may promote overdiagnosis. It reinforces the practice of dealing with disease by treatment of symptoms, and diverts interest from prevention.

Although the cost of prescription drugs represents only 7 percent of our total health-care expense, the influence of the drug industry is largely responsible for skyrocketing medical costs. Doctors and drug companies are getting rich at our expense. Americans deserve the right to make informed decisions about their health care. Unfortunately, most Americans do not realize that there are natural alternatives to drugs and surgery that will produce better results at a fraction of the cost.

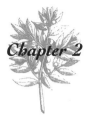

Chapter 2

NATURAL MEDICINE:
A RATIONAL ALTERNATIVE

> Nature is doing her best each moment to make us well. She exists for no other end. Do not resist. With the least inclination to be well, we should not be sick.
>
> —Henry David Thoreau

A *paradigm* refers to a model used to explain events. As our understanding of the environment and the human body evolves, new paradigms are developed. Most evident is the paradigm shift occurring in physics. The classical cause-and-effect views of Descartes and Newton were replaced by quantum mechanics, Einstein's theory of relativity, and the theoretical physics of Stephen Hawking.

In physics, the major paradigm shift was away from the view that for every action there is an equal and opposite reaction. Instead, the contemporary view incorporates possibilities rather than certainties. The new paradigm also takes into consideration the tremendous interconnectedness of the universe. In other words, it takes a more holistic view in place of a reductionist view.

Historically, paradigm shifts in medicine have lagged behind those in physics. While the old paradigm viewed the body basically as a machine, the new paradigm focuses on the interconnectedness of body, mind, emotions, social factors, and the environment in determining the status of health. Rather than relying on drugs and surgery, the new model utilizes natural, noninvasive techniques to promote health and healing. The relationship between the physician and patient is also evolving. The era of the physician as a demigod is over. The era of self-empowerment is beginning.

Old Paradigm

Biomechanical view that the body is a machine

The body and mind are essentially separate entities

Emphasis on eliminating disease

Treatment of symptoms

Specialization at the expense of holistic thinking

High technology, heroic measures

Physician should be emotionally neutral, detached

Physician is the all-knowing authority

Physician is in control of patient's health decisions

Focus on objective information (how the patient is doing based on charts, statistics, tests results, etc.)

New Paradigm

Holistic view concerned with the whole patient

The body and mind are interconnected

Emphasis on achieving health

Treatment is designed to address underlying illnesses

An integrated approach in treatment

Focus on diet, life-style, and preventive measures

Physician's caring and empathy are critical to healing

Physician is a partner in the healing process

Patient is in charge of his or her health-care choices

Focus on subjective information (how the patient is feeling)

Naturopathy

At the forefront of the natural medicine movement is naturopathy, a method of healing that employs various natural means to empower an individual to achieve health. In addition to providing recommendations on life-style, diet, and exercise, naturopathic physicians may elect to utilize a variety of natural healing techniques, including clinical nutrition, herbal medicine, homeopathy, Oriental medicine and acupuncture, hydrotherapy, physical medicine including massage and therapeutic manipulation, counseling and other psychotherapies, and minor surgery.

The modern naturopathic physician provides all phases of primary health care. He or she is trained to be the doctor first seen by the patient for general (nonemergency) health care. Some naturopathic physicians choose to emphasize a particular healing technique, while others are more eclectic and utilize a number of techniques. Some naturopaths elect to specialize in particular medical fields such as pediatrics, natural childbirth, and physical medicine.

Although the terms *naturopathy* and *naturopathic medicine* were not used until the late nineteenth century, their roots go back thousands of years. Drawing from the healing wisdom of many cultures, including India (Ayurvedic), China (Taoist), and Greece (Hippocratic), naturopathic medicine is a system of medicine founded on the four time-tested medical principles discussed below. These principles also define the philosophy and foundation of natural medicine, whether they are utilized by a naturopath (N.D.), medical doctor (M.D.), osteopath (D.O.), chiropractor (D.C.), or any other health-care provider.

Principle One: The Healing Power of Nature

The human body has considerable power to heal itself. The role of the physician is to facilitate and enhance this process. There is increasing evidence to support the contention that the healing process is best enhanced with the aid of natural nontoxic therapies. Of particular interest is the tremendous healing power of the mind.

In the last few years, a stack of best-sellers have explored the links among mind, emotions, and health. Among them: *Head First: The Biology of Hope and the Healing Power of the Human Spirit* by the late Norman Cousins; *Love, Medicine, and Miracles* by Bernie Siegel, M.D.; and *Quantum Healing: Exploring the Frontiers of Mind-Body Medicine* by Deepak Chopra, M.D. Within conventional medicine circles it is becoming increasingly understood that the faith, hope, and beliefs of the patient may be the most significant aspects of any treatment.

The ability of the mind to affect the process of virtually every disease has been well documented, and the internal mechanisms and pathways by which the mind can positively or negatively affect healing processes and the immune system have received considerable attention in the scientific literature.[1,2] As the body of knowledge documenting the critical importance of the patient's psyche on the therapeutic environment has grown, the healing potential of the human mind has become increasingly important for all schools of medicine.

Principle Two: First, Do No Harm

As Hippocrates said, "Above all else, do no harm." Unfortunately, these words are not being heeded. Not only is it simply a matter of a drug or surgery being potentially harmful, but inappropriate medications or procedures can cause problems as well. In other words, since doctors and nurses are human, errors can occur that cause harm. In fact, iatrogenic illness—the creation of additional problems resulting from treatment by a physician or surgeon—is becoming a major health problem in the United States.[3,4]

In one study, 36 percent of 815 patients admitted consecutively to the general medical service of one hospital experienced illnesses during their stay caused by previous medical treatment.[5] The iatrogenic disease threatened the life of or produced major disability in 9 percent of all persons admitted, and resulted in death in 2 percent. The investigators concluded that the risk of iatrogenic disease during hospitalization is far from trivial, as at least one third of the patients seen suffered some ill effect that was caused by hospital medical treatment.

What makes these mishaps particularly sad is that there is often an effective, natural, nontoxic therapy for a particular illness. Unfortunately, not enough physicians and patients are aware of these alternatives.

Principle Three: Identify and Treat the Cause

The treatment of the underlying causes of a disease is of vital importance, far more than simply suppressing its symptoms. As shown throughout Section Two of this book, more and more evidence is accumulating that many drug treatments are effective only in suppressing symptoms. Because they do not address causes, the disease process progresses.

Many drugs actually have side effects that promote the very disease they are trying to treat. Drugs used in psychiatry often cause psychiatric illness; drugs used in the treatment of heart-rate abnormalities can lead to those same abnormalities; aspirin use in arthritis treatment is associated with greater joint destruction; and drugs prescribed to prevent heart disease by lowering blood pressure have actually been shown to increase the likelihood of a heart attack.

The search for a cause must include not only the physical, but also the mental and emotional factors. While most diseases affecting Americans can be traced back to diet and life-style (i.e., cigarette smoking, alcohol use, exercise or lack thereof, sleeping habits, sexual activity), there is almost always a mental and/or emotional component as well. The individual must be viewed as a whole entity comprising a complex interaction of physical, mental-emotional, spiritual, and social factors.

Principle Four: The Physician as Teacher

The primary meaning of the word *doctor* is teacher. The physician's role is to teach patients about achieving health and avoiding disease. Thomas Edison said, "The doctor of the future will give no medicine, but will interest his patient in the care of the human frame, in diet and in the cause and prevention of disease."

Conventional medical doctors simply do not have the time to teach. A typical first office visit lasts less than seven minutes. Seven minutes is usually only enough time to make a quick diagnosis and write a prescription. In contrast, a typical first office visit with a naturopathic doctor takes one hour. Making a careful assessment of health status and diagnosing disease is only one part of the examination. Since naturopathic physicians consider teaching one of their primary goals, the time devoted to discussing and explaining principles of health is one of the aspects that sets naturopaths apart from conventional medical doctors.

Another contrast is the tremendous difference in the nutrition education of a naturopathic doctor (N.D.) compared with a medical doctor (M.D.). While an N.D. has over 138 course hours in nutrition, the typical M.D. has less than 4 hours of nutritional training. The majority of medical schools in the United States do not even have a required course in nutrition.

In a 1985 report, the National Research Council's Committee on Nutrition in Medical Education cited an insufficient number of hours devoted to nutrition and inconsistency in the scope and depth of topics included in nutrition courses in medical schools. The committee concluded that nutrition studies in education programs at American medical schools were largely inadequate to meet the demands of the medical profession.[6] Conventional medical doctors know very little about nutrition, especially the therapeutic use of foods, vitamins, and minerals. Given the importance of nutrition in the prevention of disease and maintenance of health, this inadequacy is inexcusable.

In Conclusion

To the uninformed, naturopathic medicine as well as the entire concept of natural medicine appears to be a fad that will soon disappear. To the informed, naturopathic medicine is the medicine of the future.

Many medical organizations that in the past have spoken out strongly against naturopathic medicine now endorse recommendations naturopaths have been making for decades. For example, naturopaths have long extolled the value of eating more high-fiber foods; reducing the intake of refined sugars, fats, and food additives; exercising on a regular basis; taking nutritional supplements; and reducing stress.

The adoption of naturopathy into conventional medicine illustrates the paradigm shift occurring in medicine. What was once scoffed at is now becoming generally accepted as effective treatment. In fact, in most instances the natural alternative offers significant benefit over standard medical practices. There remains little doubt that in the future, many of the concepts, philosophies, and practices of natural medicine will be incorporated into conventional medical practice.

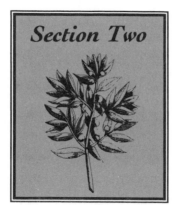

Common Drugs and Their Natural Alternatives

"Is there really a safer, more effective natural alternative to my drug?" Most likely, the answer is *yes*. The following section details the most common health conditions facing Americans, and how natural alternatives compare to standard drug therapy. If you elect to use any of the natural alternatives recommended in this section, it is important to follow these guidelines:

- Do *not* self-diagnose. Proper medical care is critical to good health. If you have symptoms suggestive of an illness discussed in this section, please consult a physician, preferably a naturopath, holistic M.D. or osteopath, chiropractor, or other natural-health-care specialist.

- If you are currently on prescription medication, you absolutely *must* work with your doctor before discontinuing any drug.

- If you wish to try the natural approach, discuss it with your physician. Since your physician is most likely unaware of the natural alternatives available, you may need to educate him or her. Take this book along with you to the doctor's office. The natural alternatives being recommended are based upon published studies in medical journals. Key references are provided if your physician wants additional information.

- The description and side effects of each drug discussed in this section can be found in the *Physician's Desk Reference*. This large book, updated annually, contains information on all prescription drugs and is available at all public libraries, physicians' offices, and pharmacies. Before you elect to take any drug, you must weigh the benefits against the risks. If you need help understanding the drug, talk it over with your doctor or pharmacist.

- Although effective on their own, many natural alternatives, such as nutritional supplements and herbs, work even better if they are part of a comprehensive natural treatment plan that focuses on diet and life-style factors. See a naturopathic physician to discuss how to integrate these supplements into a holistic program for staying healthy.

One question that may come up while reading this section is: If these natural substances are so effective, why aren't they marketed as drugs? There is a simple answer to this question: money. Because these natural products cannot be patented, there is no financial incentive for drug companies to market them or do research on them. A drug company could spend hundreds of millions of dollars to get a natural substance approved as a drug, but once approved, because there is no patent on the natural product, another company could market the identical product without having to spend a dime on getting the drug approved. Obviously, this situation must be remedied, like so many other of our health-care problems.

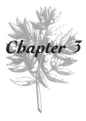

Chapter 3

ACNE MEDICATIONS

Acne is the most common of all skin problems. It occurs mostly on the face and, to a lesser extent, on the back, chest, and shoulders. Acne occurs in two forms: acne vulgaris—affecting the hair follicles and oil-secreting glands of the skin and manifesting as blackheads (comedones), whiteheads (pustules), and inflammation (papules); and acne conglobata—a more severe form, with deep cyst formation and subsequent scarring.

Acne has its origin in the pores of the skin. A skin pore consists of a canal through which a hair follicle passes. Glands known as sebaceous glands produce sebum, a mixture of oils and waxes that lubricate the skin and prevent the loss of water. Sebaceous glands are found in highest concentration on the face, but also on the back, chest, and shoulders. Acne affects the areas of skin that have sebaceous glands.

Acne is most common at puberty. Typical teenage outbreaks of acne are due to the fact that certain hormones stimulate changes in the skin that can lead to acne. The male sex hormone testosterone is the major hormonal factor in acne. Although men have higher levels of testosterone than women, during puberty there is an increase of testosterone in both sexes, making girls just as susceptible to acne in this age group.

Testosterone causes the sebaceous glands to enlarge and produce more sebum. In addition, the cells that line the skin pores produce more keratin, a sulfur-containing protein that forms the chemical basis of nails and hair. The increased secretion of both sebum and keratin can lead to blockage of the pore and the formation of a blackhead. With the blockage of the pore, bacteria are allowed to overgrow and release enzymes that break down sebum and promote inflammation. This forms what is known as a whitehead or pimple.

Although acne is considered to be a male hormone–dependent condition, excessive secretion of male hormones is not necessarily the cause, since there is only a poor correlation between blood levels of these hormones and the severity of the disease. What appears to be more important is that the skin of patients with acne shows greater activity of an enzyme (5-alpha-reductase) that converts testosterone to dihydrotestosterone, a more potent form of the hormone.

Common Drugs Used for Acne

TOPICAL TREATMENTS

Some general guidelines are appropriate when using topical preparations for the treatment of acne. First of all, make sure the skin is clean and dry. Start treatment slowly to determine the skin's tolerance by applying small amounts to small areas of the affected skin. Skin irritation due to topical treatment of acne is quite common; even the weaker over-the-counter preparations can cause irritation. If topical treatment results in a rash or irritation, consult your physician or dermatologist.

Chemical terms with some brand names in parentheses follow.

Benzoyl peroxide (e.g., Oxy-5, Oxy 10, Clearasil, Benoxyl-5, Benoxyl-10)
Benzoyl peroxide is by far the most popular topical treatment for mild to moderate acne. It is available without prescription. Although the exact action of benzoyl peroxide is not known, it is thought to work as a skin antiseptic that keeps the growth of bacteria down. Benzoyl peroxide is most effective in superficial pimples that are inflamed. In order to be effective, benzoyl peroxide preparations must be applied on a daily basis.

Side effects: The primary side effects of benzoyl peroxide preparations are a tendency to dry out the skin and/or cause redness and peeling.

Use of the drug can also cause a burning or stinging sensation when applied, and some people develop an allergic rash.

TOPICAL ANTIBIOTICS

Tetracycline (Topicycline), Erythromycin (A/T/S, Erycette, EryDerm), and Clindamycin (Cleocin T)
These preparations are used to keep the bacteria under control in the treatment of mild to moderate acne. They are available by prescription only. If applied on a regular basis, they can prevent pimple formation. Usually it will take a period of three to four weeks to produce significant improvement.

Side effects: Topical antibiotic preparations can cause dryness, skin tenderness, itching, redness, and burning sensations. Some people can develop an allergic rash. In rare instances, diarrhea may occur.

Tretinoin or Retinoic Acid (Retin-A)
Retin-A is a synthetic form of vitamin A that is used in the topical treatment of moderate to severe acne. It is available by prescription only. Retin-A works by decreasing keratin formation by the cells that line the skin pore, thus preventing the blockage of sebum and subsequent pimple formation. Retin-A is a harsh medicine that is very difficult to work with (see side effects below). It may also cause an initial worsening of the condition and often takes up to twelve weeks before improvement is noticeable. Once improvements are established, a maintenance regimen with less frequent applications can be instituted.

Side effects: The major side effects of Retin-A are skin drying and irritation. In fact, these side effects are rarely avoidable. Symptoms can often be quite severe (a chemical burning of the skin can occur) and require discontinuation of the medication. For this reason, it is best to follow the doctor's recommendation of carefully introducing Retin-A by starting at the lowest concentration. Applying more Retin-A than needed does not produce any better clinical response, and will most likely cause marked redness, peeling, or severe skin damage.

INTERNAL TREATMENTS

Tetracycline (Achromycin)

Tetracycline has become the "drug of choice" of most dermatologists in the treatment of acne. It is generally thought to have fewer side effects and to yield better results than other antibiotics. When tetracycline cannot be used due to intolerance or pregnancy, erythromycin is prescribed. In similar fashion to the topical antiseptics discussed above, tetracycline improves acne by preventing the overgrowth of bacteria in the skin pore. Tetracycline is most effective for the more superficial forms of acne affecting the face.

Side effects: The most common side effect is overgrowth of *Candida albicans* and other yeast in the gastrointestinal and genitourinary tract. This can result in the appearance of symptoms attributed to systemic candidiasis (see page 90), as well as in yeast infections of the mouth, intestinal tract, rectum, and/or vagina. Tetracylcine is often prescribed along with an antifungal agent (amphotericin B) to prevent yeast overgrowth.

Additional side effects and/or adverse reactions are also consistent with other antibiotics. They include allergic reactions; nausea, diarrhea, and vomiting; loss of appetite; and colitis. In rare instances, tetracycline can lead to anemia and low white blood cell and platelet levels.

Tetracylcine is not used during pregnancy or lactation, or in children under eight years of age because it interferes with tooth development. Use of tetracylcine in these cases can result in permanent discoloration and/or malformation of teeth.

Isotretinoin or Isotretinoic Acid (Accutane)

Isotretinoin is another synthetic derivative of vitamin A, but unlike tretinoin (Retin-A), isotretinoin or Accutane is used internally. Because of its high rate of toxicity, Accutane is reserved for the treatment of severe acne that has not responded to other conventional medicines. Accutane should not be used to treat mild to moderate acne. Its primary action in the treatment of severe acne is to inhibit the formation of sebum. Usually Accutane must be used continuously for five to six months before results are apparent. Like Retin-A, Accutane may cause an initial worsening.

Side effects: It is extremely important that individuals taking Accutane be closely monitored by their physicians and follow dosage recommendations exactly. Because Accutane can cause serious birth defects, it must not be used during pregnancy. Women taking Accutane must use two forms of birth control, such as diaphragm and condom, simultaneously.

In virtually every patient, Accutane will cause dryness of the nose and mouth, chapped lips, dry skin and itching, peeling of the palms of the hands and soles of the feet, and elevations of blood cholesterol and triglyceride levels. Women will usually experience vaginal drying and changes in the menstrual cycle. Other side effects, although less common, include allergic reactions, decreased libido, liver damage, thinning of hair, muscular and joint aches, abnormal bone development, and many others.

Dietary Factors in Treating Acne

A healthful diet rich in natural whole foods like vegetables, fruits, whole grains, and beans is the first recommendation for treating acne. All refined and/or concentrated sugars must be eliminated from the diet. Foods containing trans-fatty acids, such as milk, milk products, margarine, shortening, and other synthetically hydrogenated vegetable oils, as well as fried foods, must be avoided. Chocolate can produce a double whammy in that it is high in both sugar and fats. Milk should be avoided not only because it contains trans-fatty acids, but also because it may contain trace levels of hormones. And, finally, foods high in iodized salt should be eliminated, as some people are quite sensitive to the iodine, a known cause of acne.

Other General Recommendations

1. Avoid medications that may cause acne: anabolic steroids such

as testosterone, corticosteroids, progesterone, and drugs containing bromides or iodides.

2. Avoid exposure to or ingestion of oils and greases.

3. Avoid the use of greasy creams or cosmetics.

4. Wash your pillowcase regularly in chemical-free (no added colors or fragrances) detergents.

5. Remove excess sebum and oil from the face by washing thoroughly twice daily (more if necessary).

Natural Alternatives to Acne Medications

For additional help, there are alternatives to the current topical and internal compounds used in the treatment of acne. Several substances below have demonstrated results comparable to prescription and over-the-counter drugs in clinical studies. However, rather than rely exclusively on any one natural approach, a more comprehensive approach should be used. Such an approach is discussed below under Final Comments. The focus of a natural approach is healing from the inside out, rather than using topical preparations alone.

INTERNAL TREATMENTS

Zinc
The first natural alternative is the essential mineral zinc. Zinc is vitally important in the health of the skin. It is involved in local hormone activation; the formation of vitamin A–binding protein; wound healing; immune system activity; inflammation control; and tissue regeneration. In relation to acne, low levels of zinc increase the conversion of testosterone to its more active form (dihydrotestosterone, DHT), while high concentrations of zinc significantly inhibit this reaction. The conversion of testosterone to DHT is the underlying factor in the development of acne. Not surprisingly, serum zinc levels are lower in thirteen- and fourteen-year-old males than in any other age group.[1]

Several double-blind studies have demonstrated the effectiveness of zinc in the treatment of acne. In fact, these studies have shown zinc to yield similar results to tetracycline in superficial acne and superior results in deeper acne.[2,3,4] Although there are some studies of zinc in acne patients in which improvements of this magnitude were not obtained,[5] the inconsistency of the results can be explained by differences in dosages or the form of zinc used. For example, studies using zinc citrate or zinc gluconate show improvements similar to tetracycline, while those using plain zinc sulfate have shown fewer beneficial results, because zinc sulfate is poorly absorbed.

Although some people in studies showed dramatic improvement immediately, the majority usually required twelve weeks of supplementation before good results were achieved. There have been no studies to date using zinc picolinate or zinc monomethionine. These forms of zinc are more effectively absorbed than the forms of zinc used in the positive studies and, therefore, may produce even better effects. A safe and effective dose for zinc is 30 to 45 milligrams per day.

Vitamin A

Vitamin A, like the synthetic version Accutane, has been shown in many studies to reduce sebum production and other factors that contribute to pimple formation. Like Accutane, vitamin A has been shown to be effective in treating acne, but must be used at high, potentially toxic, dosages, i.e., 100,000 to 400,000 International Units (IUs) per day for five to six months.[6] Therefore, as with Accutane, the use of vitamin A in these high doses poses significant risk. High-dose vitamin A treatment should not be used without the close supervision of a medical professional.

In monitoring for vitamin A toxicity, laboratory tests appear unreliable until obvious toxicity symptoms are apparent. The first significant toxic symptom is usually headache followed by fatigue, emotional instability, and muscle and joint pain. Chapped lips (cheilitis) and dry skin (xerosis) will generally occur in the majority of patients, particularly in dry or cold weather. Because high doses of vitamin A during pregnancy can cause birth defects, women of child-bearing age should use birth control during vitamin A treatment and should continue using birth control for at least one month after treatment has stopped.

High doses of vitamin A may not be necessary if other nutritional factors like zinc and vitamin E are included. These nutrients work with vitamin A in promoting healthy skin. A safe recommendation for vitamin

A in the treatment of acne is less than 25,000 IUs per day. Pro-vitamin A (beta-carotene) does not appear to be effective in acne, but can be used to support healthy skin.

Chromium and High-Chromium Yeast

Several studies have suggested that acne is a result of impaired sugar metabolism and/or insulin insensitivity of the skin.[7,8] To measure the ability of the body to handle sugar, a glucose tolerance test is performed. The subject is given a soda containing glucose, and then has blood drawn at regular intervals to measure changes in the level of glucose or blood sugar. If blood sugar control mechanisms are working properly, the body will efficiently keep the glucose levels within the proper range. If not, faulty sugar metabolism is the cause. Although blood levels of glucose during glucose tolerance tests are normal in acne patients, repetitive skin biopsies reveal that their skin's glucose tolerance is significantly impaired.[9] One researcher discussing the role of glucose tolerance in acne coined the term "skin diabetes" to describe the disorder of acne. Considering the known detrimental effects of refined sugar, its intake should be strictly eliminated.

To further improve blood sugar control, it is important to have adequate levels of chromium. Chromium functions in the "glucose tolerance factor," a critical enzyme system involved in blood sugar regulation. Considerable evidence now indicates that chromium levels are a major determinant of how sensitive cells throughout the body are to the hormone insulin.[10] Insulin signals the uptake of blood sugar by the cells, including skin cells. Without chromium, the insulin will not be effective and will lead to impaired glucose tolerance. Low chromium levels may contribute to acne. In one study, high-chromium yeast was reported to produce rapid improvement in patients with acne.[11] Although double-blind studies have yet to be done to document this effect, chromium is a safe nutritional supplement that should be used in patients with acne. A safe and effective dosage is 1 tablespoon of high-chromium nutritional yeast or 200 micrograms of chromium bound to either chromium polynicotinate or picolinate.

Selenium and vitamin E

Dietary antioxidants like selenium and vitamin E are also important in acne, as acne patients have been shown to have significantly decreased levels of antioxidant enzymes.[12] The level of these critical enzymes normalizes when vitamin E and selenium are supplemented in the diet. The acne of both men and women improves with this treatment. This improvement is probably due to inhibition of the formation of toxic fatty acid derivatives in the sebum.

A diet rich in plant foods should provide adequate levels of a wide range of antioxidants, including vitamin E and selenium. However, if additional support is needed, take 200 to 400 IUs of vitamin E and 200 micrograms of selenium per day.

Vitamin B_6

Women with premenstrual aggravation of acne are often responsive to vitamin B_6 supplementation, reflecting its role in the normal metabolism of hormones.[13] A safe and effective dosage for vitamin B_6 in this case would be 50 milligrams three times a day. It may be best to take this in a formula containing the other B vitamins to provide additional support.

TOPICAL TREATMENTS

A variety of topical gels, ointments, and creams, available in health-food stores, can be used in the treatment of acne. The goal of these preparations is the same as for benzoyl peroxide; that is, to reduce the bacteria level and reduce inflammation. Although there are many possibilities to choose from, the most popular formulas are those that feature either tea tree oil or sulfur.

Tea Tree Oil

Melaleuca alternifolia, or "tea tree," is a small tree native to only one area of the world: the northeast coastal region of New South Wales, Australia. The leaves—the portion of the plant used medicinally—are the source of a valuable therapeutic oil.

Tea tree oil possesses significant antiseptic properties, and is regarded by many as the ideal skin disinfectant. This claim is supported by its efficacy against a wide range of organisms, and its good penetration and lack of irritation to the skin. The therapeutic uses of tea tree oil are based largely on its antiseptic and antifungal properties.

In a study conducted at the Royal Prince Hospital in New South Wales, Australia, a 5-percent tea tree oil solution was shown to demonstrate beneficial effects similar to those of 5-percent benzoyl peroxide in acne, but with substantially fewer side effects.[14] However, this 5-percent tea tree oil solution is probably not strong enough for moderate to severe acne. Stronger solutions (up to 15 percent) should provide even better results. Numerous studies have shown that tea tree oil is extremely safe for use as a topical antiseptic.

In addition to acne, tea tree oil has been used in the treatment of: athlete's foot, boils, burns, carbuncles, impetigo, infections of the nail bed, insect bites, ringworm, and vaginal infections. Many products based on tea tree oil exist in the marketplace, including toothpastes, shampoos and conditioners, hand and body lotions, creams, soaps, gels, liniments, and nail polish removers.

Sulfur

Products containing sulfur for the treatment of skin disorders have been around for thousands of years. Sulfur is a topical antiseptic just like benzoyl peroxide, but not as potent or irritating. Although sulfur-containing formulas are still around, their use has been replaced by newer compounds like benzoyl peroxide. This doesn't mean that sulfur is not effective. In fact, preparations containing 3 to 10 percent sulfur have produced such good results and are so widely accepted as therapeutic that the Food and Drug Administration (FDA) has approved sulfur as a safe and effective acne treatment. Sulfur-containing products for the treatment of acne are available in health-food stores as well as drugstores.

Final Comments

The most effective acne-treatment program is one that involves:

Removing excess sebum from the skin
Preventing overgrowth of bacteria
Preventing those factors that lead to closure of the skin pore
Supporting the body nutritionally through diet and supplementation

All of these goals can be achieved utilizing a natural approach. And, while medications may work in achieving the first three goals, they do not achieve the final goal, as they do not support the body nor address the imbalances that lead to acne. If electing to use the natural approach, it is very important that the following be done:

1. Follow the dietary recommendations given above.
2. Thoroughly cleanse the face daily with sulfur or soaps containing tea tree oil or a suitable alternative.
3. Take zinc, vitamin A, vitamin E, selenium, and vitamin B$_6$ at the recommended levels.
4. Utilize topical creams or ointments as directed.

The natural program that I am most familiar with is the Derma-Klear Acne Treatment program. It is manufactured by Enzymatic Therapy and is available at health-food stores. This complete program provides a cleanser, topical cream, and a nutritional supplement.

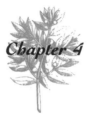

Chapter 4

ANGINA MEDICATIONS

Angina is the term used to describe a squeezing or pressurelike pain in the chest. The pain may radiate to the left shoulder blade, left arm, or jaw. The pain typically lasts for one to twenty minutes. Angina is caused by an insufficient supply of oxygen to the heart muscle. Since physical exertion and stress cause an increased need for oxygen by the heart, they are often preceding factors.

Angina is most often a result of atherosclerosis, which is fully discussed in Chapter 9, "Cholesterol-Lowering Medications." The primary cause of atherosclerosis is the buildup of cholesterol-containing plaque, which progressively narrows and ultimately blocks the blood vessels supplying the heart—the coronary arteries. This blockage results in a decreased blood and oxygen supply to the heart tissue. When the flow of oxygen to the heart muscle is substantially reduced, or when there is an increased need for oxygen by the heart, the result is an attack of angina.

A special type of angina exists that is not related to a buildup of plaque on the coronary arteries. It is known as Prinzmetal's variant angina, and is caused by spasm of a coronary artery. This form of angina is more apt to occur at rest, may occur at random times during the day or night, and is more common in women under age fifty. It usually responds to magnesium supplementation (see below).

Leading Angina Medication

Nitroglycerin (e.g., Nitro-Bid, Nitrostat, Minitran)
Nitroglycerin has been the treatment of choice for angina since the drug's introduction to medicine in 1847. Nitroglycerin has historically been given in little pills under the tongue (sublingual), but is now available in a variety of different forms including skin patches.

Nitroglycerin is remarkably effective in relieving an acute angina attack. It causes immediate dilation of the blood vessels of the heart and reduces oxygen demand. Typically, nitroglycerin will stop an angina attack in one to three minutes.

Nitroglycerin is probably best reserved as a treatment for acute attacks. Although there are long-acting forms of nitroglycerin, use of these forms will lead to the development of tolerance; that is, the drug will no longer be effective.

Side effects: Headaches occur in over 50 percent of patients taking nitroglycerin. Other common side effects include: rapid heart rate, palpitations, low blood pressure, and flushing of the face. It can also cause what are known as transient ischemic attacks. These periods of decreased blood flow to the brain can lead to temporary speech impairment, confusion, or paralysis.

OTHER ANGINA MEDICATIONS

Beta-blockers and calcium channel blockers are often used in treating angina. These drugs are discussed in detail in Chapter 8, "Blood Pressure–Lowering Medications."

Dietary and Life-style Factors in Treating Angina

The dietary and life-style recommendations given in Chapter 9, "Cholesterol-Lowering Medications," and Chapter 8, "Blood Pressure–Lowering Medications," are appropriate here as well. Especially important is a diet rich in fresh fruits and vegetables or their fresh juice. This will provide many nutrients that nourish and protect the heart. Also important are foods rich in potassium and magnesium, like whole grains and legumes.

Since angina is known to be exacerbated by physical exertion following a meal, give your body at least one and a half hours after a meal before exercising.

Natural Alternatives to Angina Medications

Angina is a serious condition that requires strict medical supervision. The recommendations given below are specific for angina, but are meant to be part of a comprehensive plan. For example, if the angina is due to cholesterol deposits, it is important to follow those guidelines and recommendations given in Chapter 9, "Cholesterol-Lowering Medications." In severe cases, as well as in the initial stages, the prescription medications may be necessary, but eventually, the condition should be controlled via the natural measures described below.

From a natural perspective, there are two primary therapeutic goals in the treatment of angina: improving energy metabolism within the heart, and improving the blood supply to the heart. These goals are interrelated, as an increased blood flow means improved energy metabolism and vice versa.

The heart utilizes fats as its major metabolic fuel. It converts free fatty acids to energy much like the way an automobile burns gasoline. Defects in the utilization of fats by the heart greatly increase the risk of atherosclerosis, heart attacks, and angina pains. Specifically, impaired utilization of fatty acids by the heart results in accumulation of high concentrations of fatty acids within the heart muscle. This deficiency then makes the heart extremely susceptible to cellular damage, which ultimately leads to a heart attack.

Carnitine, pantethine, and coenzyme Q_{10} (CoQ_{10}) are essential compounds in normal fat and energy metabolism and are of extreme benefit to sufferers of angina. These nutrients prevent the accumulation of fatty acids within the heart muscle by improving the conversion of fatty acids and other compounds into energy. Pantethine is discussed on page 138.

Carnitine and CoQ_{10} are discussed below, along with magnesium and two herbs—hawthorn and khella—all of which have an effect in improving heart function in individuals with angina.

Carnitine

Carnitine, a vitaminlike compound, stimulates the breakdown of long-chain fatty acids by the energy-producing units in cells—the mitochondria. Carnitine is essential in the transport of fatty acids into the mitochondria. A deficiency in carnitine results in a decrease in fatty acid concentrations in the mitochondria and reduced energy production. A deficiency of carnitine in the heart would be similar to trying to run an automobile without a fuel pump. There may be plenty of fuel, but no way to get it to the engine.

Normal heart function is critically dependent on adequate concentrations of carnitine. While the normal heart stores more carnitine than it needs, a heart without a good supply of oxygen cannot store enough carnitine. Decreased carnitine leads to decreased energy production in the heart and increased risk for angina and heart disease. Since angina patients have a diminished supply of oxygen, carnitine supplementation makes good sense.

Several clinical trials have demonstrated that carnitine ameliorates angina and heart disease.[1] Supplementing the diet with carnitine normalizes heart carnitine levels and allows the heart muscle to utilize its limited oxygen supply more efficiently, translating to an improvement in cases of angina. Improvements have been noted in exercise tolerance and heart function. The results indicate that carnitine is an effective alternative to drugs in cases of angina. The dosage used in these studies has typically been 300 milligrams of L-carnitine three times daily. It is important to use L-carnitine versus D,L-carnitine, which is a mixture of the D and L forms of carnitine. The body uses L-carnitine but the D actually interferes with L-carnitine.

By improving fatty acid utilization and energy production in the heart muscle, carnitine also prevents the production of toxic fatty acid metabolites.[2] These compounds are extremely damaging as they disrupt cellular membrane structures. These changes in the properties of cell membranes throughout the heart are thought to contribute to impaired contraction of the heart muscle and increased susceptibility to irregular beats, and eventual death of heart tissue. Supplementing the diet with carnitine increases heart carnitine levels and has been shown to prevent the production of fatty acid metabolites that can damage the heart.[3] Carnitine also lowers triglycerides and total cholesterol levels while raising HDL-cholesterol. As discussed in Chapter 9, "Cholesterol-Lowering Medications," all of these effects are important in preventing a heart attack.

Coenzyme Q_{10}

Coenzyme Q_{10} (CoQ_{10}), also known as ubiquinone, is an essential component of the mitochondria—the energy-producing units of the body's cells. Although CoQ_{10} can be synthesized within the body, deficiency states have been reported. Deficiency could be a result of impaired CoQ_{10} synthesis due to deficiencies of essential vitamins and minerals, a genetic or acquired defect in CoQ_{10} synthesis, or increased tissue needs.

Cardiovascular diseases including angina, hypertension, mitral valve prolapse, and congestive heart failure are examples of diseases that require increased tissue levels of CoQ_{10}.[4] In addition, the elderly in general may have increased CoQ_{10} requirements as the age-related decline of CoQ_{10} levels within the body may be partly responsible for the deterioration of the immune system.

CoQ_{10} deficiency is common in individuals with heart disease. Heart tissue biopsies in patients with various heart diseases showed a CoQ_{10} deficiency in 50 to 75 percent of cases.[4,5] Being one of the most metabolically active tissues in the body, the heart may be unusually susceptible to the effects of CoQ_{10} deficiency. Accordingly, CoQ_{10} has shown great promise in the treatment of heart disease and angina.

In one study, twelve patients with angina were treated with CoQ_{10} (150 milligrams per day for four weeks) in the most strict type of scientific study (a double-blind, crossover trial).[6] Compared with placebo, CoQ_{10} reduced the frequency of angina attacks by 53 percent. In addition, there was a significant increase in treadmill exercise tolerance (time to onset of chest pain and time to development of electrocardiogram abnormalities) during CoQ_{10} treatment. The results of this study and others suggest that CoQ_{10} is a safe and effective treatment for angina pectoris.

Like carnitine and pantethine, CoQ_{10} also exerts a beneficial effect on blood triglyceride and cholesterol levels. CoQ_{10} has also been shown to lower blood pressure in cases of high blood pressure.

Magnesium

A magnesium deficiency has been shown to produce spasms of the coronary arteries, and is thought to be one cause of heart attacks brought on by coronary artery spasm rather than atherosclerosis. Several reports have suggested that magnesium should be the treatment of choice for Prinzmetal's variant angina (see above).[7] Furthermore, it has been observed that individuals dying suddenly of heart attacks have significantly lower levels of magnesium in their heart, as well as of potassium, than matched controls.

Magnesium administration has been found to be helpful in the management of angina, irregular heartbeat, and other cardiovascular diseases. A good therapeutic dose is 250 milligrams of magnesium three to four times daily. A soluble form of magnesium such as magnesium aspartate or citrate is the preferred form, since it is better absorbed as well as being better tolerated than magnesium oxide or sulfate.[8]

Hawthorn (Crataegus oxyacantha)

Hawthorn berry and flowering-tops extracts are widely used by physicians in Europe for their effect on the cardiovascular system. Studies have shown hawthorn extracts to be helpful in reducing angina attacks as well as lowering blood pressure and serum cholesterol levels.[9]

The beneficial effects of hawthorn extracts in the treatment of angina are a result of improvement in the blood and oxygen supply to the heart by dilating the coronary vessels, as well as improvement of the metabolic processes in the heart.

Various flavonoid components in hawthorn have been shown to inhibit constriction of vessels in a manner similar to the calcium-channel blockers; however, this is only part of the total picture. Hawthorn extracts also improve energy production within the heart as a result of the flavonoids improving the utilization of oxygen by the heart. The net result is improved heart function and an increase in the force of contraction. This is in stark contrast to beta-blockers and calcium-channel blockers, which actually reduce heart function. The effects of hawthorn also make it beneficial in cases of congestive heart failure and rhythm disturbances. In addition, the procyanidins of hawthorn are known to decrease cholesterol levels and the size of cholesterol-containing plaques in the arteries.

Hawthorn's ability to dilate coronary blood vessels has been repeatedly demonstrated in experimental studies.[10] This positive effect appears to be due to various flavonoid components in hawthorn that cause the relaxation of the smooth muscle that surrounds the artery.

Improvement in heart metabolism has also been demonstrated in humans and animals to whom hawthorn extracts have been given.[9,10] The improvement is a result not only of increased blood and oxygen supply to the heart muscle, but also of hawthorn flavonoids interacting with key enzymes.

To summarize, hawthorn extracts have exhibited a combination of effects that are a great value to sufferers of angina or other heart problems. The dosage depends on the type of preparation and source material. Standardized extracts, similar to those used in Europe, are available commercially in the United States at health-food stores. These extracts are the preferred form. The dosage for hawthorn extracts standardized to contain 1.8 percent vitexin-4'-rhamnoside or 10 percent procyanidins is 100 to 250 milligrams three times daily.

Khella (Ammi visnaga)

This ancient medicinal plant is native to the Mediterranean region, where it has been used in the treatment of angina and other heart ailments since the time of the pharaohs. Several of its components have demonstrated effects in dilating the coronary arteries. Its mechanism of action appears to be very similar to the calcium channel–blocking drugs.

Since the late 1940s, there have been numerous scientific studies on the clinical effects of khella extracts in the treatment of angina. More specifically, khellin, a derivative of the plant, was shown to be extremely helpful in relieving angina symptoms, improving exercise tolerance, and normalizing electrocardiographic tests. This is evident in the concluding statements in a study published in *The New England Journal of Medicine* in 1951: "The high proportion of favorable results, together with the striking degree of improvement frequently observed, has led us to the conclusion that khellin, properly used, is a safe and effective drug for the treatment of angina pectoris."[11]

At high doses, 120 to 150 milligrams per day, pure khellin was associated with mild side effects such as loss of appetite, nausea, and dizziness. Although most clinical studies used high dosages, several studies show that as little as 30 milligrams of khellin per day appears to offer as good results, with fewer side effects.[12]

Rather than use the isolated compound khellin, khella extracts standardized for khellin content (typically 12 percent) are the preferred form. A daily dose of such an extract would be 250 to 300 milligrams, equal to 30 to 36 milligrams of khellin. Khella appears to work very well with hawthorn extracts.

Final Comments

The effects of the natural measures recommended above have been confirmed in strict scientific studies, and these natural means are usually quite effective in most cases of angina. Since angina is a serious medical condition, it is extremely important that proper medical monitoring be performed. Do *not* take yourself off any drug prescribed by your physician. Instead, work with him or her toward eventual withdrawal from the medication. The natural approaches described above can be used alone, in combination, or along with prescription angina medications. For example, nitroglycerin can be used along with the natural approach during acute attacks. In the case of unstable angina—a more severe form of angina—along with the natural measures, calcium channel–blocking drugs like Procardia and Adalat (nifedipine) may be necessary until the condition has stabilized.

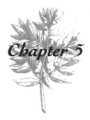

Chapter 5

ANTACIDS

Millions of people use over-the-counter antacid preparations to relieve symptoms of indigestion. The term *indigestion* is often used to describe a feeling of gaseousness or fullness in the abdomen. It can also be used to describe heartburn. Indigestion can be attributed to a great many causes, including not only increased secretion of acid but also decreased secretion of acid and other digestive juices and enzymes. Antacids are also used in the treatment of peptic ulcer (see Chapter 17, "Peptic Ulcer Medications").

Antacids work by raising the pH level, the chemical scale that measures acid levels. A substance that has a pH of 7 is neutral; anything below it is acid; anything above it is alkaline. The stomach's optimal pH range is 1.5 to 2.5, with hydrochloric acid being the primary stomach acid. Although an antacid will not neutralize all of the acid, it will typically raise the pH above 3.5. This effectively inhibits the action of pepsin, an enzyme involved in protein digestion that can be irritating to the stomach. Although raising the pH can reduce symptoms, it is important to note that hydrochloric acid and pepsin are key factors in protein digestion. If hydrochloric acid secretion is insufficient or inhibited, proper protein digestion will not occur. Therefore, it is essential to use antacids wisely and sparingly. In addition, many naturopathic physicians find that sometimes it is not too much acid, but rather a lack of acid, that is the problem. Typically, in addressing indigestion, naturopaths use measures to enhance rather than inhibit digestion. Commonly used digestive acids include hydrochloric acid and pancreatic enzyme preparations.

General Considerations

A 1983 article in the *American Journal of Gastroenterology* asked the question, "Why do apparently healthy people use antacids?"[1] The answer: reflux esophagitis, the medical term for heartburn. Heartburn is most often caused by the flow of gastric juices up the esophagus. This causes what is known as heartburn, a burning discomfort that radiates upward and is made worse by lying down.

Overeating is the most common cause of heartburn, but there are other causes as well, including obesity, cigarette smoking, and eating and drinking chocolate, fried foods, carbonated beverages (soft drinks), alcohol, and coffee. These factors either increase the pressure within the stomach, thereby causing the gastric contents to flow upward, or they decrease the tone of the sphincter between the stomach and the esophagus, which normally prevents gastric reflux into the esophagus. The first step in treating heartburn is prevention. This simply involves eliminating or reducing the causative factors.

For occasional heartburn, antacids can be used. However, they should not be abused. If heartburn is a chronic problem, it may be a sign of a hiatal hernia, an outpouching of the stomach above the diaphragm. However, it is interesting to note that only 5 percent of patients with hiatal hernias actually experience reflux esophagitis. Perhaps the most effective treatment of chronic heartburn is to utilize gravity. Simply place four-inch blocks under the bedposts at the head of the bed to prevent the backing up of gastric juices. This elevation of the head is very effective in many cases.

Another recommendation to heal the esophagus is the use of deglycyrrhizinated licorice or DGL (see page 208). Although DGL is primarily used for treating peptic ulcers, I have used it clinically with success in cases of heartburn.

Common Antacid Medications

All antacids are relatively safe when used on an occasional basis for heartburn or indigestion. Taken regularly, however, they can lead to malabsorption of nutrients, bowel irregularities, kidney stones, and other side effects. There are several approved types of antacids, each discussed separately below.

Aluminum-Containing Compounds

Aluminum-containing antacids include Maalox, Rolaids, Digel, Mylanta, Riopan, WinGel, Amphojel, and AlernaGel. Although these antacids are potent and effective in neutralizing acid, there are some significant long-term safety concerns. There is ever-growing evidence to indicate that aluminum may play a role in impairing mental function, and have adverse effects in diseases of the nervous system including Alzheimer's disease, dialysis dementia, Parkinson's disease, and Lou Gehrig's disease (amyotrophic lateral sclerosis).[2] Although manufacturers and the FDA tell us that the aluminum in antacids is not absorbed, this appears to be inaccurate information, as absorption studies prove otherwise, even when low-dose therapy is used.[3] Absorption of aluminum is greatly enhanced in patients with Alzheimer's disease or impaired kidney function, or when a meal contains any citrus fruit, orange juice, soda pop, or other source of citric acid. There is no reason to use the aluminum-containing antacids at this time, as the potential risk far outweighs the short-term benefit.

Sodium Bicarbonate

Sodium bicarbonate is baking soda. Alka-Seltzer is simply ordinary baking soda in an effervescent form. Although sodium bicarbonate can be useful in short-term therapy, it is not indicated for chronic or prolonged therapy, due to the risk of sodium overload. In addition, because the bicarbonate ion is rapidly absorbed, long-term administration can cause systemic alkalosis (excessive pH throughout the body). This can lead to nausea, vomiting, headache, mental confusion, and the formation of kidney stones.

Calcium Carbonate and Calcium Citrate

Tums is an example of an antacid that contains calcium carbonate. Although fast-acting and potent, calcium carbonate can produce what is known as acid rebound, three or four hours after use. This means that the body will try to overcompensate for the neutralization of gastric acid by secreting even more acid. This is not viewed as being clinically significant in the treatment of indigestion, but it may play a role in delaying ulcer healing.

Many physicians have been recommending Tums as a calcium supplement. In fact, calcium carbonate is the most widely used form of calcium supplement. While calcium carbonate is an effective antacid, there are better forms of calcium for supplementation.

In order for calcium carbonate and other insoluble calcium salts to be absorbed, they must first be solubilized and ionized by stomach acid. Unfortunately, many individuals lack sufficient stomach acid. In studies with postmenopausal women, it has been shown that about 40 percent are severely deficient in stomach acid.[4] Patients with insufficient stomach acid output can only absorb about 4 percent of an oral dose of calcium as calcium carbonate, while those with normal stomach acid can typically absorb about 22 percent.[5] Patients with low stomach-acid secretion need a form of calcium already in a soluble and ionized state, like calcium citrate, calcium lactate, or calcium gluconate. About 45 percent of the calcium is absorbed from calcium citrate in patients with reduced stomach acid, compared with 4 percent absorption for calcium carbonate. It has also been demonstrated that calcium is more absorbable from calcium citrate than from calcium carbonate in normal subjects.[6]

The strong alkaline nature of carbonate, combined with the calcium that is absorbed, greatly increases the risk of kidney stones, especially if milk products are a regular part of the diet. In contrast, the chemical nature of citrate is actually to prevent kidney stones from developing.[7] This, along with its superior absorption, clearly demonstrates that calcium citrate is much more beneficial than calcium carbonate as a calcium supplement. Calcium citrate may be the best antacid as well; it is showing impressive results as such in patients with kidney disease,[8] being better tolerated than aluminum-containing antacids. Although I am not aware of any calcium citrate preparations being marketed as antacids, calcium citrate preparations are available at health-food stores as calcium supplements. As calcium supplementation may decrease the absorption of other minerals, when an antacid effect is desired, the best recommendation may be simply to take a multimineral formula that uses minerals bound to citrate or other Krebs cycle intermediate(s). There are numerous mineral formulations in health-food stores that meet this criterion. When using a multimineral preparation as an antacid, simply gauge the dosage based on its calcium content. Take 500 to 1,000 milligrams of calcium per day.

Magnesium Compounds

Magnesium salts such as magnesium oxide, hydroxide, and carbonate often appear in aluminum-containing products. Phillips' milk of magnesia is the sole major brand that features only magnesium; it is a suspension of magnesium hydroxide in water. In addition to acting as a mild antacid, magnesium hydroxide also exerts a laxative effect. It is a safe and effective product for people with normal kidney function, though diarrhea is a definite risk.

Natural Alternatives to Antacids

Although some antacids are in essence natural products and have an appropriate use in treating occasional indigestion, in most chronic cases a more critical look at the problem of indigestion is needed. In the patient with chronic indigestion, rather than focus on blocking the digestive process with antacids, the natural approach to indigestion focuses on aiding digestion.

Digestion occurs as a result of both physical and chemical processes. The physical changes of food are brought about by grinding, crushing, and mixing of the food mass (chyme) with digestive juices during propulsion through the digestive tract. Chewing food thoroughly is the first aspect of good digestion. Not only are the mechanics effective, but the mixing of the food with saliva is also important. Saliva contains the enzyme salivary amylase (ptyalin), which breaks down starch molecules into smaller sugars.

The role of the esophagus is to transport food and liquids from the mouth to the stomach. The stomach functions primarily in the digestion of proteins and the ionization of minerals, and it secretes hydrochloric acid, various hormones, and enzymes.

Hydrochloric Acid

As stated previously, although much is said about hyperacidic conditions, probably a more common cause of indigestion is a lack of gastric acid secretion. Hypochlorhydria refers to deficient gastric acid secretion, while achlorhydria refers to a complete absence of gastric acid secretion.

There are many symptoms and signs, listed in Tables 5.1 and 5.2,

Table 5.1   Common Symptoms of Low Gastric Acidity

Bloating, belching, burning, and flatulence immediately after meals
A sense of "fullness" after eating
Indigestion, diarrhea, or constipation
Multiple food allergies
Nausea after taking supplements
Itching around the rectum

Table 5.2   Common Signs of Low Gastric Acidity

Weak, peeling, and cracked fingernails
Dilated blood vessels in the cheeks and nose
Acne
Iron deficiency
Chronic intestinal parasites or abnormal flora
Undigested food in stool
Chronic candida infections
Upper digestive tract gassiness

that suggest impaired gastric acid secretion, and a number of specific diseases, listed in Table 5.3, have been found to be associated with insufficient gastric acid output.[9]

Several studies have shown that the ability to secrete gastric acid decreases with age.[10] Low stomach acidity has been found in more than half of those over age sixty. The best method of diagnosing a lack of gastric acid is a special procedure known as the Heidelberg gastric analysis.[11] This technique utilizes an electronic capsule attached to a string. The capsule is swallowed and then kept in the stomach with the aid of the string. The capsule measures the pH of the stomach and sends a radio message to a receiver, which then records the pH level. The response to a bicarbonate challenge is the true test of the functional ability of the stomach to secrete acid.[12] In cases of hypochlorhydria, insufficient acid will be secreted to neutralize the bicarbonate. After the test, the capsule is pulled up from the stomach by the string attached to it.

Since not everyone can have detailed gastric acid analysis to determine the need for gastric acid supplementation, a practical method of determination is often used. If an individual is experiencing any of the symptoms and signs of gastric acid insufficiency listed in Tables 5.1 and

Table 5.3   Diseases Associated with Low Gastric Acidity

Addison's disease
Asthma
Celiac disease
Dermatitis herpetiformis
Diabetes mellitus
Eczema
Gallbladder disease
Graves' disease
Chronic autoimmune disorders
Hepatitis
Chronic hives
Lupus erythematosus
Myasthenia gravis
Osteoporosis
Pernicious anemia
Psoriasis
Rheumatoid arthritis
Rosacea
Sjogren's syndrome
Thyrotoxicosis
Hyper- and hypothyroidism
Vitiligo

5.2, or has any of the diseases listed in Table 5.3, the method outlined below can be employed.

Protocol for Hydrochloric Acid Supplements

1. Begin by taking one tablet or capsule containing 10 grains (600 milligrams) of hydrochloric acid (HCl) at your next large meal. If this does not aggravate your symptoms, at every meal of comparable size take one additional tablet or capsule. (One at the next meal; two at the meal after that; three at the next meal.)

2. Continue to increase the dose until you reach seven tablets, or

when you feel a warmth in your stomach—whichever occurs first. A feeling of warmth in the stomach means that you have taken too many tablets for that meal, and you need to take one tablet less for that meal size. It is a good idea to try the larger dose again at another meal to make sure that it was the HCl that caused the warmth and not something else.

3. After you have found what the largest dose is that you can take at your large meals without feeling any warmth, maintain that dose at all meals of similar size. You will need to take fewer tablets at smaller meals.

4. When taking a number of tablets or capsules, it is best to space them throughout the meal, rather than taking them all at once.

5. As your stomach begins to regain the ability to produce the amount of HCl needed to digest your food properly, you will notice the warm feeling again, and will have to cut down the dose level.

Enzymes

The pancreas produces enzymatic secretions required for the digestion and absorption of food. Each day the pancreas secretes about 1.5 quarts of pancreatic juice in the small intestine. Enzymes secreted include lipases, which digest fat; proteases, which digest proteins; and amylases, which digest starch molecules.

Pancreatin is often used by naturopathic physicians in the treatment of indigestion. The term refers to preparations of pancreatic enzymes isolated from fresh hog pancreas. Pancreatin addresses the problem of insufficient output of pancreatic enzymes. Pancreatic insufficiency is characterized by impaired digestion, malabsorption, nutrient deficiencies, and abdominal discomfort.

It is best to use a full-strength undiluted pancreatic extract (8 to 10 times *United States Pharmacopeia* [USP]), as lower-potency pancreatin products are often diluted with salt, lactose, or galactose. Take 250 to 500 milligrams of full-strength pancreatin before meals when using it as a digestive aid. Pancreatin and hydrochloric acid preparations can be used together, as long as the pancreatin is taken before the meal and the hydrochloric acid is taken during or after the meal.

Final Comments

Proper digestion is a requirement for optimum health, and incomplete or disordered digestion can be a major contributor to the development of many diseases. The problem is not only that ingestion of foods and nutritional substances is of little benefit when breakdown and assimilation are inadequate, but also because incompletely digested food molecules can be absorbed into the body, leading to the development of food allergies.

Although antacids may lead to relief of symptoms attributed to indigestion, they actually interfere with the digestive process. In many cases, the goal is to enhance digestion with the help of digestive aids like hydrochloric acid, pancreatin, and enzyme preparations.

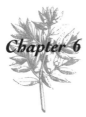

Chapter 6

ARTHRITIS MEDICATIONS

The three major forms of arthritis are osteoarthritis, rheumatoid arthritis, and gout. Each type of arthritis has its own unique features. Osteoarthritis and rheumatoid arthritis are discussed in this chapter, while gout is the topic of Chapter 14. The primary drugs used in the treatment of both osteoarthritis and rheumatoid arthritis are the so-called nonsteroidal anti-inflammatory drugs, or NSAIDs, which include aspirin.

Although these drugs are extensively used in the United States, research indicates that in the treatment of osteoarthritis and rheumatoid arthritis these drugs may be producing short-term benefit, but actually accelerating the progression of the joint destruction and causing more problems in the patient's future. Results of numerous studies have raised some interesting questions: Does medical intervention in some way promote disease progression? Can nutrition and various natural therapies enhance the body's own response to bring about improved health? The answer to both of these questions, as is evident from the information presented in this chapter, is clearly *yes*. Before providing that evidence, let's first examine the main features of osteoarthritis and rheumatoid arthritis.

Osteoarthritis

Osteoarthritis, or degenerative joint disease, is the most common form of arthritis. It is seen primarily, but not exclusively, in the elderly. Surveys have indicated that more than forty million Americans have osteoarthritis, including 80 percent of persons over the age of fifty. Under the age of forty-five, osteoarthritis is much more common in men; after age forty-five, it is ten times more common in women.[1]

The cumulative effects of decades of use of our bodies' joints leads to degenerative changes through stress on the integrity of the support structure (collagen matrix) of the cartilage. Damage to the cartilage results in the release of enzymes that destroy structural components. With aging, there is a decreased ability to restore and manufacture normal cartilage.[2,3] As we age, the number as well as the activity of important repair enzymes is greatly reduced, making the joint structures especially prone to damage.

The weight-bearing joints and joints of the hands are most often affected by the degenerative changes associated with osteoarthritis. Specifically, there is much cartilage destruction followed by hardening of the cartilage and the formation of large bone spurs in the joint margins. Pain, deformity, and limitation of motion in the joint result. Inflammation is usually minimal.[4]

The onset of osteoarthritis can be very subtle. Morning joint stiffness is often the first symptom. As the disease progresses, there is pain when the affected joint is in motion, which is made worse by prolonged activity and relieved by rest.

Rheumatoid Arthritis

Rheumatoid arthritis (RA) is a chronic inflammatory condition that affects the entire body, but especially the synovial membranes of the joints. It is a classic example of an autoimmune disease, a condition in which the body's immune system attacks the body's own tissue.

In rheumatoid arthritis, the joints typically involved are the hands and feet, wrists, ankles, and knees. Somewhere between 1 percent and

3 percent of the population is affected; female patients outnumber males almost three to one; and the usual age of onset is between twenty and forty years, although rheumatoid arthritis may begin at any age.[1]

There is abundant evidence that rheumatoid arthritis is an autoimmune reaction, where antibodies develop against components of joint tissues. Yet what triggers this autoimmune reaction remains largely unknown. Speculation and investigation have centered around genetic susceptibility, abnormal bowel permeability, life-style and nutritional factors, food allergies, and microorganisms. Rheumatoid arthritis is a multifactorial disease, in which there seem to be an interesting assortment of genetic and environmental factors that contribute to the disease process. For a full discussion of all of these factors, please consult the *Encyclopedia of Natural Medicine* (see footnote 1).

The onset of rheumatoid arthritis is usually gradual, but occasionally it can be quite abrupt. Fatigue, low-grade fever, weakness, joint stiffness, and vague joint pain may precede the appearance of painful, swollen joints by many weeks. Several joints are usually involved in the onset, typically in a symmetrical fashion: that is, both hands, both wrists, or both ankles. In about one third of persons with rheumatoid arthritis, initial involvement is confined to one or a few joints.[1]

Involved joints will characteristically be quite warm, tender, and swollen. The skin over the joint will take on a ruddy purplish hue. As the disease progresses, joint deformities result in the hands and feet.

ASPIRIN AND OTHER NSAIDS FOR ARTHRITIS

The first drug generally used in the treatment of osteoarthritis and rheumatoid arthritis is aspirin. It is an example of a nonsteroidal anti-inflammatory drug, or NSAID. Aspirin is often quite effective in relieving both the pain and the inflammation. It is also relatively inexpensive. However, since the therapeutic dose required is relatively high (2 to 4 grams per day), toxicity often occurs. Tinnitus (ringing in the ears) and gastric irritation are early manifestations of toxicity.

Other NSAIDs (or "New Sorts of Aspirin in Disguise") are often used as well, especially when aspirin is ineffective or intolerable. The following are representative of this class of drugs (generic, then some brands in parentheses):

Fenoprofen (Nalfon)

Ibuprofen (Motrin, Advil, Nuprin)

Indomethacin (Indocin, Indometh)

Meclofenamate (Meclofen, Meclomen)

Naproxen (Naprosyn)

Piroxicam (Feldene)

Sulindac (Clinoril)

Tolmetin (Tolectin)

Although these drugs have not proven to be more effective than aspirin, some may be better tolerated. However, they are also much more expensive and still carry significant risk for side effects and are, therefore, recommended only for short periods of time. In addition to being used in arthritis, NSAIDs are also used in the relief of headaches, low back pain, traumatic injury, postoperative pain, and menstrual cramps.

Although much of how NSAIDs work has not been completely established, they are known to reduce inflammation by suppressing the formation of prostaglandins and related compounds, chemicals involved in the production of inflammation and pain.

Side effects: Since the dosage of NSAIDs necessary to suppress symptoms is usually quite high, so is the rate of side effects. The most common side effects of aspirin and other NSAIDs are damage to the intestinal tract and ulcer formation. NSAID-induced peptic ulcers can be serious and life-threatening. In fact, more people die each year as a result of peptic ulcers caused by NSAIDs than from cocaine abuse.

In addition to causing ulcers, NSAIDs often cause allergic reactions such as easy bleeding and bruising, ringing in the ears, and fluid retention. More serious complications include kidney and liver damage.

NSAIDS IN ARTHRITIS: MORE HARM THAN GOOD?

One side effect of aspirin and other NSAIDs that is often not mentioned is their inhibition of cartilage repair (that is, inhibition of collagen matrix synthesis) and acceleration of cartilage destruction.[5] Since osteoarthritis is caused by a degeneration of cartilage, it appears that while NSAIDs are fairly effective in suppressing the symptoms, they may possibly worsen the condition by inhibiting cartilage formation and accelerating cartilage destruction. Simply stated, aspirin and other NSAIDs appear to suppress the symptoms but accelerate the progression of osteoarthritis. This is supported by clinical evidence as well. In an effort to evaluate the effectiveness of current drug treatment of osteoarthritis, several studies have attempted to determine the "natural course" of the disease,[3,5] that is, the course of the disease if no treatment is given. In one study of the natural course of osteoarthritis of the hip over a ten-year period, initially all subjects had changes suggestive of advanced osteoarthritis, yet the researchers reported remarkable clinical improvement and X ray–confirmed recovery of the joint space in fourteen of thirty-one hips at the end of the study.[6] The authors of the study purposely applied no therapy and regarded their results as reflecting the natural course of the disease. Nearly half of the patients had confirmed recovery without any therapy. In contrast, several studies have shown that NSAID use is associated with acceleration of osteoarthritis and increased joint destruction.[7,8,9] In other words, NSAIDs appear to promote osteoarthritis. All of the evidence seems to suggest that people would be better off without the NSAIDs for osteoarthritis.

NSAIDs present some problems in rheumatoid arthritis as well. It is generally well accepted that in the long run, standard medical therapy is of limited value in most cases of rheumatoid arthritis, as it fails to address the complexity of this disease. Furthermore, both NSAIDs and corticosteroids may actually contribute to the disease process. For example, individuals with rheumatoid arthritis have increased intestinal permeability.[10] Their intestines are too "leaky." NSAIDs have been shown to greatly increase the leakiness of the gut of rheumatoid arthritis sufferers.[11] What is the significance of this? The result of a leaky gut is an increased absorption of large dietary and bacterial molecules. Normally, these molecules are prevented from being absorbed because they are too large. In rheumatoid arthritis, however, they are absorbed into the body, leading to the formation of complexes that can be deposited in the joints. Ultimately, much inflammation and joint destruction is the result. Because aspirin and NSAIDs decrease the symptoms, yet increase gut "leakiness," the net effect is an acceleration of factors that promote the disease process.

OTHER DRUGS FOR ARTHRITIS

If NSAIDs do not offer enough benefit, more aggressive and potentially more toxic treatments are available. For example, in rheumatoid arthritis, gold salt injection aids about 60 percent of patients. However, severe side effects occur in nearly one third of patients. Other powerful drugs are used, including methotrexate, d-penicillamine, and hydroxychloroquine, but benefit often does not warrant the toxicity suffered. And, despite the fact that long-term use of corticosteroids in rheumatoid arthritis is not advised due to side effects, corticosteroids are still widely prescribed in the long-term treatment of rheumatoid arthritis.

Dietary Factors in Treating Arthritis

Diet has been strongly linked to many forms of arthritis for many years, both to cause and to cure. All sorts of specific diets have been recommended for arthritis. Since both osteoarthritis and rheumatoid arthritis are not as common in societies that eat a diet rich in natural foods, vegetables, and fiber, and low in sugar, meat, refined carbohydrates, and saturated fat, it suggests that following such a diet is indicated in the prevention and treatment of all forms of arthritis.

A diet that focuses on plant foods and features regular consumption of fresh fruit and vegetable juices will provide high levels of natural antioxidant compounds, which can protect against cellular damage, including damage to our joints. The cells throughout the human body are constantly under attack. The culprits are free radicals and pro-oxidants. These highly reactive molecules can bind to and destroy cellular components. Free-radical damage is one of the major reasons we age. Free-radical damage is also linked to osteoarthritis and rheumatoid arthritis as well as to the development of many other diseases including cancer, heart disease, cataracts, Alzheimer's, and virtually every other chronic degenerative illness.

Although the body creates free radicals during metabolic processes, the environment contributes greatly to the free-radical "load" of an individual. Cigarette smoking, for example, greatly increases an individual's free-radical load. Many of the harmful effects of smoking, whether primary or secondary, are related to the extremely high levels of free radicals being inhaled, depleting key antioxidant nutrients such as vitamin C and beta-carotene. Other external sources of free radicals include air pollutants, pesticides, anesthetics, X rays, sunlight, fried food, solvents, alcohol, and formaldehyde. These compounds greatly stress the body's antioxidant mechanisms and should be avoided as much as possible.

The joint tissues protect themselves against free radicals and oxidative damage with the help of enzymes and antioxidants from the plant foods we consume in our diets, such as carotenes, flavonoids, vitamins C and E, and sulfur-containing compounds such as legumes. A diet that focuses on fruits, vegetables, grains, beans, nuts, and seeds is the first step in giving the joints the nourishment they need to prevent damage and promote healing. Although this is a general dietary recommendation, it is an important one. Here are some more specific dietary recommendations for both osteoarthritis and rheumatoid arthritis.

Dietary Factors in Treating Osteoarthritis

Perhaps the most important dietary recommendation for individuals suffering from osteoarthritis is that they achieve normal body weight. Being overweight means increased stress on weight-bearing joints affected with osteoarthritis.

In terms of both preventing and treating osteoarthritis with diet, it is critical that one's diet be rich in whole natural foods, especially raw fruits and vegetables because of their rich source of nutrients critical to joint health, particularly antioxidant factors like vitamin C, carotenes, and flavonoids. Especially beneficial are flavonoid-rich fruits like cherries, blueberries, and blackberries. Also important are sulfur-containing foods such as legumes, garlic, onions, brussels sprouts, and cabbage, indicated by the fact that the sulfur content in fingernails of arthritis sufferers is lower than that of healthy people.[12] Normalizing the sulfur content of the nails was reported to alleviate pain and swelling of the joints, according to clinical data from the 1930s.[13] For some reason, this promising research was never pursued.

Norman Childers, Ph.D., popularized a diet in the treatment of osteoarthritis that eliminated foods from the genus *Solanaceae* (nightshade family) after finding this simple dietary elimination cured his osteoarthritis.[14] Childers developed the theory that genetically susceptible individuals might develop arthritis, as well as a variety of other complaints, from long-term, low-level consumption of alkaloids found in tomatoes, potatoes, eggplant, peppers, and tobacco. Presumably these alkaloids inhibit normal collagen repair in the joints or promote the inflammatory degeneration of the joint. To test his theory, Dr. Childers conducted an informal study of over five thousand arthritis patients who agreed to avoid eating nightshade family vegetables. Over 70 percent reported relief from aches and pains. Although it remains to be proved in a strict scientific study, Childers's diet may offer some benefit to certain individuals, and is certainly worth a try.

Dietary Factors in Rheumatoid Arthritis

The most important dietary recommendation in rheumatoid arthritis is to eliminate allergy-inducing foods, which has been shown to offer tremendous benefit to many individuals with rheumatoid arthritis.[15] An elimination or low-allergenic diet, followed by systematic reintroduction, is often an effective method of isolating offending foods. Virtually any food can aggravate rheumatoid arthritis, but the most common offending foods are wheat, corn, milk and other dairy products, beef, and nightshade-family foods.

Patients with rheumatoid arthritis have benefited from fasting. However, strict water fasting should be done only under direct medical supervision. Fasting presumably decreases the absorption of allergenic food components, although it may also impact the immune system.[16] A juice fast is safer and may actually yield better results. Please check with your doctor before starting any fast.

A recent study highlights the effectiveness of juicing as part of a healthful diet and life-style in relieving rheumatoid arthritis.[17] In a thirteen-month study conducted in Norway at the Oslo Rheumatism Hospital, two groups of patients suffering from rheumatoid arthritis were studied to determine the effect of diet on their condition. One group followed a therapeutic diet (the treatment group), the other participants (control group) were allowed to eat as they wished. Both groups started the study by visiting a "health farm," or what we in America call a spa, for four weeks.

The treatment group began its regimen by fasting for seven to ten days and then started following a special diet. Dietary intake during the fast consisted of herbal teas, garlic, vegetable broth, decoction of potatoes and parsley, and the following juices: carrots, beets, and celery. Interestingly enough, no fruit juices were allowed.

After the fast, the patients reintroduced a "new" food item every second day. If they noticed an increase in pain, stiffness, or joint swelling within two to forty-eight hours, this new food item was omitted from the diet for at least seven days before being reintroduced a second time. If the food caused worsening of symptoms after the second time, it was omitted permanently from the diet.

The results of the study indicated that short-term fasting, followed by a vegetarian diet, produced "a substantial reduction in disease activity" in many patients. The results indicated a therapeutic benefit beyond elimination of food allergies alone. The authors suggested that the additional improvements were due to changes in dietary fatty acids. Vegetarian diets are often beneficial in the treatment of allergic and inflammatory conditions as a result of decreasing the availability of arachidonic acid—a fatty acid found exclusively in animal products—which is converted in the body to compounds that promote inflammation.

Another important way of decreasing the inflammatory response of rheumatoid arthritis is the consumption of cold-water fish such as mackerel, herring, sardines, and salmon. These fish are rich sources of eicosapentaenoic acid (EPA), which competes with arachidonic acid for prostaglandin and leukotriene production. The net effect of consumption of these fish or fish oil supplements is a significantly reduced inflammatory/allergic response in some cases. Several clinical studies have demonstrated a therapeutic effect in rheumatoid arthritis by supplementing the diet with EPA (1.8 grams daily).[18] However, supplementation may not be necessary if a serving of one of these cold-water fish is consumed at least once daily. For vegetarians, flaxseed oil, canola oil, and evening primrose oil supplementation may provide similar benefit to EPA, although the research behind this recommendation is not as solid.[19] Nonetheless, it must be kept in mind that a vegetarian diet alone is therapeutic for many rheumatoid arthritis sufferers.

There are other special foods that offer benefit to the sufferer of rheumatoid arthritis. Several bioflavonoids (pigments found in plants) have demonstrated effects in experimental studies indicating they may be beneficial to individuals with rheumatoid arthritis.[20] Good sources of the most beneficial flavonoids are cherries, other berries, and citrus fruits. Fresh pineapple may also offer some benefit due to the presence of bromelain (discussed below), a well-accepted anti-inflammatory enzyme. During flare-ups, fresh pineapple juice, along with some fresh ginger, may help because of their anti-inflammatory properties. Ginger inhibits the manufacture of inflammatory compounds; it contains an anti-inflammatory enzyme similar to bromelain. In one clinical study, seven patients with rheumatoid arthritis for whom conventional drugs had provided only temporary or partial relief were treated with ginger.[21] One patient took 50 grams per day of lightly cooked ginger, while the remaining six people took either 5 grams of fresh or 0.1 to 1 gram of powdered ginger daily. All patients reported substantial improvement, including pain relief, joint mobility, and decrease in swelling and morning stiffness.

Natural Alternatives to Arthritis Medications

While the dietary recommendations above are often quite therapeutic on their own, there is still much that can be done to relieve osteoarthritis and rheumatoid arthritis. Of particular importance is supplying adequate levels of antioxidant nutrients like selenium, manganese, vitamins C and E, and those nutrients important in the manufacture of joint substances, especially: niacinamide, pantothenic acid, vitamin B_6, and zinc. But, before we look at these nutrients, the first substance I want to discuss is glucosamine, because it is a classic example of how a natural substance improves a condition by addressing the underlying cause and supporting the body's ability to heal itself.

Glucosamine Sulfate
Glucosamine, a naturally occurring substance found in high concentrations in joint structures, appears to be nature's best remedy for osteoarthritis. In the body, the main action of glucosamine on joints is to stimulate the manufacture of cartilage components. In other words,

glucosamine is responsible for stimulating the manufacture of substances necessary for joint repair. This action alone suggests a therapeutic role in osteoarthritis. But there is much more. Glucosamine has also been shown to exert a protective effect against joint destruction and, when given orally as glucosamine sulfate, it is selectively taken up by joint tissues to exert a powerful therapeutic effect in osteoarthritis.[22]

Numerous double-blind studies have shown that glucosamine sulfate produces much better results compared with NSAIDs and placebos in relieving the pain and inflammation of osteoarthritis[23]—this, despite the fact that glucosamine sulfate exhibits no analgesic or pain-relieving effects.[22] While NSAIDs offer purely symptomatic relief and may actually promote the disease process, glucosamine sulfate addresses the cause of osteoarthritis. By getting at the root of the problem, glucosamine sulfate not only alleviates the symptoms, including pain, it also helps the body repair damaged joints. This is outstanding, but what is even more outstanding is the safety and the lack of side effects associated with oral glucosamine sulfate. In contrast, the side effects and risks associated with NSAIDs currently used in the treatment of osteoarthritis are significant. The therapeutic margin, a measure of safety, is ten to thirty times more favorable for glucosamine sulfate than for commonly used NSAIDs.[22]

One thing that must be pointed out is that the benefits of glucosamine are more obvious the longer it is used. Because glucosamine sulfate is not a pain-relieving substance per se, it takes a while longer to produce results. But once it starts working, it will produce much better results compared with NSAIDs. For example, in one study that compared glucosamine sulfate with ibuprofen, pain scores decreased faster in the first two weeks in the ibuprofen group; however, by week four, the group receiving the glucosamine sulfate was doing significantly better than the ibuprofen group.[24] This is demonstrated in the graph on page 76.

Glucosamine sulfate products are available at health-food stores or through nutritionally oriented physicians. Be sure to use glucosamine sulfate rather than glucosamine hydrochloride or N-acetyl-glucosamine, because the scientific studies were performed with the sulfate form. The standard dose for glucosamine sulfate is 500 milligrams three times per day. As mentioned earlier, glucosamine sulfate is extremely well tolerated. In addition, there are no contraindications or adverse interactions with these drugs. Glucosamine sulfate may cause some gastrointes-

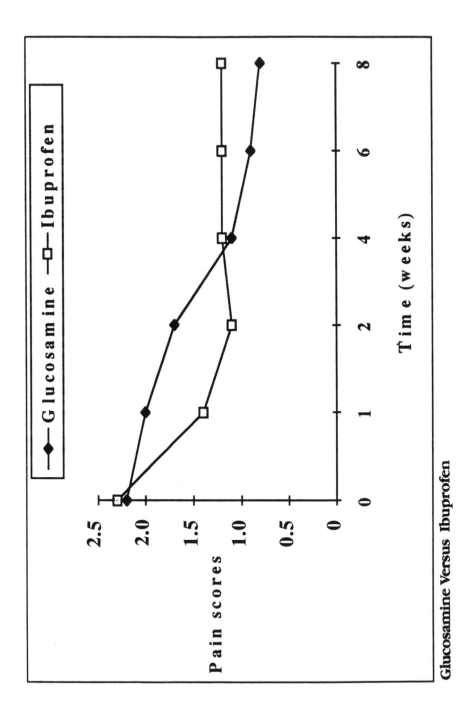

Glucosamine Versus Ibuprofen

tinal upset (nausea, heartburn, etc.) in rare instances. If this occurs, try taking it during meals or using DGL (see page 208).

ANTIOXIDANT NUTRIENTS

As much of the joint destruction in both osteoarthritis and rheumatoid arthritis is due to free-radical and oxidative damage, antioxidant nutrients are vitally important. A number of individual antioxidant nutrients have been shown to be of significant clinical benefit in both osteoarthritis and rheumatoid arthritis. Several of these nutrients are discussed below. In addition to possessing antioxidant activity, these nutrients are also critical in the manufacture of joint structures.

Vitamin C

Vitamin C functions as an important antioxidant and is an essential nutrient for the manufacture of many joint components, especially collagen. Several studies have demonstrated that vitamin C has a positive effect on cartilage and joint repair.[25] Deficient vitamin C intake is common in the elderly, resulting in altered collagen synthesis and compromised connective tissue repair. The white blood cell and plasma concentrations of vitamin C are significantly decreased in arthritis patients, indicating an increased need for vitamin C.[26]

While there are relatively high amounts of vitamin C present in broccoli, brussels sprouts, cabbage, citrus fruits, tomatoes, berries, and other vegetables, patients with arthritis will require much more. They will need at least 500 to 1,000 milligrams three times daily. It may be necessary to gradually increase vitamin C intake to these levels because some people may experience stomach upset, gas, and/or diarrhea with high doses of vitamin C. Supplementing vitamin C in the diet increases antioxidant activities, decreases histamine levels, and provides some anti-inflammatory action.[27]

Selenium and Vitamin E

A clinical trial using 600 IUs of vitamin E in patients with osteoarthritis demonstrated significant benefit from the vitamin E.[28] The benefit was thought to be due to vitamin E's antioxidant and membrane stabilizing actions. Later studies have shown that vitamin E has an ability to inhibit the enzymatic breakdown of cartilage as well as to stimulate cartilage synthesis.[29]

In rheumatoid arthritis, one clinical study indicated that vitamin E combined with selenium had a positive effect.[30] Vitamin E works together with selenium in antioxidant mechanisms. Selenium levels are low in patients with rheumatoid arthritis.[31] Low selenium levels in joint tissues may be a significant factor contributing to the inflammatory process in rheumatoid arthritis. Selenium plays an important role as an antioxidant and serves as the mineral cofactor in the free-radical scavenging enzyme glutathione peroxidase. This enzyme is also important in reducing the production of inflammatory compounds that cause much of the damage to tissues seen in rheumatoid arthritis. A deficiency of selenium would result in even more significant damage.

Supplementing the diet with 50 to 200 micrograms of selenium and 200 to 400 IUs of vitamin E daily appears to be appropriate, based on increased demand for antioxidant support and the positive results of clinical studies.

Zinc

Zinc is required for the manufacture of many joint structures and is also an antioxidant. It functions in the antioxidant enzyme superoxide dismutase (copper-zinc SOD), an important protector against cellular damage. Zinc levels are typically reduced in patients with rheumatoid arthritis, and several studies have been done using zinc sulfate in the treatment of the disease, with some of the studies demonstrating a slight therapeutic effect.[32] Better results may be obtained by using a more absorbable form of zinc like zinc picolinate, citrate, or monomethionine. The dosage for zinc is 30 to 45 milligrams per day. In addition, good dietary sources of zinc are whole grains, nuts, and seeds.

Manganese

Manganese also functions in the antioxidant enzyme superoxide dismutase (manganese SOD), which is deficient in patients with rheumatoid arthritis.[33] Manganese supplementation has been shown to increase SOD activity, indicating increased antioxidant activity. A good dosage for a manganese supplementation is 5 to 15 milligrams per day. Good dietary sources include nuts, whole grains, dried fruits, and green leafy vegetables. Meats, dairy products, poultry, and seafood are considered poor sources of manganese.

Pantothenic Acid

Studies have shown that deficiency of pantothenic acid in the rat causes a pronounced failure of cartilage growth that eventually produces lesions similar to osteoarthritis. Low pantothenic acid levels are implicated in the development of human osteoarthritis and rheumatoid arthritis, as whole-blood pantothenic acid levels have been reported to be lower in rheumatoid arthritis patients compared with normal controls.[34] In addition, disease activity was inversely correlated with pantothenic acid levels; that is, the lower the level of pantothenic acid, the more severe the symptoms. Correction of low pantothenic acid levels to normal brings about some alleviation of symptoms.[35]

Clinical improvement in osteoarthritis has been reported with the daily supplementation of 12.5 milligrams of pantothenic acid.[36] Results often took seven to fourteen days to manifest themselves. Better and quicker results may be produced by using higher dosages, such as those used in rheumatoid arthritis. For example, in one double-blind study, patients receiving 2 grams of calcium pantothenate daily noted improvements in duration of morning stiffness, degree of disability, and severity of pain.[35]

Although pantothenic acid has shown good clinical results, a diet rich in pantothenic acid may produce similar benefits. Good dietary sources of pantothenic acid are whole grains and legumes. Pantothenic acid is supplied in most multivitamin formulas.

Niacinamide

Dr. William Kaufman has reported very good clinical results in reducing pain and improving joint range of movement in the treatment of hundreds of patients with rheumatoid and osteoarthritis using high-dose niacinamide (that is, 900 to 4,000 milligrams in divided doses daily).[37] However, niacinamide at this high dose can result in significant side effects (glucose intolerance, liver damage), and should therefore be monitored by a physician.

Methionine

The essential amino acid methionine, administered as S-adenosyl-methionine (SAM), was shown to be superior to ibuprofen (Motrin) in the treatment of osteoarthritis in a double-blind clinical trial.[38] The positive effect in this trial is consistent with several other clinical studies.[39] SAM has also been shown to exert an antidepressant activity in patients with rheumatoid arthritis. Although SAM is not available in the United States, an equivalent amount of methionine (250 to 500 milligrams of L-methionine three times daily) may produce similar results. But, the best recommendation may be to eat more methionine- and sulfur-rich foods like legumes, nuts, seeds, and whole grains.

Bromelain

Bromelain refers to a mixture of enzymes found in pineapples. Bromelain was introduced as a medicinal agent in 1957, and since that time, over two hundred scientific papers on its therapeutic applications have appeared in medical literature.[40] Bromelain has been reported in these scientific studies to exert a wide variety of beneficial effects, including reducing inflammation in cases of arthritis, sports injury, or trauma, and prevention of swelling (edema) after trauma or surgery.

Several mechanisms may account for bromelain's anti-inflammatory effects, including the inhibition of pro-inflammatory compounds. Bromelain also blocks the production of kinins, the compounds produced during inflammation that increase swelling and cause pain.

Although most studies have utilized commercially prepared bromelain, it is conceivable that drinking fresh pineapple juice could exert similar effects. The standard dosage of bromelain is based on its m.c.u. (milk clotting unit) activity. The most beneficial range of activity appears to be 1,800 to 2,000 m.c.u. The dosage for this range would be 400 to 500 milligrams three times daily on an empty stomach.

Curcumin

Curcumin is the yellow pigment of turmeric (*Curcuma longa*), and it appears to be one of nature's most potent anti-inflammatory agents. Its mechanism of action is discussed in more detail beginning on page 162. In short, although curcumin has some direct anti-inflammatory effects, it is also thought to enhance the body's own anti-inflammatory mechanisms.[41] Clinical studies have substantiated curcumin anti-inflammatory effects, including a significant beneficial effect in rheumatoid arthritis. In one study, curcumin was compared to phenylbutazone, a very potent NSAID that has fallen out of favor because of frequent side effects.[42] The improvements in the duration of morning stiffness, walking time, and joint swelling were comparable in both groups.

A major fact that must be pointed out is that while curcumin has an anti-inflammatory effect similar to phenylbutazone and various NSAIDs, it does not possess any significant toxicity. The standard dosage for curcumin is 400 milligrams three times daily. Many commercial preparations combine curcumin with bromelain, as the two agents appear to work well together, and bromelain may increase the absorption of curcumin.

Final Comments

Let me summarize some clear recommendations in terms of where to start with nutritional and herbal supplements for arthritis, and how physical therapy might also be of help.

OSTEOARTHRITIS

High-potency multiple vitamin and mineral supplement

Antioxidant supplement that will provide higher levels of some of the nutritional antioxidants, including vitamin C

Glucosamine sulfate, 500 milligrams three times daily

RHEUMATOID ARTHRITIS

High-potency multiple vitamin and mineral supplement

Antioxidant supplement that will provide higher levels of some of the nutritional antioxidants, including vitamin C

EPA, 1.8 grams each day

Bromelain and curcumin

PHYSICAL THERAPY

In addition, various physical therapy modalities (exercise, heat, cold, diathermy, ultrasound, etc.) performed by physical therapists, naturopathic physicians, and chiropractors are often very beneficial in improving joint mobility and reducing pain in sufferers of arthritis. The importance of physical therapy appears to be quite significant, especially when administered regularly by a trained professional. Much of the benefit of physical therapy is thought to be a result of achieving a proper water content within the joint capsule.

Clinical and experimental studies seem to indicate shortwave diathermy may be of the greatest benefit.[43] Combining shortwave diathermy therapy with periodic ice massage, rest, and appropriate exercise appears to be the most sensible approach. Proper exercise includes isometric exercises and swimming. These types of movement increase circulation to the joint and strengthen surrounding muscles without placing too much strain on the joint.

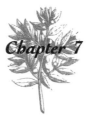

ASTHMA, HAY FEVER, AND ANTIHISTAMINE MEDICATIONS

The number of Americans suffering from allergies, asthma, and hay fever has risen dramatically over the last fifteen years. Some possible reasons include: increased stress on the immune system due to the greater chemical pollution in our air, water, and food; earlier weaning and earlier introduction of solid foods to infants; food additives; and genetic manipulation of plants, resulting in food components with greater allergenic tendencies. Probably all of these reasons and a few others have contributed to the increased frequency and severity of allergies. It is currently estimated that over forty million, or 25 percent of Americans suffer from asthma and other allergies.[1]

What Is an Allergy?

A classic allergic reaction starts when a foreign substance such as pollen, dust, animal dander, or food is attacked and then bound by a specific type of antibody produced by the body, known as IgE (immunoglobulin E). The substance bound to the allergic antibody is the "antigen" or "allergen." The IgE-antigen complex then binds to specialized white blood cells known as "mast cells" and "basophils." This binding causes the release of substances such as histamine, that cause swelling and inflammation. A variety of allergic symptoms may result, depending on the location of the mast cell: In the nasal passages, it causes sinus congestion; in the bronchioles, asthma; in the skin, hives and eczema; in the lining of the joints, arthritis; in the intestinal tract, inflammation with resulting diarrhea; and in the brain, headaches.

Asthma is an allergic disorder characterized by spasm of the bronchial tubes and excessive excretion of a viscous mucus in the lungs, which can lead to difficulty in breathing. It strikes as recurrent attacks that range from mild wheezing to a life-threatening inability to breathe.

Hay fever (seasonal allergic rhinitis) is an allergic reaction of the nasal passages and airways to airborne pollens. Ragweed pollen accounts for about 75 percent of the hay fever in the United States. Other significant pollens inducing hay fever include various grass and tree pollens. If the hay fever develops in spring, it is usually due to tree pollens. If it develops in summer, grass and weed pollens are usually the culprits. Hay fever symptoms that persist year-round are known as perennial allergic rhinitis. This may or may not be due to pollens.

Asthma, Hay Fever, and Allergy Medications

Since asthma is the most serious of the conditions being discussed in this chapter, it will receive the most attention. And rightfully so. Asthma is a major health problem in the United States that is getting worse, much worse. During the 1980s, the death rate for asthma more than doubled.[2] The obvious question is: Are the current medicines being used to treat asthma responsible for this effect? This is a difficult question to ponder, because there are many factors to consider, but there is evidence to support an affirmative answer. Foremost in the link between medical treatment and asthma mortality is the increased reliance on multiple prescriptions. Although these medicines may provide immediate short-term benefit, for the long term they may be causing more health problems. It is, therefore, vitally important to address underlying factors in asthma, rather than relying on a prescription. The following drug categories will be discussed:

Antihistamines

Bronchodilators

Cromolyn
Xanthine preparations
Corticosteroids

ANTIHISTAMINES

Antihistamines are big business in the United States, as these drugs dominate both the over-the-counter and prescription markets. In addition to being used in allergies, antihistamines are used as nasal decongestants and for the treatment of insomnia and peptic ulcers.

Over-the-Counter Antihistamines
Common OTC antihistamine ingredients used for allergies and hay fever include (with some brand names in parentheses after each):

Brompheniramine (Dimetapp, Dimetane, Drixoral)

Chlorpheniramine (Allerest, Chlor-Trimeton, Coricidin, Triaminic Allergy)

Diphenhydramine (Benadryl)

Phenyltoloxamine (Sinutab)

Over-the-counter antihistamines often contain a mixture of an antihistamine along with a nasal decongestant like pseudoephedrine, phenylpropanolomine, or phenylephrine. Nasal decongestants are discussed in Chapter 10, "Common Cold Medications." Although OTC antihistamines and nasal decongestants are often used in self-treating allergies, they offer only limited benefit. Antihistamines do not block the release of histamine. Instead, they block the action of histamine at receptor sites. Since histamine functions in the brain to maintain alertness, most antihistamines produce drowsiness. Although many OTC antihistamines contain stimulants to prevent that effect, the use of OTC antihistamines in allergic disorders has been replaced by two prescription antihistamines, Seldane and Hismanal, which do not produce drowsiness (see below).

Side effects: Drowsiness is the primary side effect with most antihistamines, especially those without stimulants. The warning on the product not to drive or operate heavy machinery should be taken quite seriously. As little as 50 milligrams of diphenhydramine (Benadryl) may produce an impairment in driving similar to a 0.1-percent blood alcohol content, the standard for drunk driving.[3] Other possible side effects include allergic reactions, headache, nausea, and drying of the nose, mouth, and throat.

Prescription Antihistamines

Seldane (terfenadine) was the first nonsedating antihistamine to hit the market. It was quickly followed by Hismanal (astemizole). Although both antihistamines work in a manner similar to that of other antihistamines, they are more specific for cells outside the brain so they do not produce drowsiness. Although an advantage over other antihistamines, Seldane and Hismanal have their own risks. As of May 1992, 127 serious cardiovascular events, including 15 deaths, have been linked to Seldane or Hismanal.[4] This prompted the FDA to recommend that the manufacturers of the drugs (Marion Dow and Janssen) issue warnings to physicians about possible side effects. The drugs have been given a "black box" designation by the FDA. The warning that these drugs can produce serious adverse side effects if used in doses in excess of manufacturer's recommendation—or if used in patients with significant liver dysfunction or in patients taking the drugs ketoconazole or erythromycin—must appear within heavy black lines on the product label to signify the seriousness of the side effects. Thus, the designation "black box" is given.

Side effects: In addition to possible serious side effects, both Seldane and Hismanal tend to dry out the body's mucous membranes, causing dry nose, mouth, or throat. Other possible side effects include allergic reactions, nausea, indigestion, vomiting, increased appetite, weight gain, headache, nervousness, and fatigue.

BRONCHODILATORS

These medications stimulate beta receptors on cells much like the body hormone adrenaline and are therefore known as beta-agonists. The effect of these drugs on asthma is to relax the bronchial muscles and open up the airways rapidly during a mild to moderate asthma attack.

Beta-agonists are available in both inhaler (aerosol) and pill form. However, the aerosol form is preferred because it is less likely to cause side effects. Examples of this class of asthma medication are:

Albuterol (Ventolin, Proventil)
Isoetharine (Bronkometer, Bronkosol)
Isoproterenol (Isuprel, Medihaler-Iso)
Metaproterenol (Alupent, Metaprel)
Pirbuterol (Maxair)
Terbutaline (Brethine, Bricanyl)

In most cases of an acute asthma attack, these medications are extremely effective. However, amelioration lasts only three to six hours at the most. The result is an increased reliance on the inhaler, which can result in reduced effectiveness over time as well as an increased risk for side effects. These drugs are, therefore, best reserved for acute asthmatic attacks or as directed by a physician.

Side effects: The aerosols will almost always produce dryness or irritation of the mouth or throat, but they are much less likely to produce other side effects as do the pill forms. Because these drugs bind to the same receptors as adrenaline, they can cause some of the same effects. In addition to the desired effect of relaxing the airways, these drugs can lead to an increased heart rate and blood pressure as well as insomnia and feelings of anxiety. The increases in heart rate and blood pressure can lead to serious consequences. Other side effects of beta-agonists include headache, dizziness, muscle cramps, nausea, and heart palpitations.

CROMOLYN

Cromolyn (Intal, Nasalchrom) is a synthetic derivative of a natural compound, khellin, originally isolated from the plant *Ammi visnaga*. Native to the Mediterranean and used by the ancient Egyptians to treat asthma and angina, *Ammi visnaga* was discussed in Chapter 4, "Angina Medications." Cromolyn is similar in structure and activity to many natural compounds, including bioflavonoids like quercetin (discussed below).

Cromolyn, also known as cromolyn sodium or disodium chromogly-cate, works by inhibiting the release of histamine and other allergic compounds from mast cells. Therefore, it is viewed as a preventive measure rather than a treatment for an acute asthma attack. In other words, it will not reverse an allergic reaction once it is under way.

Available for use in capsules, eye drops, inhalation aerosols, pow-ders, and nasal solutions, cromolyn is a prescription drug; your physician can help you determine which form and dosage are best. Because cromo-lyn is not absorbed that well (less than 1 percent) by mouth, it is best used by local administration. That is, for allergic rhinitis, cromolyn should be administered to the lining of the nasal passages; for asthma, it must come in contact with the lining of the bronchioles. Cromolyn is prescribed for use in asthma, hay fever, perennial allergic rhinitis, and allergic reactions in the outer lining of the eye (conjunctivitis). It is especially useful in preventing asthma triggered by exercise.

Side effects: Although the aerosol does not taste very good, cromolyn is otherwise extremely well tolerated. Side effects are rare (fewer than one in ten thousand), but can include bronchospasm, coughing or wheezing, joint swelling and pain, skin rash or hives, and nausea. A severe allergic reaction (anaphylaxis) is rare.

XANTHINE PREPARATIONS

Xanthine preparations usually refer to those brand drugs that con-tain theophylline: Bronkodyl, Elixophyllin, Somophyllin-T, Slo-bid, Slo-Phyllin, Theo-Dur, Theo-24, Theobid, Theolair, and Uniphyl. These products may contain theophylline alone or in combination with ephed-rine (discussed later in this chapter) to enhance the bronchodilator effects; guaifenesin to thin the mucus secretions; or phenobarbital to reduce anxiety.

Theophylline is a member of the methylxanthines, a group of closely related alkaloids that also includes caffeine and theobromine. Like cro-molyn, which was derived from an ancient medicinal plant, methylxan-thines were discovered from research into medicinal plants. Theophylline is found in the leaves of tea (*Camellia sinensis*). Caffeine is also found in tea, as well as in coffee beans (*Coffea arabica*) and cola nuts (*Cola acuminata*). Theobromine is found in the seeds of cocoa (*Theobroma cacao*).

While these plants have been used for thousands of years in treating asthma, modern theophylline-containing preparations have been used extensively in the treatment of asthma for over fifty years. Theophylline preparations work by causing the relaxation of the muscles in the bronchial tubes and of the blood vessels in the lungs. This relaxation results in relief of asthma, expanded lung capacity, and improved lung circulation. Although of unquestioned benefit in relieving asthma, theophylline use carries some problems.

Theophylline has a very narrow margin of safety. This means that the margin or difference between a therapeutic dose and a toxic dose is quite small. The narrow margin of safety requires strict medical supervision and periodic determination of the level of theophylline in the blood. Side effects due to theophylline are assured, especially in children. The long-standing practice of using theophylline as a first-line treatment of asthma in the United States is coming to an end. Most other parts of the world utilize theophylline only for the relief of an acute asthma attack.

Side effects: Theophylline can produce effects similar to drinking too much coffee: nervousness, insomnia, rapid heart rate, nausea, and increased urination. Due to the dosage requirements, these symptoms almost always appear. In children especially, theophylline will most always produce restlessness, hyperactivity, poor concentration, headache, or an upset stomach. If theophylline levels are too high, even more significant symptoms will appear, including severe anxiety, disturbed heart rate, and seizures.

CORTICOSTEROIDS

Although oral corticosteroids have long been employed in the treatment of chronic asthma, the development of steroid-containing inhalers is changing the way the medicine is being delivered to the body. Due to the toxicity problems with theophylline and oral corticosteroids like prednisone, the use of inhaled corticosteroids has increased substantially in recent years. Examples of some popular steroid inhalers include beclomethasone (Beclovent, Beconase, Vanceril); flunisole (AeroBid); and triamcinolone (Azmacort).

Corticosteroids are thought to work in asthma by reducing the production of allergic and inflammatory compounds. Compared with the pill form, the inhaled form offers the advantage of acting on the lining of the respiratory tract, thereby significantly reducing some of the side effects of oral corticosteroids. Like cromolyn, steroid inhalers are only useful in preventing an asthma attack; they are not effective during an acute attack. Although the steroid inhalers are safer than the pill forms, their use is associated with common side effects. Therefore, it appears that cromolyn is a better choice of prevention. Like cromolyn, steroid inhalers are also used in the treatment of allergic rhinitis.

The current medical consensus is that oral corticosteroids should not be used routinely in asthma.[1] However, during episodes of severe worsening, they may offer substantial benefit. Usually the dosage is at a high level for a short period of time and then abruptly halted. For example, 30 milligrams of prednisone are given twice daily for five days and then halted if control over the asthma is restored. Although it is still widely prescribed by many physicians, the use of long-term oral corticosteroids is to be avoided. For a more detailed discussion of oral corticosteroids see Chapter 11, "Corticosteroids."

Side effects: Since the side effects of oral corticosteroids are given in Chapter 11, this discussion shall focus on the side effects of steroid inhalers. The most common complication of steroid inhalers is an overgrowth of the common yeast *Candida albicans*. This growth can lead to thrush, or candida infection of the mouth. Thrush is characterized by the appearance of sore, creamy-yellow patches. To reduce the risk of developing thrush, it is often recommended that "spacers" be used. Spacers are simple devices that fit onto the inhaler to provide a chamber or space from which the medicine can be inhaled gradually. This allows the medicine to be inhaled into the lungs more effectively, and cuts down on the accumulation in the mouth, tongue, and throat. Rinsing the mouth out with water after every use of a steroid inhaler is very important.

Other side effects of steroid inhalers include allergic reactions, dryness of mouth, hoarseness, and sore throat. Because these drugs suppress the immune system, they should not be used during any sort of infection.

Long-term use may increase the likelihood of developing a respiratory tract infection.

Systemic effects are usually only minimal if the inhaler is being used as prescribed. With inappropriate use and overuse, however, systemic side effects identical to those of oral corticosteroids may result.

Dietary and Life-style Factors in Treating Asthma, Hay Fever, and Allergies

The natural approach to treating asthma, hay fever, and allergies is first to reduce the allergic threshold. Allergens can be viewed as straws on a camel's back. Adding enough straws to the camel's back will ultimately cause it to break. Similarly, increasing the exposure to allergens will ultimately cause symptoms. There are two primary weapons in reducing the allergic threshold: the reduction of airborne and of food allergens.

Along with adopting a diet low in allergens, a healthful life-style can significantly reduce allergies. In a recent study of 706 Japanese factory workers, it was demonstrated that a healthful life-style reduced immunoglobulin E (IgE) levels, while an unhealthful life-style resulted in elevated IgE levels.[5] Life-style factors that tended to result in elevated IgE levels included poor dietary habits, alcohol consumption, cigarette smoking, and increased feelings of stress.

AVOIDING AIRBORNE ALLERGENS

Airborne allergens such as pollen, dander, and dust mites are often difficult to avoid entirely, but measures can be taken to reduce exposure. Eliminating dogs, cats, carpets, rugs, upholstered furniture, and other surfaces where allergens can collect is a great first step. If these measures can't be taken entirely, make sure that the bedroom is as allergy-proof as possible. Encase the mattress in an *allergen-proof* plastic; wash sheets, blankets, pillowcases, and mattress pads every week; consider using bedding material made from Ventflex, a special hypoallergenic synthetic material; install an air purifier. The best air purifiers are HEPA (high-efficiency particulate-arresting) filters, which can be attached to central heating and air-conditioning systems. These units are available from suppliers of heating and air-conditioning units. Portable HEPA air purifiers are less effective, but may still provide good results, and typically cost between three hundred and five hundred dollars.

If rugs and upholstery are in the house, it is important to use a vacuum cleaner that has an efficient filtering system, such as those that trap dust in water or HEPA filters. Since most vacuum cleaners do not trap all the material they collect, they actually spread allergens through the air. Vacuum cleaners with efficient filtering units are the only types an allergic person should use.

All of these special products are available from supply houses that deal specifically in products designed for allergy sufferers. Two sources are:

Allergy Control Products
89 Danbury Road
Ridgefield, CT 06877
(800) 422-DUST

National Allergy Supply
4579 Georgia Highway 120
Duluth, GA 30136
(800) 522-1448

FOOD ALLERGIES

Food allergies undoubtedly play a major role in determining an individual's "allergic threshold." Eliminating food allergens is very effective in treating most allergic conditions, including asthma, hay fever, allergic rhinitis, eczema, and hives.[6,7,8] Follow recommendations given in Chapter 22 (page 266).

The importance of eliminating food additives from the diet of allergy sufferers cannot be overstated. Food additives such as yellow dye #5 (tartrazine) and benzoates increase the production of a compound that then increases the number of mast cells in the body.[9] A person with more mast cells in the body will typically be more prone to allergies. Food additives appear to be a major factor in many allergies. Colorings (azo dyes), flavorings (salicylates, aspartame), preservatives (benzoates, nitrites, sorbic acid), synthetic antioxidants (hydroxytoluene, sulfite, gallate), and emulsifiers/stabilizers (polysorbates, vegetable gums) have all been shown to produce allergies and play a role in many cases of asthma.[10]

An important way of decreasing the allergic response is by decreasing the intake of animal fats while simultaneously increasing the consumption of omega-3 oils found in certain vegetable oils such as flaxseed oil, and cold-water fish such as mackerel, herring, sardines, and salmon. The net effect of this simple dietary change is a significantly reduced inflammatory/allergic response, to be discussed in detail in Chapter 11, "Corticosteroids."

VEGETARIAN DIET

A vegetarian diet is being shown to help in treating many chronic allergic or inflammatory diseases, including asthma. For example, one long-term trial of a vegan diet (elimination of all animal products) provided significant improvement in 92 percent of the twenty-five treated patients who completed the study (nine patients dropped out within the first two months).[11]

The diet excluded all meat, fish, eggs, and dairy products. Drinking water was limited to spring water (chlorinated tap water was specifically prohibited), and coffee, ordinary tea, chocolate, sugar, and salt were excluded. Herbal spices were allowed, and water and herbal teas were allowed up to one and a half liters per day. Vegetables used freely were lettuce, carrots, beets, onions, celery, cabbage, cauliflower, broccoli, nettles, cucumber, radishes, Jerusalem artichokes, and all beans except soybeans and green peas. Potatoes were allowed in restricted amounts. A number of fruits were also used freely: blueberries, cloudberries, raspberries, strawberries, black currants, gooseberries, plums, and pears. Apples and citrus fruits were not allowed, and grains were either restricted or eliminated.

The beneficial effects of this dietary regime are probably related to two areas: (1) the elimination of common food allergens, and (2) an altered fatty-acid metabolism. The allergic compounds that trigger asthma are derived from arachidonic acid, a fatty acid found exclusively in animal products. By eliminating the dietary source of these allergic compounds, an allergic reaction is greatly reduced. In addition, several of the foods consumed (e.g., onions and berries) have exerted anti-asthmatic effects in experimental studies. Onions are particularly beneficial.[12]

One key point that needs to be made is the importance of maintaining the diet for at least one year. In the above study, while 72 percent of the patients responded within four months, one year of therapy was required before a full 92 percent of patients responded. The results are most obvious over a long period of time. In addition to being effective against asthma, the researchers also found a reduction in the tendency to infectious disease.

Natural Alternatives to Asthma, Hay Fever, and Antihistamine Medications

In addition to reducing the allergic threshold, eliminating allergy-inducing foods, and following a vegetarian diet, there are several natural substances that exert important antiallergy effects. Foremost are antioxidant nutrients, vitamin C, quercetin and other bioflavonoids, vitamin B_{12}, vitamin B_6, and the herb *Ephedra sinica*.

ANTIOXIDANTS

Vitamin C and several other nutrients, such as vitamin E and selenium, have demonstrated significant antiallergy effects in experimental and clinical studies. Much of this activity appears to be due to their ability to function as antioxidants. An antioxidant is a substance that prevents damage to cells by free radicals or pro-oxidants. Strictly speaking, a "free radical" is a molecule that contains a highly reactive unpaired electron, while a "pro-oxidant" is a molecule that can promote oxidative damage. Although the body's own generation of free radicals is important, the environment contributes greatly to the free-radical "load" of an individual. External sources of free radicals include primary and secondary cigarette smoke, chemotherapeutic drugs, air pollutants, pesticides, anesthetics, X rays, sunlight, fried food, solvents, alcohol, and formaldehyde. These compounds greatly impair the body's antioxidant mechanisms, thereby increasing the likelihood of developing allergies. When mast cells are exposed to free radicals and pro-oxidants, they become quite fragile and much more likely to release histamine and other inflammatory compounds.

Vitamin C and other antioxidants are thought to provide important defenses against allergies and asthma, since oxidizing agents can both stimulate constriction of the lungs and increase allergic reactions to other agents. Both treated and untreated asthmatic patients have been shown to have significantly lower levels of vitamin C in the blood and white blood cells.[13] Furthermore, vitamin C has been shown to inhibit bronchial constriction in both normal and asthmatic subjects.[14,15] Vitamin C appears to normalize fatty acid metabolism and reduce histamine production. As an antioxidant and mast-cell stabilizer, vitamin C also reduces histamine secretion. It also functions in the detoxification of histamine. Supplementing the diet with vitamin C has been shown to lower blood histamine levels in double-blind studies.[16] This effect may explain some of the positive results of vitamin C supplementation in clinical studies in asthma and other allergic conditions. A good therapeutic dose of vitamin C in cases of allergies is 500 to 1,000 milligrams three to four times daily. Carotenes, vitamin E, and selenium are also important due to their powerful antioxidant activity.

QUERCETIN AND OTHER FLAVONOIDS

Flavonoids are compounds responsible for many of the colors of fruits and flowers. Flavonoids are also responsible for many of the medicinal effects of foods and herbs. Quercetin is the flavonoid that typically displays the highest degree of activity in models of allergy and inflammation.[17]

Quercetin exerts effects similar to cromolyn. Unlike antihistamine drugs, which block the binding of histamine to cellular receptors, quercetin has been shown to actually inhibit the release of histamine and other inflammatory mediators from mast cells. By inhibiting the release of histamine and other inflammatory compounds from mast cells, quercetin greatly reduces the allergic/inflammatory response.

Quercetin has further antiallergy action due to its potent antioxidant activity and its ability to inhibit the formation of inflammatory compounds like leukotrienes.[18] These compounds are a thousand times more potent in stimulating inflammatory processes than histamine.

Quercetin appears to have a very strong affinity for mast cells, as demonstrated in experimental studies in animals.[19] However, like cromolyn, quercetin is not absorbed that well. Combining quercetin with an equal amount of bromelain, the anti-inflammatory enzyme from pineapple, may increase its absorption. Bromelain has been shown to increase the absorption and tissue concentrations of a variety of compounds and may produce a similar effect with quercetin.[20] A good dosage for quercetin is 250 to 500 milligrams five to ten minutes before meals.

VITAMIN B_{12}

Jonathan Wright, M.D., believes, "B_{12} therapy is the mainstay in childhood asthma."[21] In one clinical trial, weekly intramuscular injections of 1,000 micrograms of vitamin B_{12} produced definite improvement in asthmatic patients. Of twenty patients, eighteen showed less shortness of breath during exertion, as well as improved appetite, sleep, and general health.[22] Vitamin B_{12} appears to be especially effective in sulfite-sensitive individuals. It offers the best protection when given orally prior to eating sulfites, having demonstrated better results compared with several drugs, including cromolyn.[23] The mode of action is the formation of a sulfite-cobalamin complex, which blocks sulfite's effect. Oral supplementation with 1 to 3 milligrams of vitamin B_{12} daily may provide similar benefit to the injectable form.

VITAMIN B_6

Children with asthma have been shown to have a defect in tryptophan metabolism, and reduced platelet transport of serotonin. Tryptophan is converted to serotonin, a known broncho-constricting agent in asthmatics. Double-blind clinical studies have shown that patients benefit from either a tryptophan-restricted diet or vitamin B_6 supplementation to correct the blocked tryptophan metabolism.[24]

In another study, pyridoxal phosphate (the active form of vitamin B_6) levels in fifteen adult patients with asthma were significantly lower than in sixteen controls.[25] Oral supplementation with 50 milligrams of vitamin B_6 twice daily resulted in a dramatic decrease in frequency and severity of wheezing and asthmatic attacks. Although all patients reported benefit, in seven of the patients, supplementation failed to produce a substantial elevation of the pyridoxal phosphate, suggesting that some patients may need even more vitamin B_6, or they may need to take the active pyridoxal-5-phosphate form.

EPHEDRA SINICA

The Chinese have long treasured ephedra, or mahuang, for allergy, asthma, hay fever, colds, and inflammatory conditions.[26] In fact, the medicinal use of ephedra can be traced back to over five thousand years ago. Its use in modern medicine began in 1923 with the "discovery" of the alkaloid compound ephedrine. Synthetic manufacture of ephedrine began shortly thereafter (1927). Synthetic ephedrine and related compounds are still widely used in many prescription medications for asthma, emphysema, hay fever, and nasal congestion. There are, however, other components in the crude plant besides ephedrine that possess significant anti-inflammatory and antiallergy activities.[27]

Ephedra can produce the same side effects that ephedrine can, that is, increased blood pressure and heart rate, insomnia, and anxiety. But, according to the American Pharmaceutical Association, "There is far more discussion of ephedrine tachyphylaxis (rapid decrease in effectiveness) or tolerance than is evidenced as a significant problem in the scientific literature."[28] A 1977 study of ephedrine therapy in asthmatic children published in the *Journal of the American Medical Association* (JAMA) concluded: "Ephedrine is a potent bronchodilator that, in appropriate doses, can be administered safely along with therapeutic doses of theophylline without the fear of progressive tolerance or toxicity."[29]

The FDA advisory review panel on nonprescription drugs recommended that ephedrine not be taken by patients with heart disease, high blood pressure, thyroid disease, diabetes, or difficulty in urination due to enlargement of the prostate gland. Nor should ephedrine be used in patients on antihypertensive or antidepressant drugs.

The ancient herbal treatment of asthma and hay fever involves the use of ephedra in combination with herbal expectorants. Expectorants are herbs that modify the quality and quantity of secretions of the respiratory tract resulting in the expulsion of secretions and improvement in respiratory tract function. Examples of commonly used expectorants include: lobelia (*Lobelia inflata*), licorice (*Glycyrrhiza glabra*), and grindelia (*Grindelia camporum*).

The optimum dosage of ephedra depends on the alkaloid content in the form used. The average total alkaloid content of *Ephedra sinica* is 1 to 3 percent. When used in the treatment of asthma, the ephedra dose should have an ephedrine content of 12.5 to 25.0 milligrams and be taken two to three times daily. For the crude herb, an equal dose would be 500 to 1,000 milligrams three times per day. Standardized preparations are often preferred, as they have more dependable therapeutic activity.

While ephedra and its alkaloids have proven to be effective in the treatment of mild to moderate asthma and hay fever, the therapeutic effect of ephedra may diminish if used over a long period of time due largely to weakening of the adrenal gland caused by ephedrine. Use ephedra in combination with the above-mentioned herbs and with nutrients that support the adrenal glands, such as vitamin C, magnesium, zinc, vitamin B_6, and pantothenic acid.

Final Comments

While most allergies are not life-threatening, asthma can be a serious medical emergency. Proper medical care is essential. In severe cases, the best treatment is a combined approach using natural measures to reduce the allergic threshold and prevent acute attacks, along with proper drug treatment of acute attacks. Here is my view of the hierarchy of medical treatment of asthma, hay fever, and allergic rhinitis:

1.   Avoid airborne allergens, and allergy-proof the house.

2. Eliminate food allergies and food additives from diet.

3. Follow a vegetarian diet.

4. Support the body's antiallergy mechanisms with vitamin C, other antioxidants, quercetin, vitamin B_{12}, and vitamin B_6.

5. Use cromolyn, inhaled for asthma, intranasally for hay fever and allergic rhinitis.

6. Take ephedra-based herbal products.

7. Use bronchodilators (asthma only).

8. Employ inhaled corticosteroids (intranasally for hay fever and allergic rhinitis).

9. Use theophylline-containing products.

10. Take oral corticosteroids.

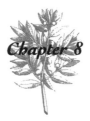

Chapter 8

BLOOD PRESSURE-LOWERING

MEDICATIONS

Each time the heart beats, it sends blood coursing through the arteries. The peak reading of the pressure exerted by this contraction is the systolic pressure. Between beats, the heart relaxes and blood pressure drops. The very lowest reading is referred to as the diastolic pressure. A normal blood pressure reading for an adult is: 120 (systolic) / 80 (diastolic).

High blood pressure or hypertension refers to a reading of greater than 140/90. An elevated blood pressure is one of the major risk factors for a heart attack or stroke. Since heart disease and strokes account for more than 43 percent of all deaths in the United States, it is very important to keep the blood pressure in the normal range. Over sixty million Americans have high blood pressure. Approximately 38 percent of black adults have high blood pressure—a higher rate than for white adults (29 percent).

High blood pressure is divided into different levels: Borderline (120–160/90–94); Mild (140–160/95–104); Moderate 140–180/105–114); and Severe (160 + /115 +). Although physicians are primarily concerned with diastolic pressure (the second number in the blood pressure reading), systolic pressure is also an important factor. The following measurement shows how high in millimeters (mm) applied pressure will cause mercury (Hg) to rise on a measuring instrument. Individuals with a normal diastolic pressure (less than 82 mm Hg) but elevated systolic pressure (more than 158 mm Hg) have a twofold increase in their cardiovascular death rates when compared with individuals who have normal systolic pressures (less than 130 mm Hg).

Drug Versus Nondrug Therapy

Since over 80 percent of patients with high blood pressure are in the borderline-to-moderate range, most cases of high blood pressure can be brought under control through changes in diet and life-style. In fact, in head-to-head comparisons, many nondrug therapies, such as diet, exercise, and relaxation techniques, have proved superior to drugs in cases of borderline-to-mild hypertension. These nondrug therapies are discussed in detail below.

Another strike against prescription drugs is the increasing evidence indicating that they may be doing more harm than good. Specifically, in some people, these drugs may be producing the very thing they are trying to prevent: a heart attack. Several well-designed, long-term clinical studies have found that people taking the blood pressure–lowering drugs (most often, diuretics and/or beta-blockers) actually suffer from unnecessary side effects including an *increased* risk for heart disease. The reason is obvious when the side effects of the drugs, discussed below, are examined in close detail.

Virtually every medical authority (textbooks, organizations, journals), including the Joint National Committee on Detection, Evaluation and Treatment of High Blood Pressure, has recommended that nondrug therapies be used in the treatment of borderline-to-mild hypertension in place of drugs. According to several clinical studies, the drugs carry with them no real benefit, yet possess significant risks. The two most definitive trials, the Australian and Medical Research Council trials, as well as five other large trials, including the famous Multiple Risk Factor Intervention Trial (MRFIT), have shown the drugs offer no benefit in protecting against heart disease in borderline-to-moderate hypertension.[1–7] Opposed to these seven negative trials, there are two that found treatment was somewhat effective.[8,9] However, upon further examination, both of these studies were found to be flawed. The European Working Party on Hypertension in the Elderly Trial was relatively small, and in the Hypertension Detection and Follow-up Program, there was an inadequate control group.

The most startling conclusion to draw is that these studies compared drug treatment with no treatment (placebo). If the natural alternatives outlined in this chapter were compared with standard drug treatment in borderline-to-moderate hypertension in clinical trials, there is little doubt

Table 8.1 Effect of Drug Treatment Versus Placebo—Summary of Trials

Trial	No. of Subjects	Entry DBP (mm Hg)	Incidence CHD Events Treatment	Control	% Difference
Showing no or negative benefit					
VA	380	90 to 114	11	13	13
USPHS	389	90 to 115	7	6	−17
Oslo	785	90 to 109	20	13	−54
Australian	3,427	95 to 109	33	33	0*
MRFIT	7,012	90+	115	124	5
MPPCDM	1,222	95+	19	9	−111
MRC	17,354	90 to 109	222	234	12
Showing benefit					
EWPHE	840	90 to 119	7	16	56
HDFP	7,825	90 to 104	86	107	20

Includes either mortality alone or morbidity plus mortality when data for both are given.
*Intention to treat.
CHD = coronary heart disease; DBP = diastolic blood pressure; EWPHE = European Working Party High Blood Pressure in the Elderly; HDFP = Hypertension Detection and Follow-up Program; MPPCDM = Multifactorial Primary Prevention of Cardiovascular Diseases in Middle-Aged Men; MRC = Medical Research Council; MRFIT = Multiple Risk Factor Intervention Trial. USPHS = United States Public Health Service; VA = Veterans Administration.

that the natural approach would yield substantial benefit. Here is a quote from an article examining drug treatment in hypertension that appeared in the *American Journal of Cardiology*. It is consistent with current medical opinion: "Few patients with uncomplicated marginal hypertension require drug treatment . . . there is little evidence these patients [with marginal hypertension] will achieve enough benefit to justify the costs and adverse effects of antihypertensive drug treatment."[10]

Despite substantial evidence and expert medical opinion, blood pressure–lowering drugs are still among the most widely prescribed drugs in America. Why? According to an article in the *Journal of the American Medical Association*, "Treatment of hypertension has become the leading reason for visits to physicians as well as for drug prescriptions."[11] In other words, blood pressure–lowering drugs are big business to the drug companies and to physicians. Yearly sales of blood pressure medications are estimated to be greater than ten billion dollars. Since it is estimated that approximately 50 percent of patients with high blood pressure are in the borderline-to-mild range, if doctors prescribed non-drug protocols that have been recommended by the authorities, it could mean a loss of greater than five billion dollars to the drug companies each year, as well as a substantial financial loss to physicians.

Blood Pressure–Lowering Medications

For many years, the drug of first choice for high blood pressure was a thiazide diuretic, alone or in combination with a beta-blocker. As mentioned above, due to lack of effectiveness in reducing the cardiovascular death rate, and side effects noted in numerous studies, this approach is being challenged. Nonetheless, the most popular drug therapy of high blood pressure still involves the use of a diuretic and/or some type of medication designed to relax the arteries, such as beta-blockers, calcium channel blockers, and ACE (angiotensin-converting enzyme) inhibitors.

When a diuretic or any of these other drugs is used alone, it is referred to as a "step-one" drug. Thiazide diuretics are still the most popular step-one drugs, but may soon be displaced by calcium channel blockers or ACE inhibitors. Beta-blockers are not suitable as step-one drugs due to their known side effects. A step-two drug utilizes two medications; a step-three uses three; and a step-four drug is composed of four medications. Physicians are instructed by the medical experts to utilize single therapies prior to combinations of medicines.

There are other types of blood pressure–lowering medications that can be used as step-three or step-four drugs, including those that act on the brain, such as clonidine (Catapres), methyl-dopa (Aldomet), and reserpine (Serpasil). Some others that are potent dilators of the blood vessels are minoxidil (Loniten) and hydralazine (Apresoline), but these drugs have fallen out of favor with the development of the calcium channel blockers and ACE inhibitors. Nonetheless, these drugs may be appropriate in certain situations, as determined by your physician.

DIURETICS

Diuretics lower blood pressure by reducing the volume of fluid in the blood and body tissues by promoting the elimination of salt and water through increased urination. Blood pressure is similar to water pressure through a garden hose. If the amount of water flowing through the hose is increased, the water flows from the hose with greater pressure. The increased pressure is due to a greater amount or volume of water being forced through the hose. Diuretics work by reducing the fluid volume being forced through the arteries, and by relaxing the smaller arteries of the body, allowing them to expand and increase the total fluid capacity of the arterial system—similar to directing some of the water from the garden hose to other hoses. The net result of diuretics is lower pressure due to reduced volume in an expanded space.

There are three major types of diuretics: thiazides, loop diuretics, and potassium-sparing diuretics. Here are some examples in each category, generic name followed by brand:

Thiazide Diuretics
Bendroflumethiazide (Corzide, Naturetin, Rauzide)

Benzthiazide (Exna)

Chlorothiazide (Aldoclor, Diuril)

Chlorthalidone (Thalitone)

Hydrochlorothiazide (Esidrix, Thiuretic)

Hydroflumethiazide (Diucardin)

Polythiazide (Renese)

Loop Diuretics
Bumetanide (Bumex)

Furosemide (Lasix)

Potassium-Sparing Diuretics
Amiloride (Midamor)

Spironolactone (Alatone, Aldactone)

Triamterene (Dyrenium)

The thiazide diuretics are often the first drugs used in treating mild-to-moderate high blood pressure. They are more effective in lowering blood pressure than the loop and potassium-sparing diuretics. As a result, thiazide diuretics can be used at lower dosages than the other drugs. Since they can be used at lower dosage levels, they are safer.

Because the thiazide diuretics tend to potentiate the effectiveness of other blood pressure–lowering drugs, they are often combined in one pill with other diuretics, beta-blockers, drugs that dilate the arteries (vasodilators), or ACE inhibitors. However, physicians are urged by the medical experts to try a single ingredient before combining medications. This recommendation holds true whether the first drug used is a diuretic, beta-blocker, calcium channel blocker, or ACE inhibitor. Here are some brand name examples of some combination products:

ACE Inhibitor and Hydrochlorothiazide
Capozide

Vaseretic

Beta-blocker and Hydrochlorothiazide
Inderide

Tenoretic

Normozide

Side effects: Thiazide diuretics cause the loss of potassium and magnesium from the body. Each of these minerals has been shown to exert blood pressure–lowering effects and prevent heart attacks. The drugs also increase cholesterol and triglyceride levels, increase the viscosity of the blood, raise uric acid levels, and increase the stickiness of the platelets, making them likely to aggregate and form clots. These factors may explain why thiazide diuretics may actually increase the risk of dying from a heart attack or stroke. Thiazide diuretics also worsen blood sugar control, making them difficult for diabetics to use safely.

The typical side effects of these drugs are lightheadedness; increased blood sugar levels; increased uric acid levels and aggravation of gout; and muscle weakness and cramps caused by low potassium levels. Decreased libido and impotence are also reported. Less frequent side effects include allergic reaction, headache, blurred vision, nausea, vomiting, and diarrhea.

Dosage recommendation given for the diuretic must be followed carefully. Often it is recommended to consume a diet rich in potassium and magnesium or take these minerals in supplement form. If taking a diuretic, check with your physician on the advisability of this recommendation.

BETA-BLOCKERS

Beta-blockers are drugs that block the binding of adrenaline on a type of cellular receptor known as a beta-receptor. This blocking results in both a reduced heart rate and a reduced force of contraction of the heart, as well as a relaxation of the arteries. Returning to our model of blood pressure and the garden hose, how do you increase the water pressure in a garden hose? By either turning up the faucet, or reducing the diameter of the hose by pinching it off a bit or putting your thumb over the opening. Beta-blockers work by simultaneously turning down the faucet and increasing the diameter of the hose. Some common beta-blockers are (generic name followed by brand name):

Acebutolol (Sectral)

Atenolol (Tenormin)

Carteolol (Cartrol)

Labetalol (Normodyne, Trandate)

Metoprolol (Lopressor)

Nadolol (Corgard)

Penbutolol (Levatol)

Pindolol (Visken)

Propanolol (Inderal)

Timolol (Blocadren)

In addition to their use for high blood pressure, beta-blockers are also used in treating angina and certain rhythm disturbances of the heart. Because heart function is reduced, there is a decreased need for oxygen and angina is relieved. In the long term, however, this inhibition of heart function can lead to heart failure. That is to say, once again, the drug actually produces the very condition it is designed to treat.

Side effects: Beta-blockers produce some significant side effects in many patients. Because the amount of blood being pumped by the heart is reduced in a more relaxed arterial system, it is often difficult to get enough blood and oxygen to the hands, feet, and brain. Some typical symptoms in users of beta-blockers are cold hands and feet, nerve tingling, impaired mental function, fatigue, dizziness, depression, lethargy, reduced libido, and impotence. Beta-blockers also raise cholesterol and triglyceride levels considerably. Elevations of cholesterol and triglycerides by beta-blockers may explain some of the negative effects in the clinical studies that failed to demonstrate any significant benefit of beta-blockers in reducing mortality from cardiovascular disease.

A beta-blocker should not be discontinued suddenly. Stopping the medication suddenly can produce a withdrawal syndrome consisting of headache, increased heart rate, and dramatic increase in blood pressure. When attempting to discontinue the medication, it is important to work with a physician to reduce the dosage gradually before stopping it entirely.

CALCIUM CHANNEL BLOCKERS

Calcium channel–blocking drugs represent a higher sophistication in the drug approach to high blood pressure. These drugs, along with the ACE inhibitors, will likely take over the top spots in the drug treatment of high blood pressure currently held by diuretics and beta-blockers because they are better tolerated. However, if these drugs provide any significant benefit in reducing cardiovascular mortality (fatal heart attacks and strokes), the primary goal of blood pressure–lowering (antihypertensive) therapy remains to be proven.

These drugs work by blocking the normal passage of calcium through certain channels in cell walls. Since calcium is required for nerve transmission and muscle contraction, the effect of blocking the calcium channel is to slow down nerve conduction and inhibit the contraction of the muscle. In the heart and vascular system, blocking calcium channels results in reducing the rate and force of contraction, relaxing the arteries, and slowing the nerve impulses in the heart. In our garden-hose model, calcium channel blockers work along the same lines as the beta-blockers. Among today's leading calcium channel blocking drugs are (generic name followed by some brand names):

Diltiazem (Cardizem)
Isradipine (DynaCirc)
Nicardipine (Cardene)
Nifedipine (Adalat, Procardia)
Verapamil (Calan, Isoptin, Verelan)

Side effects: Although much better tolerated than beta-blockers and diuretics, calcium channel blockers still produce some mild side effects including constipation, allergic reactions, fluid retention, dizziness, headache, fatigue, and impotence (about 20 percent of users). More serious side effects include disturbances of heart rate or function, heart failure, and angina.

ACE INHIBITORS

ACE (angiotensin-converting enzyme) inhibitors prevent the formation of active angiotensin, a substance that increases both the fluid volume and degree of constriction of the blood vessels. In our garden-hose model, angiotensin would have an effect similar to pinching off the hose while turning up the faucet full blast. By inhibiting the formation of this compound, ACE inhibitors relax the arterial walls and reduce fluid volume.

Unlike the beta-blockers and calcium channel blockers, however, ACE inhibitors actually improve heart function and increase blood and oxygen flow to the heart, liver, and kidneys. The actions of ACE inhibitors indicate that these drugs may actually reduce cardiovascular mortality. However, because ACE inhibitors were introduced to the market in 1979 and are fairly new drugs compared with the other antihypertensive drugs, the long-term effects on cardiovascular mortality are not yet known. ACE inhibitors include (generic name followed by some brand names):

Captopril (Capoten)
Enalapril (Vasotec)

Lisinopril (Prinivil, Zestril)

Ramipril (Altace)

Side effects: ACE inhibitors are generally very well tolerated, but share many of the same side effects as the other antihypertensives including dizziness, lightheadedness, and headache. The most common side effect is the development of a dry nighttime cough. ACE inhibitors can also cause the body to retain potassium, which can lead to heart problems and kidney problems, so potassium levels and kidney function must be monitored.

Captopril is not tolerated as well as the newer ACE inhibitors. It has some side effects not noted with the others, such as disturbances in the sense of taste, skin rashes, and impaired manufacture of blood cells due to suppression of the bone marrow. All of the ACE inhibitors appear to be capable of producing a severe allergic reaction that can be life-threatening.

Dietary and Life-style Factors in Treating High Blood Pressure

High blood pressure is closely related to life-style and dietary factors. Some of the important life-style factors that may cause high blood pressure are coffee consumption, alcohol intake, lack of exercise, stress, and smoking. Some of the dietary factors include: obesity; too much sodium and not enough potassium (high sodium to potassium ratio); low-fiber, high-sugar diet; high saturated fat and low essential fatty acids intake; and a diet low in calcium, magnesium, and vitamin C. Several of these dietary and life-style factors will be discussed in greater detail below.

Besides attaining healthy body weight, perhaps the most important dietary recommendation is to increase the consumption of plant foods in the diet. Vegetarians generally have lower blood pressure levels and a lower incidence of high blood pressure and other cardiovascular diseases than nonvegetarians.[12] While dietary levels of sodium do not differ significantly between these two groups, a vegetarian's diet typically contains more potassium, complex carbohydrates, essential fatty acids, fiber, calcium, magnesium, and vitamin C, and less saturated fat and refined carbohydrate. All these factors have a favorable influence on blood pressure.

Since the health of the artery is critical to maintaining normal blood pressure, it is very important to prevent atherosclerosis, or hardening of the arteries. Using our garden-hose model, if the hose loses its elasticity and becomes hard, it will not expand slightly to relieve an increase in water pressure. As a result, the pressure exerted against the walls of the hose is increased. When the arteries become hard due to the buildup of plaques containing cholesterol, blood pressure rises. Therefore, it is critical to reduce the risk factors for atherosclerosis. Chapter 9, "Cholesterol-Lowering Medications," provides information on natural methods to keep the arteries free from cholesterol buildup.

DIETARY FACTORS

High blood pressure is another of the many diseases or syndromes associated with the so-called civilized or Western diet rich in sugar, protein, and fat. High blood pressure is found almost entirely in developed countries. People living in remote areas of China, the Solomon Islands, New Guinea, Panama, Brazil, and Africa show virtually .no evidence of high blood pressure, nor do they experience a rise in blood pressure with advancing age.[18] Furthermore, when racially identical members of these societies migrate to less remote areas and adopt a more "civilized" diet, the incidence of high blood pressure increases dramatically.

Obesity
Obesity is a major causative factor in high blood pressure. Weight reduction should be the primary therapeutic goal for decreasing high blood pressure in the overweight individual.

Potassium and Sodium
The balance of potassium and sodium is extremely important to human health. Numerous studies have demonstrated that a diet low in potassium and high in sodium plays a major role in the development of cardiovascular disease (heart disease, high blood pressure, strokes) and

cancer.[19,20,21] Conversely, a diet high in potassium and low in sodium can help prevent these diseases; and in the case of high blood pressure, it can be therapeutic.

Excessive consumption of dietary sodium chloride (table salt), coupled with diminished dietary potassium, is a common cause of high blood pressure. However, sodium restriction alone does not improve blood pressure control in most people—it must be accompanied by a high potassium intake.[22] In fact, in most people with high blood pressure, potassium supplementation produces better blood pressure–lowering effects than avoidance of sodium. Nonetheless, it is the balance of potassium intake to sodium intake that is important; sodium intake must be decreased.

In our society, only 5 percent of sodium intake comes from the natural ingredients in food. Prepared foods contribute 45 percent of our sodium intake; 45 percent is added in cooking; and another 5 percent is added as a condiment. All that the body requires in most instances is the salt that is supplied in the food (or 5 percent of current sodium intake).

Most Americans have a potassium-to-sodium (K:Na) ratio of less than 1:2. In other words, most people ingest twice as much sodium as potassium. Researchers recommend a dietary potassium-to-sodium ratio of greater than 5:1 to maintain good health. This ratio is ten times higher than the average intake. However, even this may not be optimal. A natural diet rich in fruits and vegetables can produce a K:Na ratio greater than 100:1, as most fruits and vegetables have a K:Na ratio of at least 50:1. For example, here are the average K:Na ratios for several common fresh fruits and vegetables:

Apples, 90:1
Bananas, 440:1
Carrots, 75:1
Oranges, 260:1
Potatoes, 110:1

The estimated safe and adequate daily dietary intake of potassium, as set by the Committee on Recommended Daily Allowances, is 1.9 grams to 5.6 grams. If body potassium requirements are not being met through diet, supplementation is essential to good health. Patients with

Table 8.2   Potassium/Sodium Content of Selected Foods and Juices

Food	Portion Size	Potassium (milligrams)*	Sodium (milligrams)*
Fresh Vegetables			
Asparagus	½ cup	165	1
Avocado	½	680	5
Carrot, raw	1	225	38
Corn	½ cup	136	trace
Lima beans, cooked	½ cup	581	1
Potato	1 medium	782	6
Spinach, cooked	½ cup	292	45
Tomato, raw	1 medium	444	5
Fresh Fruits			
Apple	1 medium	182	2
Apricots, dried	¼ cup	318	9
Banana	1 medium	440	1
Cantaloupe	¼ melon	341	17
Orange	1 medium	263	1
Peach	1 medium	308	2
Plums	5	150	1
Strawberries	½ cup	122	trace
Unprocessed Meats			
Chicken, light meat	3 ounces	350	54
Lamb, leg	3 ounces	241	53
Roast beef	3 ounces	224	49
Pork	3 ounces	219	48
Fish			
Cod	3 ounces	345	93
Flounder	3 ounces	498	201
Haddock	3 ounces	297	150
Salmon	3 ounces	378	99
Tuna, drained solids	3 ounces	225	38

*1,000 milligrams equals 1 gram.

high blood pressure, the elderly, and athletes often require additional
potassium. Potassium salts are commonly prescribed by physicians in

the dosage range of 1.5 grams to 3.0 grams per day. However, potassium salts can cause nausea, vomiting, diarrhea, and ulcers. These effects are not seen when potassium levels are increased through the diet, only highlighting the advantages of using fresh fruit or vegetable juices, foods, or food-based potassium supplements to meet the human body's high potassium requirements.

Can you take too much potassium? Of course, but most people can handle any excess of potassium. The exceptions are people with kidney disease or patients on certain medications including ACE inhibitors. These people do not handle potassium in the normal way and are likely to experience heart disturbances and other consequences of potassium toxicity. They need to restrict their potassium intake and follow the dietary recommendations of their physicians.

Sugar

Sucrose—common table sugar—elevates blood pressure. The most plausible explanation appears to involve increased adrenaline production resulting in increased blood vessel constriction and increased sodium retention. In contrast to refined sugar, diets rich in complex-carbohydrate, high-fiber foods actually lower blood pressure.

Omega-3 Fatty Acids

The omega-3 fatty acids are special oils found in cold-water fish such as salmon, mackerel, and herring, and in some vegetable oils (most notably, flaxseed oil). As well as lowering cholesterol (see Chapter 9, "Cholesterol-Lowering Medications," for a more detailed discussion), these natural oils also decrease blood pressure.

Numerous double-blind studies have demonstrated that either fish oil (EPA or eicosapentaenoic acid) supplements or linolenic acid from flaxseed oil are very effective in lowering blood pressure.[23,24] Although the fish oils are more effective than flaxseed oil, because the dosage of fish oils used in the studies was quite high (e.g., equal to one hundred fish oil capsules), flaxseed oil is the better choice for lowering blood pressure, especially when cost effectiveness is considered. One tablespoon per day is all that is required. For best results, the flaxseed oil should definitely be cold-processed (produced without the aid of heat) and used as a salad dressing or food supplement.

Special Foods

Special foods for people with high blood pressure include: celery, garlic, and onions; nuts and seeds or their oils for their essential fatty acid content; cold-water fish (salmon, mackerel, etc.); green leafy vegetables as a rich source of calcium and magnesium; whole grains and legumes for their fiber; and foods rich in vitamin C such as broccoli and citrus fruits.

Celery is a particularly interesting recommendation for high blood pressure. Two researchers at the University of Chicago Medical Center have performed studies on a compound found in celery, 3-n-butyl phthalide, and found that it can lower blood pressure. In animals, a very small amount of 3-n-butyl phthalide lowered blood pressure by 12 to 14 percent and also lowered cholesterol by about 7 percent. The equivalent dose in humans can be supplied in about four ribs of celery. The research was prompted by one researcher's father, who, after eating a quarter-pound of celery every day for one week, observed his blood pressure dropped from 158 over 96 to a normal reading of 118 over 82. The celery prescription of four ribs per day is certainly worth a try.

Garlic is another beneficial food for lowering blood pressure. Although most recent research has focused on the cholesterol-lowering properties, garlic preparations have also been shown to decrease blood pressure.[25] Garlic has been reported to lower the systolic pressure by 20 to 30 mm Hg and the diastolic by 10 to 20 mm Hg in 40 percent of patients in as little time as one week.[26] However, to achieve the blood pressure–lowering properties of garlic, it appears that garlic must be ingested in large quantities (the equivalent to three or more cloves per day). Rather than relying solely on commercial garlic and onion products (pills, capsules, tablets, etc.), garlic and onion should be used liberally in the diet.

LIFE-STYLE FACTORS

Caffeine

While the effects of long-term caffeine consumption on blood pressure have not yet been clearly determined, studies of the short-term effects consistently show that the intake of caffeine (found in coffee, tea, chocolate, and cola) causes a rise in blood pressure. One large study (6,321 adults) demonstrated a small but statistically significant elevation in blood pressure when comparing those who drank five or more cups of coffee a day with noncoffee drinkers.[13]

Alcohol

Even moderate amounts of alcohol produce elevations in blood pressure in some people, and chronic alcohol consumption is one of the strongest predictors (sodium consumption being the other) of high blood pressure.[14] Abstinence or restricting alcohol intake to one ounce of alcohol daily (this roughly correlates to two ounces of liquor, four ounces of wine, or twelve ounces of beer) is definitely a good idea when an individual has high blood pressure.

Smoking and Heavy Metals

Cigarette smoking is a well-documented contributor to high blood pressure. Smokeless tobacco, that is, snuff, chewing tobacco, and plug, also induces high blood pressure via its nicotine and sodium content. People who smoke also tend to eat more high-sugar foods and drink more coffee and alcohol, all of which increase blood pressure.

The hypertensive response to nicotine results from its ability to stimulate the adrenal gland, which causes increased adrenaline secretion. Furthermore, cigarette smokers are known to have higher body concentrations of lead and cadmium and lower concentrations of vitamin C than nonsmokers.

Chronic exposure to lead and cadmium from environmental sources, including drinking water, is associated with increased cardiovascular mortality. Elevated blood-lead levels have been found in a significant number of individuals with high blood pressure.[15] Cadmium has also been shown to increase blood pressure. Studies have shown blood cadmium levels three to four times higher in people with high blood pressure than in people with normal blood pressure.[16]

Stress

Stress can be a causative factor of high blood pressure. Relaxation techniques such as biofeedback, self-hypnosis (autogenics), transcendental meditation, yoga, progressive muscle relaxation, and hypnosis have all been shown to have some value in lowering blood pressure.[17] Although the effect is only modest, a stress reduction technique is a beneficial component in a natural blood pressure–lowering program. See page 225 for a description of a popular relaxation technique.

Exercise

People who exercise regularly have lower blood pressure and better cardiovascular function. Exercise is strongly indicated in the treatment of high blood pressure, since it reduces stress and blood pressure.[17] Any exercise program should, of course, be carefully designed, taking into consideration an individual's cardiovascular condition. The question "How to design an exercise program?" is answered in Chapter 23, "The Importance of Exercise."

Natural Alternatives to Blood Pressure–Lowering Drugs

There are numerous natural substances that can serve as alternatives to blood pressure–lowering drugs. However, these natural alternatives are most effective when they are part of a comprehensive program that focuses on diet and life-style.

Vitamin C

There is an inverse relationship between serum vitamin C levels and blood pressure in men with hypertension; that is, the lower the vitamin C level, the higher the blood pressure.[27] Whether this is due to better dietary habits or a blood pressure–lowering effect of vitamin C has yet to be determined. My belief is that it is a combination of both.

Vitamin C is also important in helping the body eliminate heavy metals like lead and cadmium. As mentioned earlier, chronic exposure to lead and cadmium from environmental sources, including drinking water and cigarette smoke, is associated with increased cardiovascular mortality. Elevated blood-lead levels have been found in a significant number of hypertensive patients.

Calcium and Magnesium Supplements

Population studies indicate that calcium and magnesium may offer some protection against the development of high blood pressure and heart disease.[28,29] These data led to several clinical studies designed to determine the blood pressure–lowering effect of supplemental calcium or magnesium.[30,31] The results of these studies indicate that some people will respond to calcium or magnesium supplementation. As this is a safe therapy, it is certainly worth a try as a step-one medication. The dosage for calcium is 1,000 to 1,500 milligrams per day. For magnesium the dosage is 500 to 1,000 milligrams per day. Use forms of calcium or magnesium that are highly absorbable, like citrate, aspartates, or Krebs-cycle intermediates.

Hawthorn (Crataegus Oxyacantha)

As discussed in Chapter 4, "Angina Medications", hawthorn extracts are widely used by physicians in Europe and Asia to reduce blood pressure, angina attacks, and serum cholesterol levels. The mild blood pressure–lowering effects of hawthorn extracts have been demonstrated in many experimental and clinical studies.[32,33] Hawthorn's action in lowering blood pressure is quite unique, in that it does so through a combination of many diverse actions. Specifically, it dilates the larger blood vessels, inhibits ACE similarly to the drug captopril, increases the functional capacity of the heart, and possesses mild diuretic activity.

The dosage of hawthorn depends on the type of preparation and source material. Standardized extracts available in American health-food stores are the preferred form for medicinal purposes. The dosage for a hawthorn extract (standardized to contain 1.8 percent vitexin-4'-rhamnoside or 10 percent procyanidins) would be 100 to 250 milligrams three times daily. Unlike synthetic drugs, hawthorn extracts are without side effects and are extremely well tolerated.

The blood pressure–lowering effects of hawthorn extracts generally require up to two weeks before manifesting themselves. It appears this time is necessary to achieve adequate tissue concentrations of the flavonoids.

Final Comments

High blood pressure should not be taken lightly. By keeping your blood pressure in the normal range, you can increase not only the length of your life, but also the quality. This statement is especially true if natural measures rather than drugs are used to attain proper blood pressure. Here are eight concise guidelines for achieving these goals.

FOR MILD HYPERTENSION (140–160/90–104)

1. Reduce excessive weight.
2. Eliminate salt (sodium chloride) intake.
3. Follow a healthful life-style. Avoid alcohol, caffeine, and smoking.
4. Exercise and use stress-reduction techniques.
5. Follow a high-potassium diet rich in fiber and complex carbohydrates.
6. Increase dietary consumption of celery, garlic, and onions.
7. Reduce or eliminate the intake of animal fats while increasing the intake of vegetable oils.
8. Supplement the diet with the following:
     Calcium—1,000 to 1,500 milligrams per day
     Magnesium—500 milligrams per day
     (*Note*: An ionized source of calcium and magnesium is most beneficial, e.g., citrates, orotates, aspartates, or Krebs-cycle chelates.)
     Vitamin C—1 to 3 grams per day
     Zinc (picolinate)—15 to 30 milligrams per day
     Flaxseed oil—1 tablespoon per day

If after following the above recommendations for a period of three to six months, blood pressure has not returned to normal, please consult a physician for further nondrug recommendations.

FOR MODERATE HYPERTENSION (140–180/105–114)

1. Employ all the measures above.
2. Take hawthorn extracts at the dosage recommended above.
3. Take Coenzyme Q_{10}—20 milligrams three times daily.

Follow these guidelines for three months. If blood pressure has not dropped below 140/105, you will need to work with a physician to select the most appropriate medication. If a prescription drug is necessary, calcium channel blockers or ACE inhibitors appear to be the safest.

FOR SEVERE HYPERTENSION (160+/115+)

1. Consult a physician immediately.

Employ all the measures above. A drug may be necessary to achieve initial control. When satisfactory control over the high blood pressure has been achieved, work with the physician to taper off the medication.

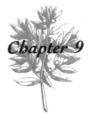

Chapter 9

CHOLESTEROL-LOWERING

MEDICATIONS

Cholesterol-lowering drugs are used in the treatment and prevention of heart disease. *Heart disease* is a term that is often used to describe a disease of the heart's blood vessels. These blood vessels are also called the coronary arteries. Coronary arteries supply the heart muscle with vital oxygen and nutrients. If the blood flow through these arteries is restricted or blocked, severe damage or death to the heart muscle often occurs. This results in what is known as a "heart attack." In most cases, the condition that blocks the blood and oxygen supply is atherosclerosis, or hardening of the artery walls due to a buildup of plaque containing cholesterol, fatty material, and cellular debris.

Atherosclerosis and its complications are the major causes of death in the United States and have reached epidemic proportions throughout all of the Western world. Heart disease accounts for 36 percent of all deaths among Americans and ranks as our number-one killer; stroke, another complication of atherosclerosis, is the third most common cause of death. In light of the fact that atherosclerosis is largely a disease of diet and life-style, it appears that many of these deaths could be significantly delayed[1] and the illnesses preceding them considerably reduced.

Cholesterol and Atherosclerosis

Foremost in the prevention and treatment of heart disease is the reduction of blood cholesterol levels. The evidence overwhelmingly demonstrates that elevated cholesterol levels greatly increase the risk of death due to heart disease.[1] The first step in reducing the risk for heart disease is keeping your total blood cholesterol level below 200 mg/dl (milligrams per deciliter).

Not all cholesterol is bad; it serves many vital functions in the body, including the manufacture of sex hormones and bile acids. Without cholesterol, many body processes would not function properly. Cholesterol is transported in the blood by molecules known as lipoproteins. Cholesterol bound to low density lipoprotein, or LDL, is often referred to as the "bad" cholesterol, while cholesterol bound to high-density lipoprotein, or HDL, is referred to as the "good" cholesterol. LDL cholesterol increases the risk for heart disease, strokes, and high blood pressure, while HDL cholesterol actually protects against heart disease.[2]

LDL transports cholesterol to the tissues. HDL, on the other hand, transports cholesterol to the liver for metabolism and excretion from the body. Therefore, the HDL-to-LDL ratio largely determines whether cholesterol is being deposited into tissues or broken down and excreted. The risk for heart disease can be reduced dramatically by lowering LDL cholesterol while simultaneously raising HDL cholesterol levels. Research has shown that for every 1-percent drop in the LDL cholesterol level, the risk for a heart attack drops by 2 percent. In addition, for every 1-percent increase in HDL levels, the risk for a heart attack drops 3 to 4 percent.[2]

In addition to keeping an eye on your cholesterol level, also keep the level of triglycerides (another blood fat or lipid that increases the risk for heart disease) in the proper range.

Dietary Cholesterol

Dietary cholesterol is a major risk factor in developing atherosclerosis. The evidence is substantial. However, several studies have shown that a lower dietary cholesterol intake was associated with up to a 37 percent lower risk of death from any cause, or an increased life expectancy of roughly 3.4 years.[3]

Although dietary cholesterol intake is an important contributor to atherosclerosis, most of the cholesterol in the body is actually manufac-

Table 9.1 Recommended Blood Cholesterol and Triglyceride Levels

Total cholesterol—less than 200 milligrams per deciliter
LDL cholesterol—less than 130 milligrams per deciliter
HDL cholesterol—greater than 35 milligrams per deciliter
Triglycerides—50 to 150 milligrams per deciliter

tured in the liver. Reducing dietary cholesterol alone is not always sufficient to lower blood cholesterol levels. As will be discussed, there are other important dietary factors.

COMMON CHOLESTEROL-LOWERING DRUGS

In an attempt to reduce blood cholesterol levels, many physicians are ignoring the need to give dietary recommendations and are instead utilizing drugs as the primary treatment. Using drugs before diet is clearly not the best approach, in terms of both effectiveness and cost. In fact, the "Report of the National Cholesterol Education Program Expert Panel on Detection, Evaluation, and Treatment of High Cholesterol in Adults" states clearly: "Dietary therapy is the primary cholesterol-lowering treatment."[4]

Several of the more popular drugs are discussed below.

HMG CoA Reductase Inhibitors
The drugs lovastatin (Mevacor), pravastin (Pravachol), and simvastatin (Zocor) are widely used to lower blood cholesterol levels. They work by inhibiting the enzyme (HMG CoA reductase) that is required in the manufacture of cholesterol in the liver. Unfortunately, in doing so these drugs also block the manufacture of other substances necessary for body functions, such as coenzyme Q_{10} (see page 52). The long-term safety or effectiveness of these drugs has not been determined. Their expense, questionable safety, and the effectiveness of natural alternatives indicate that they should not be used. Unfortunately, they are the most widely prescribed drugs for lowering cholesterol levels. Why? Effective marketing to physicians coupled with an unwillingness by patients to make the necessary diet and life-style changes. For the doctor, it is easier to spend a few seconds writing a prescription than to take the time to educate

the patient. And, many patients would much rather solve their problem by taking pills than by taking personal responsibility for their own health.

Side effects: The main side effect of these drugs is liver damage. In fact, due to the seriousness of the possible adverse effects on the liver it is necessary to have periodic blood tests to determine if the drug is harming the liver. Other side effects of HMG CoA reductase inhibitors include: muscle breakdown, muscle pain, nausea, diarrhea, flatus, abdominal pain, headache, and skin rash.

Bile Acid–Sequestering Resins

Cholestyramine (Questran) and colestipol (Colestid) are resinous powders that mix with water. They work to lower cholesterol by binding to bile acids in the intestines. Since cholestyramine and colestipol are not absorbed, the bile acid–resin complex is then excreted. As cholesterol is required to manufacture bile acids, more body cholesterol is used for bile acid synthesis. The result: lower cholesterol levels.

Unfortunately, there are some problems with cholestyramine and colestipol, such as the fact that they actually increase cholesterol synthesis, interfere with normal fat and fat soluble–vitamin absorption, and are associated with a long list of possible side effects. In addition, in order to lower cholesterol levels significantly, the dosage must be high (five to six packets per day). This means a cost of well over one hundred dollars per month. There are natural alternatives that are safer and more effective than these drugs.

Side effects: Cholestyramine and colestipol, like other cholesterol-lowering drugs, have numerous side effects. The most common one is constipation. If taken for any prolonged period of time, that is, longer than two months, deficiencies of fat-soluble vitamins (A, D, E, and K) will almost always begin to manifest themselves (night blindness, bleeding disorders, bone abnormalities). Less frequent side effects include abdominal discomfort, flatulence, nausea and vomiting, and gastrointestinal bleeding.

Fibric Acid Derivatives

Clofibrate (Atromid-S) and gemfibrozil (Lopid) are nearly identical drugs that lower cholesterol, but have a greater effect on triglycerides, another blood fat that increases the risk for heart disease. The mechanism of action of both drugs is poorly understood. They inhibit the release of LDL by the liver. Since the liver cannot release the LDL into the blood, LDL levels will drop. In other words, these drugs trap the cholesterol in the liver and gallbladder. This produces an obvious complication: gallstones.

Once widely used, clofibrate has fallen out of favor due to its side effects, limited effect on cholesterol levels, and lack of effectiveness in reducing fatal heart attacks. In fact, there is more evidence indicating clofibrate may actually lead to premature death. For example, the World Health Organization conducted a large study that demonstrated there was a 36-percent higher mortality rate in patients receiving clofibrate than in a placebo-treated group.[5] It appears that clofibrate lowered the cholesterol but increased the risk of dying prematurely from cancer, complications from gallbladder surgery (clofibrate causes gallstones), and from other conditions directly related to use of the drug. Gemfibrozil, due to its close similarity to clofibrate, is thought to produce similar negative effects.

Based on the results of several long-term studies, there is little reason to use clofibrate or gemfibrozil, especially since effective, safe, natural alternatives exist.

Side effects: The list of side effects due to clofibrate and gemfibrozil is quite long. Both are extremely toxic to the body. As mentioned above, the major side effect is the development of gallstones. Their use is also associated with nausea, gastrointestinal upset and distress, flulike symptoms, headache, dizziness, muscle cramps, skin rash, and numerous other side effects.

Dietary and Life-style Factors in Lowering Cholesterol

The most important first approach to lowering a high cholesterol level is to follow a healthful diet and life-style. The dietary changes are simple: Eat less saturated fat and cholesterol by reducing or eliminating the amounts of animal products in the diet; increase consumption of fiber-rich plant foods (fruits, vegetables, grains, and legumes); and lose weight, if necessary. Life-style changes include: Get regular aerobic exercise; stop smoking; and reduce or eliminate consumption of coffee (both caffeinated and decaffeinated).

A number of medical organizations have developed more specific guidelines for Americans to follow to reduce the risk for heart disease. Here are the six key recommendations of the U.S. Surgeon General, American Heart Association, and the National Research Council's Committee on Diet and Health:[1]

1. Reduce total fat intake to 30 percent or less of calories; reduce saturated fat intake to less than 10 percent of calories; reduce the intake of cholesterol to less than 300 milligrams daily (see Tables 9.2 and 9.3).

2. Eat five or more servings daily of a combination of vegetables and fruits, especially green and yellow vegetables and citrus fruits.

3. Increase the intake of fiber and complex carbohydrates by eating six or more servings daily of a combination of breads, cereals, and legumes.

4. Maintain protein intake at moderate levels.

5. Balance food intake and physical activity to maintain appropriate body weight.

6. Limit the intake of alcohol, refined carbohydrates (sugar), and salt (sodium chloride).

CHOLESTEROL AND SATURATED AND UNSATURATED FATS

The first step in reducing blood cholesterol levels through diet is to reduce the amount of cholesterol in the diet. As evident in Table 9.2, cholesterol is found only in animal foods. Many medical experts recommend eliminating entirely from the diet foods high in cholesterol when blood cholesterol levels are elevated to concentrations above 200 milligrams per deciliter. This recommendation is extremely sound, but it is simply the first step.

Table 9.2 Cholesterol Content of Selected Foods, in Milligrams (mg) per 3½-oz (100-g) Serving*

Animal Food

Type	Cholesterol
Egg, whole	550
Kidney, beef	375
Liver, beef	300
Butter	250
Oysters	200
Cream cheese	120
Lard	95
Beefsteak	70
Lamb	70
Pork	70
Chicken	60
Ice cream	45

Plant Food

Type	Cholesterol
All grains	0
All vegetables	0
All nuts	0
All seeds	0
All fruits	0
All legumes	0
All vegetable oils	0

*1,000 milligrams equal 1 gram.

In fighting high cholesterol levels, the amount of saturated fat in the diet must also be reduced. Saturated fats are typically animal fats (like butter) that are semisolid to solid at room temperature. In contrast, vegetable fats are liquid at room temperature and are referred to as unsaturated fats or oils. Unsaturated oils may be either monounsaturated or polyunsaturated, depending on the number of unsaturated chemical bonds. Considerable evidence shows that a diet rich in saturated fats and low in unsaturated fats leads to elevated LDL cholesterol levels and an increased risk for heart disease. Saturated fats apparently tell the liver to make more cholesterol, while unsaturated fats have the opposite effect. Remember that most of the cholesterol in the body is not from the diet; it is manufactured in the liver.

Table 9.3 Percentage of Calories as Fat

Meats			
Sirloin steak, hipbone, lean		T-bone steak, lean	
without fat	83%	without fat	82%
Pork sausage	83%	Porterhouse steak,	
		lean without fat	82%

Meats (cont.)

Bacon, lean	82%
Rib roast, lean without fat	81%
Bologna	81%
Country-style sausage	81%
Spareribs	80%
Frankfurters	80%
Lamb rib chops, lean without fat	79%
Duck meat, without skin	76%
Salami	76%
Liverwurst	75%
Rump roast, lean without fat	71%
Ham, lean without fat	69%
Stewing beef, lean without fat	66%
Goose meat, without skin	65%
Ground beef, fairly lean	64%
Veal breast, lean without fat	64%
Leg of lamb, lean without fat	61%
Chicken, dark meat without skin, roasted	56%
Round steak, lean without fat	53%
Chuck rib roast, lean only	50%
Chuck steak, lean only	50%
Sirloin steak, hipbone, lean only	47%
Turkey, dark meat without skin	47%
Lamb rib chops, lean only	45%
Chicken, light meat without skin, roasted	44%

Fish

Tuna, chunk, oil-packed	63%
Herring, Pacific	59%
Anchovies	54%
Bass, black sea	53%
Perch, ocean	53%
Caviar, sturgeon	52%
Mackerel, Pacific	50%
Sardines, Atlantic, in oil, drained	49%
Salmon, sockeye (red)	49%

Vegetables

Mustard greens	13%
Kale	13%
Beet greens	12%
Lettuce	12%
Turnip greens	11%
Mushrooms	8%
Cabbage	7%
Cauliflower	7%
Eggplant	7%
Asparagus	6%
Green beans	6%
Celery	6%
Cucumber	6%
Turnip	6%
Zucchini	6%
Carrots	4%
Green peas	4%
Artichokes	3%
Onions	3%
Beets	2%
Chives	1%
Potatoes	1%

Legumes

Tofu	49%
Soybean	37%
Soybean sprouts	28%
Garbanzo bean	11%
Kidney bean	4%
Lima bean	4%
Mungbean sprouts	4%
Lentil	3%
Broad bean	3%
Mung bean	3%

TO LOWER CHOLESTEROL, REDUCE ANIMAL-PRODUCT INTAKE

Since animal products are the primary sources of both saturated fats and cholesterol, it is obvious that the intake of animal products must be limited in order to prevent or reverse atherosclerosis. Another reason to reduce the intake of animal foods is that the body handles plant proteins differently from animal proteins. Diets made up of vegetable proteins have been shown to lower cholesterol levels, while diets containing equivalent amounts of milk protein or other animal proteins actually raise cholesterol levels. The bottom line: To reduce cholesterol levels and the risk for atherosclerosis, animal products must be substantially reduced, while plant foods must be substantially increased.

Omega-3 Fatty Acids

Possible exceptions to the recommendation of reducing the intake of animal foods are cold-water fish such as salmon, mackerel, and herring, which provide oils known as omega-3 fatty acids. These beneficial oils have been shown in hundreds of studies to lower cholesterol and triglyceride levels.[6]

The omega-3 fatty acids are being recommended to treat or prevent not only high cholesterol levels, but also high blood pressure, other cardiovascular diseases, cancer, autoimmune diseases like multiple sclerosis and rheumatoid arthritis, allergies and inflammation, eczema, psoriasis, and many other illnesses.[6] Although the majority of studies on omega-3 oils have utilized fish oils (eicosapentaenoic acid [EPA] and docosahexanoic acid [DHA]), flaxseed oil may offer similar benefit because it contains linolenic acid, an omega-3 oil that the body can convert to EPA. Linolenic acid exerts many of the same effects as EPA, as well as several on its own.

While there exists a substantial body of evidence documenting the beneficial effects of increasing the intake of fish oils in lowering blood cholesterol levels,[6,7] the question remains whether the fish oils should be taken as a supplement or through increased consumption of fish in the diet. In an effort to resolve this question, a recent study on twenty-five men with high cholesterol levels over a five-week period compared the effects of eating an equivalent amount of fish oil from whole fish versus a fish-oil supplement.[8] Although total cholesterol levels were unchanged in both groups, both fish and fish-oil supplements lowered triglycerides and raised HDL-cholesterol.

However, dietary fish produced some additional benefits over the fish-oil supplements. One key benefit of fish oils is their ability to reduce the "stickiness" of platelets and prevent clot formation. When platelets adhere to each other or aggregate to form a clot, this clot can get stuck in small arteries and produce a heart attack or stroke. In the above study, dietary fish produced a much greater effect than the fish-oil supplement on reducing platelet stickiness. These findings suggest that while both fish consumption and fish-oil supplementation produce desirable effects on lipids and lipoproteins, fish consumption is more effective in improving several other factors involved in cardiovascular disease.

If cold-water fish are not readily available, I recommend supplementing the diet with either fish oils or flaxseed oil. The dosages found to be effective when using fish-oil supplements range from 5 to 15 grams of omega-3 fatty acids per day. Since most commercial products contain 500 milligrams of omega-3 fatty acids per capsule, this means a daily dose of 10 to 30 capsules. Although this can be expensive, it is still much less expensive than some cholesterol-lowering drugs, and is certainly much safer. Flaxseed oil may indeed be the most advantageous oil for medical use, especially when cost effectiveness is considered. One tablespoon per day is all that is required. For best results, the flaxseed oil should definitely be cold-processed (processed without the aid of heat) to reduce rancidity. Flaxseed oil can be used as a salad dressing or food supplement, but loses its beneficial qualities when cooked.

Nuts and Seeds

Another way of increasing the intake of health-promoting oils is to increase the consumption of nuts and seeds. As more Americans are seeking healthier food choices, nut and seed consumption is on the rise. Nuts and seeds are rich in many important nutrients like vitamin E, zinc, magnesium, and vitamin B_6.

Because of the high oil content of nuts and seeds, one would suspect that the frequent consumption of nuts would increase the rate of obesity. But in a study of 26,473 Americans, it was found that the people who consumed the most nuts were the least obese.[9] A possible explanation is that the nuts produced satiety, a feeling of appetite satisfaction. This same study also demonstrated that higher nut consumption was associated with a protective effect against heart attacks (both fatal and nonfatal).

Nuts and seeds, due to their high oil content, are best purchased and stored in their shells. Make sure the shells are free from splits,

Figure 9.1   *Cis* Versus *Trans*

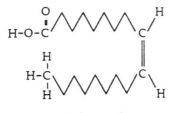
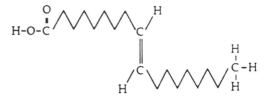

cis-fatty acid

The H's are on the same side of the
double bond, forcing the molecule
to assume a horseshoe shape.

trans-fatty acid

The H's are on opposite sides of
the double bond, forcing the
molecule into an extended position.

cracks, stains, holes, or other surface imperfections. Do not eat or use moldy nuts or seeds, as they can contain toxic substances. Also avoid limp, rubbery, dark, or shriveled nut meats. Store nuts and seeds with shells in a cool, dry environment. If whole nuts and seeds with their shells are not available, make sure the nut meat is stored in airtight containers in the refrigerator or freezer. Crushed, slivered, and other pieces of nut are most often rancid. If a recipe calls for these, prepare your own from the whole nut.

What About Margarine?

During the process of manufacturing margarine and shortening, vegetable oils are "hydrogenated." This means that a hydrogen molecule is added to the natural unsaturated fatty acid molecules of the vegetable oil to make it more saturated. Hydrogenation changes the structure of the natural fatty acid to many "unnatural" fatty acid forms, as well as from the *cis* to the *trans* configuration (see Figure 9.1). The result is that the vegetable oil is now solid or semisolid.

Researchers and nutritionists have debated the health effects of margarine since it was first developed. Although many Americans assume they are doing their body good by consuming margarine rather than butter and saturated fats, they are actually doing harm. Margarine and other hydrogenated vegetable oils (like shortenings) not only raise LDL cholesterol, they also lower the protective LDL cholesterol level and interfere with essential fatty-acid metabolism.[10] They may even cause certain cancers. Although butter may be better than margarine because it is more "natural," they both need to be restricted in a healthful

Table 9.4   Food Choices for Lowering Cholesterol

Eat Less of These	*Substitute with These*
Red meats	Fish and white meat of poultry
Hamburgers and hot dogs	Soy-based alternatives
Eggs	Tofu, egg substitutes
High-fat dairy products	Lowfat or nonfat dairy products
Butter, margarine, lard, and other saturated fats	Vegetable oils
Ice cream, pies, cake, cookies	Fruits
Refined cereals, white bread	Whole grains, whole wheat bread
Fried foods, fatty snack foods	Vegetables, fresh salads
Salt and salty foods	Low sodium, light salt
Coffee and soft drinks	Herbal teas, fresh fruit, and vegetable juices

diet. For cooking, use oils that hold up well to heat, like canola oil or olive oil.

EVEN SIMPLE FOOD CHOICES ARE IMPORTANT

The importance of even simple alterations in diet can be quite significant. In one study, two medium-size carrots were added daily to the breakfast of normal subjects.[11] After three weeks, there was an 11-percent reduction in cholesterol levels. Table 9.4 details some simple food choices that can lead to dramatic changes in your cholesterol levels and level of health.

In another example of how simple food choices affect cholesterol levels, an evaluation of data from the National Health and Nutrition Examination Survey II (a national survey of the nutritional and health practices of Americans) disclosed that serum cholesterol levels are lowest among adults eating whole grain cereal for breakfast.[12] Although those individuals who consumed other breakfast foods had higher blood cholesterol levels, levels were highest among those who typically skipped breakfast.

Thanks to an explosion of marketing information, most Americans are aware of the cholesterol-lowering effects of oats. Since 1963, there have been more than twenty major clinical studies examining the effect of oat bran on cholesterol levels.[13] Various oat preparations containing either oat bran or oatmeal have been studied, including cereals, muffins, breads, and entrees. The overwhelming majority of the studies demonstrated a very favorable effect on cholesterol levels. In individuals with high cholesterol levels (above 220 milligrams per deciliter), the consumption of the equivalent of 3 grams of water-soluble oat fiber typically lowers total cholesterol by 8 to 23 percent. The lowering of total cholesterol by oat fiber is highly significant. Remember, other studies suggest that each 1-percent drop in total blood cholesterol level brings a 2-percent decrease in the risk of developing heart disease. Three grams of fiber would be provided by approximately one bowl of ready-to-eat oat bran cereal or oatmeal. Although oatmeal's fiber content (7 percent) is less than that of oat bran (15 to 26 percent), it has been determined that the polyunsaturated fatty acids from the oatmeal contribute as much to the cholesterol-lowering effects of oats as the fiber content. Although oat bran has a higher fiber content, oatmeal is higher in polyunsaturated fatty acids. Therefore, oat bran and oatmeal are equally effective. Although individuals with high cholesterol levels will see significant reductions with frequent oat consumption, individuals with normal or low cholesterol levels will see little change.

A variety of other water-soluble fibers have been shown to lower cholesterol levels, including psyllium, guar gum, and pectin. Eating a diet rich in whole grains, legumes (beans), and fresh fruit can provide high levels of these water-soluble fiber compounds. Although supplementing the diet with additional fiber is becoming quite popular as a recommendation, it appears that eating foods rich in these water-soluble fibers makes more sense, both from a healthful and a financial perspective.

As an illustration, let's examine the effect of pectin, a remarkable type of fiber found in fresh fruits such as pears, apples, grapefruit, and oranges. Pectin has been shown to exert a number of beneficial effects, including lowering cholesterol levels. In most of the cholesterol-lowering studies, supplementing the diet with 15 grams of pectin produced a 10-percent drop in cholesterol levels.[14] Many people are buying high-priced drugs to get this kind of drop in cholesterol levels. Since 15 grams of fiber is the amount of pectin in approximately two servings of fruit rich in pectin, eating two servings per day could lower the risk for heart disease by 20 percent. In addition to pectin, these fruits would also provide important vitamins and minerals that can protect against heart disease.

Reversing Heart Disease

More and more evidence is accumulating that shows an increased HDL-to-LDL ratio is not only protective against heart disease, but can also dramatically reverse the blockage of clogged arteries. The best illustration is the now famous Lifestyle Heart Trial conducted by Dr. Dean Ornish.[15] In this study, subjects with heart disease were divided into a control group and an experimental group. The control group received regular medical care, while the experimental group was asked to eat a lowfat vegetarian diet for at least one year. The diet included fruits, vegetables, grains, legumes, and soybean products. Subjects were allowed to consume as many calories as they wished. No animal products were allowed except egg white and one cup per day of nonfat milk or yogurt. The diet contained approximately 10 percent fat, 15 to 20 percent protein, and 70 to 75 percent carbohydrate, which was predominantly complex carbohydrate from whole grains, legumes, and vegetables.

The experimental group was also asked to perform stress-reduction techniques such as breathing exercises, stretching exercises, meditation, imagery, and other relaxation regimens for an hour each day, and to exercise at least three hours a week. At the end of the year, the subjects in the experimental group showed significant overall regression of atherosclerosis of the coronary blood vessels. In contrast, subjects in the control group who were being treated with regular medical care and following the standard American Heart Association diet actually showed progression of their disease. The control group actually got worse. Ornish states: "This finding suggests that conventional recommendations for patients with coronary heart disease (such as a 30 percent fat diet) are not sufficient to bring about regression in many patients."

Although most authorities now agree that the level of blood cholesterol is largely determined by the dietary intake of total calories of cholesterol, saturated fat, and polyunsaturated fat, the results of Ornish's study and others suggest that many factors are important. Strict vegetarianism may not be as important as consuming a diet high in fiber and complex carbohydrates, low in fat, and low in cholesterol; but it is well established that vegetarians have a much lower risk of developing heart disease, and a vegetarian diet has been shown to be quite effective in lowering cholesterol levels and reducing the risk for atherosclerosis.[16] Such a diet is rich in a number of protective substances such as fiber, essential fatty acids, vitamins, and minerals including potassium and magnesium.

Other Recommendations

Quit smoking! Statistical evidence reveals a three-to-fivefold increase in the risk of heart disease in smokers compared with nonsmokers. The more cigarettes smoked and the longer the period of years smoked, the greater the risk of dying from a heart attack or stroke.

Exercise! Many studies have shown a direct relationship between physical activity and cholesterol levels. Physical exercise is also associated with a decreased risk of heart disease and stroke.

Natural Alternatives
to Cholesterol-Lowering Drugs

When there is a need for support additional to the dietary and lifestyle practices that can lower cholesterol levels, it simply makes more sense to use safer and more effective natural alternatives. To illustrate the effectiveness of several natural compounds versus the drugs discussed above, I have graphed the average effect on total cholesterol and triglyceride levels of the natural substances discussed below compared with the drugs. The values provided in the graphs below are based on using standard dosage schedules for the drugs and supplements. As is apparent, the natural substances are as effective in improving cholesterol and triglyceride levels as the drugs. It should be pointed out that while lovastatin produced the greatest decrease in total cholesterol levels (34 percent), its effect on raising HDL is less than that of the natural substances. When evaluating overall effectiveness, both LDL and HDL cholesterol levels must be taken into consideration. When you look at the cost, safety, and effectiveness, it is clear that the natural alternatives presented here are substantially superior to standard drug therapy. Once again, keep in mind that the natural alternatives discussed below are, just like the drugs, still best utilized in a comprehensive program that stresses a healthful diet and life-style.

Niacin

Niacin, or vitamin B_3, has long been used to lower cholesterol levels. In fact, niacin is recommended by the National Cholesterol Education Program as the first "drug" to use to lower blood cholesterol levels.[4] Unlike the drugs discussed above, niacin has actually been shown to lower cholesterol levels safely and to extend life. Niacin was the only substance to demonstrate a decreased mortality in the landmark Coronary Drug Project.[17] Its effects are long lasting, as demonstrated in a follow-up study to the Coronary Drug Project, which showed that the long-term death rate for coronary patients treated with niacin was actually 11 percent lower than for the group receiving a placebo, even though most of the patients had discontinued the niacin treatment many years earlier.[18]

So why isn't niacin used more to lower cholesterol? The dose required (1 gram three times per day) often results in flushing of the skin, stomach irritation, ulcers, liver damage, fatigue, and other side effects. Because of these side effects, it is recommended that niacin therapy for lowering cholesterol levels be supervised by a physician. Despite this recommendation, it is a known fact that many people are self-medicating with niacin. One of the big reasons is a financial one. A monthly dose of niacin costs about ten dollars, while a month's supply of cholestyramine and lovastatin will usually cost well over one hundred dollars.

Some people combat the acute reaction of skin flushing after taking niacin by using "sustained-release," "timed-release" or "slow-release" niacin products. These formulations allow the niacin to be absorbed gradually, thereby reducing the flushing reaction. However, while these forms of niacin reduce skin flushing, they actually have proven to be more toxic to the liver.[19] Certainly people should not self-medicate with timed-release or slow-release niacin products.

The safest form of niacin at present is known as inositol hexaniacinate. This form of niacin has long been used in Europe to lower cholesterol levels and also to improve blood flow. It yields slightly better results than standard niacin, but is much better tolerated, both in terms of flushing and, more important, long-term side effects.[20,21,22] In fact, in one study it was reported that in 153 patients treated with inositol hexaniacinate at dosages ranging from 600 to 1,800 milligrams per day, no patients reported any side effects or adverse reaction.[20] Based on this study and others, it appears that if people choose to self-medicate with niacin, the preferred form is inositol hexaniacinate at a dosage of 600 to 1,800 milligrams per day. Inositol hexaniacinate is available at health-food stores.

Gugulipid

Gugulipid is the standardized extract of the mukul myrrh tree (*Commiphora mukul*) that is native to India. The active components of gugulipid are two compounds, Z-guggulsterone and E-guggulsterone. Several clinical studies have confirmed that gugulipid has an ability to lower both cholesterol and triglyceride levels.[23,24] Typically, cholesterol levels will drop 14 to 27 percent in a four- to twelve-week period, while triglyceride levels will drop from 22 to 30 percent.

The effect of gugulipid on cholesterol and triglyceride levels is comparable to that of lipid-lowering drugs. While those drugs are associated with some degree of toxicity, gugulipid is without side effect. Safety studies in rats, rabbits, and monkeys have demonstrated it to be nontoxic. It is also considered safe to use during pregnancy.

The mechanism of gugulipid's cholesterol-lowering action is its ability to increase the liver's metabolism of LDL-cholesterol; guggulsterone increases the uptake of LDL-cholesterol from the blood by the liver.

The dosage of gugulipid is based on its guggulsterone content. Clinical studies have demonstrated that gugulipid extracts standardized to contain 25 milligrams of guggulsterone per tablet given three times per day is an effective treatment for elevated cholesterol levels, elevated triglyceride levels, or both.

Garlic and Onions

Garlic and onions exert numerous beneficial effects on the cardiovascular system, including lowering blood lipids and blood pressure. Numer-

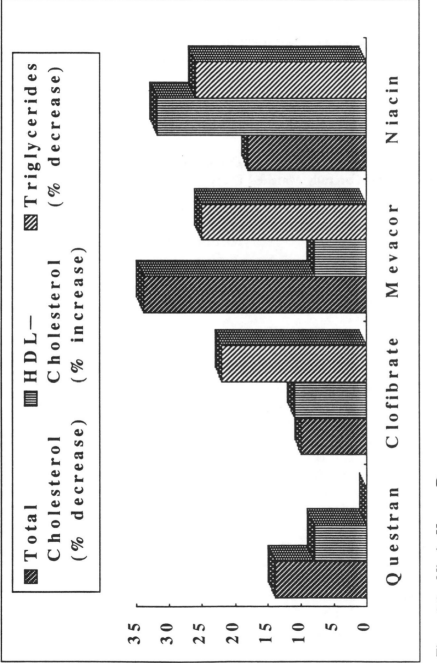

Figure 9.2 Niacin Versus Drugs

ous studies have demonstrated that both garlic and onions are effective in lowering LDL-cholesterol and triglycerides while simultaneously raising HDL-cholesterol levels.[25] In a 1979 population study, researchers studied three groups of vegetarians in the Jain community of India who consumed differing amounts of garlic and onions.[26] As is evident in the table below, the most favorable effects were observed in the group that consumed the largest amount of garlic and onions. The study is especially significant because the subjects had nearly identical diets except in garlic and onion ingestion.

Table 9.5 Effects of Garlic and Onion Consumption on Serum Lipids Under Carefully Matched Diets

Garlic/Onion Consumption Level (grams per week)	Cholesterol Level (milligrams per deciliter)	Triglyceride (milligrams per deciliter)
Garlic 50 g/wk onion 600 g/wk	159 mg/dl	52 mg/dl
Garlic 10 g/wk onion 200 g/wk	172 mg/dl	75 mg/dl
No garlic or onions	208 mg/dl	109 mg/dl

The equivalent of one clove of garlic or half an onion per day will produce good results (10 to 15 percent reduction in total cholesterol levels) in most people; others may require more. Although best raw, even cooked garlic or onion produces some beneficial effects. You can also supplement your diet by using one of the wide variety of garlic forms on the market, including so-called deodorized garlic products. Use well-respected brands like Kwai, Garlicin, and Kyolic, available at health-food stores and many drugstores.

Pantethine

Pantethine is the stable form of pantetheine, the active form of vitamin B$_5$ or pantothenic acid. Pantothenic acid is the most important component of coenzyme A (CoA). This enzyme is involved in the transport of fats to and from cells, as well as to the energy-producing compartments within the cell. Without CoA, the cells of our body would not be able to utilize fats as energy.

For some reason, pantethine has significant lipid-lowering activity, while pantothenic acid has very little (if any) effect in lowering cholesterol and triglyceride levels. Pantethine administration (standard dose, 900 milligrams per day) has been shown to reduce significantly serum triglyceride and cholesterol levels while increasing HDL-cholesterol levels.[26,27] These effects are most impressive when its toxicity (virtually none) is compared with conventional lipid-lowering drugs. Pantethine's mechanism of action is due to its ability to inhibit cholesterol synthesis and accelerate the utilization of fat as an energy source. There appears to be no toxicity or side effects from pantethine.

Because pantethine is expensive compared with other natural alternatives given, I do not recommend it to everyone. It does have its place, however. As is evident in Figure 9.3, pantethine has the best effects on blood triglyceride levels. Therefore, I recommend pantethine mostly to individuals who primarily have elevated triglyceride levels.

Final Comments

A study on the cost effectiveness of lowering cholesterol revealed some interesting results.[28] The question being asked was: How many dollars must be spent on a treatment to make a person live one year longer? Here are the results:

Dietary advice	− $2,536
Niacin	− $1,234
Psyllium husk	− $642
Lovastatin	$50,510
Colestipol	$73,406
Colestyramine	$92,603
Gemfibrozil	$108,826

The figures were derived by a formula that calculated the cost of the treatment, plus the cost of any side effects, minus the cost of dealing with illnesses averted, and the extra income earned because of the illness averted. The negative numbers on the first three interventions reflect net savings because of the illnesses prevented and the extra earned income as a result. Obviously, these natural alternatives to the drugs provide much greater benefit on a cost-effectiveness basis. In other words, reducing cholesterol by changing your diet and/or taking niacin or a fiber supplement not only can save your life, it will save you a great deal of money as well.

Without question, the best approach to lowering cholesterol levels is through diet and life-style modifications. When additional support is required, there are safer and more effective natural alternatives to commonly prescribed drugs. These natural alternatives can be taken individually or in combination with one another. Figure 9.3 shows how they compare with one another.

In my clinical practice, I prescribe a formula containing both inositol hexaniacinate and gugulipid along with chromium, vitamin C, and ginger. A deficiency of chromium or vitamin C will lead to elevated cholesterol levels. Supplementation will correct this deficiency in this instance and exert a mild cholesterol-lowering effect when tissue stores of these nutrients are adequate. Ginger is included in the formula not only because of its cholesterol-lowering action, but also for its soothing effect on the gastrointestinal tract.

The goal of therapy, whether natural or synthetic, is to get blood lipid levels down into the target ranges as quickly as possible. Once the target range has been achieved, begin reducing the amount of medicine by half, or take it every other day. Recheck your cholesterol levels in one month. If they have stabilized or continued to improve, you may no longer need the medication. If the levels have started back up again, return to the previous dosage.

If you are currently on a cholesterol-lowering drug, you must consult your doctor before discontinuing the medication.

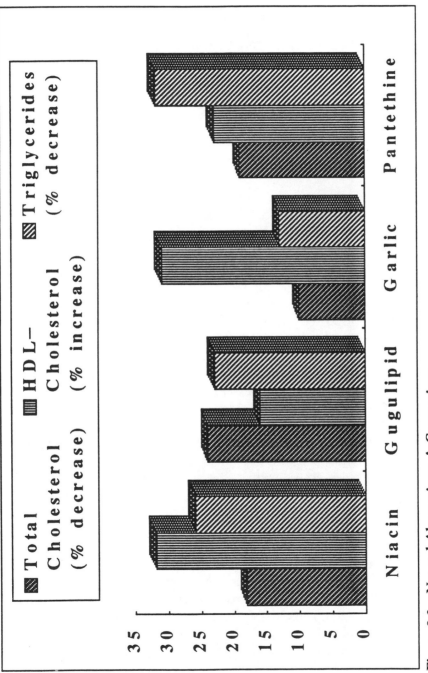

Figure 9.3   Natural Alternatives: A Comparison

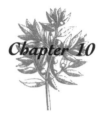

Chapter 10

COMMON-COLD

MEDICATIONS

The common cold can be caused by a wide variety of viruses that are capable of infecting the upper respiratory tract. The symptoms of a cold are well known: general malaise, fever, headache, and upper respiratory tract congestion. Initially there is a watery nasal discharge and sneezing, followed by thicker secretions containing mucus, white blood cells, and dead organisms. The throat may be red, sore, and dry.

Usually a cold can be easily differentiated from other conditions, like the flu and allergies, that have some similar symptoms. The flu (influenza) is much more severe in its symptoms and usually occurs in epidemics, so contacting the local Public Health Department is all that is needed to rule this out. Allergies may be an underlying factor in decreasing resistance and allowing a virus to infect the upper airways, but usually allergies can be differentiated from the common cold by the fact that no fever occurs with allergies, there is usually a history of seasonal allergic episodes, and there is no other evidence of infection.

Researchers tell us that it is "normal" to catch a cold four to six times per year. But, have you ever wondered why some people never seem to "catch" a cold, while others seem to suffer from a cold all the time? We are all constantly exposed to many of the viruses that can cause a cold, yet for most of us it is only when our resistance is low that we come down with the symptoms. A decrease in the effectiveness of our immune system is the major factor in catching a cold.

Getting a cold six times a year may be normal, but it certainly doesn't have to be that way. If you catch more than one or two colds a year, it is an indication that your immune system needs some support. Like

Table 10.1   Factors that Weaken the Immune System

Nutrient deficiency
Stress
Alcohol
Tobacco use
Many drugs (legal and illegal)
High blood cholesterol and triglyceride levels
Diabetes
Excessive sugar consumption
Chemical toxins
Allergies

most health conditions, it is far easier to prevent a cold than to treat a cold.

Primary prevention means building a healthy immune system. In order to have a healthy immune system, an individual must follow all the basic rules for good health (see Section Three) and avoid those factors that can weaken the immune system.

Common-Cold Medications

Most over-the-counter common-cold medications are a combination of an antihistamine and a nasal decongestant. Some also utilize antitussives (cough medicines) and/or an analgesic (aspirin or acetaminophen). Despite the widespread use of these remedies, numerous studies demonstrate they offer little else than a placebo effect. A recent study in children is a good example of the lack of effectiveness of over-the-counter cold remedies in relieving symptoms.[1]

A group of ninety-six children between the ages of six months and five years were randomly assigned to receive either an antihistamine-decongestant medication, placebo, or no treatment. The medication used in the study was Dimetapp, a combination of an antihistamine (brompheniramine) and two nasal decongestants (phenylephrine and phenyl-propranolamine). Forty-eight hours after the initial assessment, there was not a statistical advantage to any treatment. However, 71 percent of the group receiving the placebo were better, compared with 67 percent in the medication group and 57 percent of those receiving no treatment.

Antihistamines (see page 85) serve no purpose in treating the common cold because histamine itself does not play a significant role in this condition. Although some studies have shown a very small advantage over a placebo, others have not. In the positive studies, it is highly unlikely the effect was due to anything other than the medication's sedative effect, as studies using nonsedating antihistamines like Seldane (terfenadine) have shown antihistamines to be no more effective than a placebo.[2]

Another popular method of dealing with cold symptoms is to use aspirin or acetaminophen (Tylenol). However, this practice is clearly counterproductive. These drugs do not suppress the symptoms; they actually make matters worse.[3] In children, in rare instances aspirin use during a viral infection can lead to a serious condition known as Reye's syndrome, which is characterized by brain swelling, coma, and liver enlargement. Because of this possible effect of aspirin, acetaminophen is often recommended for children.

Although aspirin and acetaminophen reduce fever, in carefully controlled studies both acetaminophen and aspirin actually have been shown to increase nasal congestion and other cold symptoms.[3] Aspirin and acetaminophen have been shown to suppress the immune system. This suppression of immune function may lead to a more serious infection, and definitely increases the duration of the common cold. The use of aspirin and acetaminophen in the common cold is clearly inappropriate in most instances.

The treatments that appear to be most useful are the general and natural measures discussed below. The goal of both is to enhance the immune system. The only current over-the-counter medications that may have some benefit are appropriately used nasal decongestants.

NASAL DECONGESTANTS

Nasal decongestants can be administered either in nasal sprays, drops, or inhalers (topical); or in oral preparations (pills and liquids). Both routes usually provide immediate and dramatic decrease in nasal congestion. Unfortunately, both routes have some problems.

Topical Decongestants
Topical decongestant products feature compounds known as sympatho-mimetic amines. These molecules have the ability to bind to receptors for adrenaline and related compounds and mimic their effect. In the nasal passages, this effect is to constrict the smaller blood vessels that have become dilated during the cold. This constriction of the blood vessels leads to a reduction in the blood flow in the engorged membranes of the nasal passages and promotes drainage leading to prompt and dramatic improvements in feelings of nasal stuffiness.

Examples of compounds most often used in nasal sprays or drops include phenylephrine (Dristan, 4-Way, Neo-Synephrine, Nostril, Si-nex); oxymetazoline (Afrin, Dristan Long Lasting, Duration, 4-Way Long Lasting, Nostrilla, Sinex Long-Acting); and xylometazoline (Neo-Synephrine II). Phenylephrine produces its effect for about four hours, while oxymetazoline and xylometazoline may last five to six hours; hence, formulas containing the latter two are often referred to as long-acting. Other compounds used in topical nasal decongestants are ephedrine, naphazoline, and propylhexedrine.

Side effects: Topical nasal decongestants often cause a rebound phenomenon in which the nasal passages and sinuses become even more congested. It is for this reason that topical preparations should not be overused during a cold. It is important to follow label recommendations and never use the product for more than three or four days. With too frequent or chronic use, rebound congestion is almost assured, creating a vicious cycle of more frequent use to gain relief followed by greater rebound congestion. If nasal decongestants are used excessively, they will produce the same side effects as the oral (systemic) preparations.

Oral Decongestants
Oral decongestants also utilize sympathomimetic agents, described above. Although they cause less intense constriction of blood vessels than the topical preparations, oral decongestants possess a longer duration of action and are not associated with the rebound congestion of the topical decongestants. Unfortunately, oral decongestants do not exert their action solely on the linings of the nasal passages. This can result in side effects.

Examples of compounds used in oral decongestant products include phenylpropanolamine, phenylephrine, and pseudoephedrine. All of these substances owe their origin to ephedrine, a compound originally isolated from the Chinese medicinal plant *Ephedra sinica* (see page 97).

For the common cold, pseudoephedrine, another compound found in *Ephedra sinica*, is preferred. Unlike ephedrine, pseudoephedrine causes very little stimulatory effect. Because of this, pseudoephedrine, rather than ephedrine, is a common ingredient in many over-the-counter cold medications. The nasal decongesting effects of pseudoephedrine may be important if you absolutely have to function at work, but many natural healers view this effect as counterproductive because it more or less suppresses the symptoms.

Phenylpropanolamine and phenylephrine, synthetic drugs with actions similar to ephedrine but with fewer stimulatory effects, are used in over-the-counter cold medications.

Side effects: Because these drugs bind to the same receptors as adrenaline, they can cause feelings of anxiety and insomnia, and increases in heart rate and blood pressure. Phenylpropanolamine and phenylephrine are more likely to produce these effects than pseudoephedrine. Other side effects may include headache, dizziness, muscle cramps, nausea, and heart palpitations.

Use of oral decongestants is not indicated in patients taking monoamine oxidase (MAO) inhibitors for depression, and people with high blood pressure, hyperthyroidism, diabetes, or angina.

Dietary and Life-style Factors in Treating the Common Cold

One must keep in mind that a cold is a self-limiting illness. It will run its course. Perhaps the most important thing is to employ some general measures that will give the immune system an opportunity to fight off the infection. Employing some general measures designed to boost immune function will prevent the cold from developing into something of more significance. It will also reduce the severity and duration of the symptoms.

GET PLENTY OF SLEEP AND REST

This seems like good advice, but why? During periods of rest, relaxation, visualization, meditation, and sleep, potent immune-enhancing compounds are released, and many immune functions are greatly increased. The value of sleep and rest during a cold cannot be overemphasized.

DRINK PLENTY OF LIQUIDS

The importance of liquids is another common recommendation that needs to be explained. Maintaining good water levels throughout the body offers several benefits during a cold. For starters, when the mucous membranes that line the nose and throat get dehydrated, a much more hospitable environment for the virus exists. Consuming plenty of liquids and/or using a vaporizer maintains a moist respiratory tract that repels viral infection. Drinking plenty of liquids will also improve the function of white blood cells by decreasing the concentration of solutes in the blood.

It should be noted that the type of liquids consumed is very important. Studies have shown that consuming concentrated sources of sugars like glucose, fructose, sucrose, honey, or pasteurized orange juice greatly reduces the ability of the white blood cells to kill bacteria.[4] Sugar consumption, even if derived from "natural" sources like fruit juices and honey, should be avoided during a cold. If fruit juices are to be consumed, they should be fresh and diluted with an equal amount of water. Drinking concentrated orange juice during a cold probably does more harm than good.

Herbal teas are excellent beverage choices anytime, but especially during a cold. Teas like ginger and peppermint which promote internal warming (diaphoretic effects) are quite helpful during colds. Diaphoretic teas work to promote perspiration via warming from the inside out. Here is a great recipe, from my book *The Complete Book of Juicing*, that I call "Kill the Cold":

1-inch slice of ginger
¼ lemon
1 cup hot water

Directions: If you have a juicer, juice the ginger and lemon and add it to a cup of water. If you do not have a juicer, grate the ginger and place it in a tea strainer in a cup of hot water. Add the lemon by squeezing the juice from one half of a lemon. You may want to add some nutmeg or cardamom to the tea to give it even more benefit.

Natural Alternatives to Common-Cold Medications

In addition to the general measures discussed above, there are natural alternatives to common-cold medication that can be used to speed up recovery. With a healthily functioning immune system, a cold should not last more than three or four days. That length of time is ample for the immune system to mount a successful attack against the virus. Even utilizing a wide variety of natural healing methods, it is very difficult to completely throw off the cold within two days once it has established a firm foothold.

Many of the symptoms of a cold are a result of our body's defense mechanisms. For example, the potent immune-stimulating compound interferon released by our blood cells and other tissues during infections is responsible for many flulike symptoms. Another example is the beneficial effect of fever on the course of infection. While an elevated body temperature can be uncomfortable, suppression of fever is thought to counteract a major defense mechanism and prolong the infection. In general, fever should not be suppressed during an infection unless it is dangerously high (more than 103 degrees Fahrenheit).

Rather than suppress symptoms, most practitioners of natural medicine prefer to enhance the body's immune system. Although it is not uncommon when using natural medicines for the common-cold sufferer to experience a greater degree of discomfort, the course of the illness is generally much shorter lived.

Vitamin C
Many claims have been made about the role of vitamin C (ascorbic acid) in enhancing the immune system, especially in the prevention and treatment of the common cold. It has been over twenty years since Linus

Pauling, one of the greatest scientists of the twentieth century, wrote the book *Vitamin C and the Common Cold.*[5] Pauling based his opinion on several studies that showed vitamin C was very effective in reducing the severity of symptoms, as well as the duration of the common cold. Since 1970, there have been over twenty double-blind studies designed to test Pauling's assertion.[6] However, despite the fact that every study demonstrated that the group receiving the vitamin C had a decrease in either duration or symptom severity, for some reason, the clinical effect is still debated in the medical community.

While the vitamin C studies have consistently demonstrated results superior to over-the-counter cold medications, manufacturers of vitamin C products are prevented from making any claims for their product, while the makers of OTC common-cold medications spend hundreds of millions of dollars brainwashing the American public into believing these products are the answer to the common cold.

From a biochemical viewpoint, there is considerable evidence that vitamin C plays a vital role in many immune mechanisms. Vitamin C has been shown to increase many different immune functions, including enhancing white blood cell function and activity and increasing the levels of interferon, the body's natural antiviral compound.

Although the question of dosage has not been firmly answered, the recommendation of 500 to 1,000 milligrams of vitamin C every one to two hours during a cold seems appropriate. These high doses ensure tissue saturation of vitamin C and optimal effects on the immune system. Bioflavonoids (pigments from plants) given along with the vitamin C may produce even better effects.[7] Take at least 500 milligrams of mixed flavonoids per day when taking high doses of vitamin C for the common cold.

Zinc

Zinc is a critical nutrient for optimum immune-system function. Like vitamin C, zinc also possesses direct antiviral activity, including against several viruses that can cause the common cold. In a double-blind clinical trial, zinc gluconate lozenges significantly reduced the average duration of common colds.[8] The lozenges contained 23 milligrams of elemental zinc, which the patients were instructed to dissolve in their mouths every two waking hours after an initial double dose. After seven days, 86 percent of the thirty-seven zinc-treated subjects were symptom free, compared to 46 percent of the twenty-eight placebo-treated subjects.

The authors of the study believed that the local zinc concentration was high enough to inhibit replication of the cold viruses. Although this may account for some of the activity, the immune-enhancing effects of zinc also play a role. The use of zinc supplementation, particularly as a lozenge, appears to be of much value during a cold.

HERBS TO USE DURING A COLD

Many herbs are thought to possess direct antiviral action. However, herbs are much more than "natural" antibiotics. Several herbs have shown remarkable effects in enhancing our own immune mechanisms. Modern research is upholding what herbal practitioners have known for thousands of years: Herbs work with our bodies' systems to affect health. The following herbs represent some of the most significant enhancers of our immune system: coneflower (*Echinacea angustifolia*); goldenseal (*Hydrastis canadensis*); licorice (*Glycyrrhiza glabra*); and astragalus (*Astragalus membranaceus*). Taking these herbs individually or in combination may offer some benefit during the common cold and other infectious processes through enhancing the immune system.

Echinacea angustifolia (purple coneflower)
Perhaps the most widely used herb for enhancement of the immune system is *Echinacea angustifolia*. This perennial plant is native to the midwestern states and was used by the American Indian tribes as a "blood purifier," analgesic, antiseptic, and snake-bite remedy. Recently, this herb has been shown to have significant enhancing activity on the immune system.[9]

Echinacea has been shown to increase properdin levels. This compound is the body's natural activator of an important defense mechanism—the alternative complement pathway. This pathway is responsible for increasing nonspecific host defense mechanisms like: neutralization of viruses; destruction of bacteria; and increasing the migration of white blood cells to areas of infection.

Echinacea has other profound immunostimulatory effects. The components responsible for these effects are primarily polysaccharides that are able to bind to carbohydrate receptors on the cell surface of T-lymphocytes and other white blood cells. This binding results in nonspecific activation including increased production and secretion of interferon.

Root extracts of echinacea have also been shown to possess interferonlike activity and specific antiviral activity against influenza, herpes, and other viruses. Echinacea can be used as a general immune stimulant during infection at the following dosages three times daily:

Dried root (or as tea), 0.5 to 1 gram

Freeze-dried plant, 325 to 650 milligrams

Juice of aerial portion of *E. purpurea* stabilized in 22 percent ethanol, 1 to 2 milliliters (¼ to ½ teaspoon)

Tincture (1:5), 2 to 4 milliliters (½ to 1 teaspoon)

Solid (dry powdered) extract (6.5:1 or 3.5 percent echinacoside), 100 to 250 milligrams

Hydrastis canadensis (goldenseal)

Goldenseal is a perennial herb native to eastern North America. It was also used by Native Americans for a wide variety of conditions, including fighting infections. The activity of goldenseal has been largely attributed to its high content of biologically active alkaloids: berberine, hydrastine, and canadine.

The antibiotic activity of goldenseal's alkaloids is well documented in scientific literature. Berberine is an effective antibiotic against a wide range of harmful organisms, including: *Staphylococcal* sp.; *Streptococcus* sp.; *Chlamydia* sp.; *Corynebacterium diphtheria; Salmonella typhi; Vibrio cholerae; Diplococcus pneumonia*; and *Candida albicans*.[9]

Goldenseal has also shown remarkable immunostimulatory activity. Foremost is its ability to increase the blood supply to the spleen, thus promoting optimal activity of the spleen and the release of immune-potentiating compounds. Berberine has also been shown to be a potent activator of macrophages. These cells are responsible for engulfing and destroying bacteria, viruses, fungi, and tumor cells. Improved macrophage activity is probably the reason goldenseal produces very good effects in reducing fever.

Goldenseal can be used in the following dosage given three times a day for the common cold:

Dried root (or as tea), 1 to 2 grams

Tincture (1:5), 4 to 6 milliliters (1 to 1½ teaspoons)

Powdered solid extract (4:1), 250 to 500 milligrams

Glycyrrhiza glabra (licorice)

Licorice is a perennial herb that has been used for its medicinal properties in both Western and Eastern cultures for several thousand years. It is
reported to be especially effective in treating respiratory tract infections
(bronchitis, pharyngitis, and pneumonia).[9]

Recent scientific evidence supports licorice's use in treating upper
respiratory tract infections. Its major components have been shown to
induce interferon production.[10] This induction of interferon production
leads to significant antiviral activity, as interferons bind to cell surfaces
and stimulate the synthesis of proteins that prevent viral infection. The
major licorice components have also been shown to inhibit directly the
growth of several human viruses.

Licorice can be used at the following dosage given three times a day
for the common cold:

Dried root (or as tea), 1 to 2 grams

Tincture (1:5), 4 to 6 milliliters (1 to 1½ teaspoons)

Powdered solid extract (4:1), 250 to 500 milligrams

(*Note:* If licorice is to be used for more than two weeks, it is
necessary to increase the intake of potassium-rich foods.)

Astragalus membranaceus

The Chinese value astragalus as a specific tonic for strengthening the
body's resistance to disease. In clinical studies in China, astragalus has
been shown to reduce the frequency and shorten the course of the
common cold.[11]

While astragalus does exert some antiviral activity, its main effect is
to enhance interferon production and secretion. Astragalus can be used
at the following dosage given three times a day for the common cold:

Dried root (or as tea), 1 to 4 grams

Tincture (1:5), 2 to 6 milliliters (1 to 1½ teaspoons)

Powdered solid extract (2:1), 250 to 500 milligrams

Final Comments

Although the focus of this chapter was on the use of natural methods to assist the body in recovering from the common cold, optimum nutritional and life-style factors offer the most logical approach to treatment by their preventive effect. The old adage "An ounce of prevention is worth a pound of cure" is true for the common cold as well as for the majority of other conditions afflicting human health.

The common cold does not have to be common to you. Make having a healthy immune system a top priority in your life, and you will not be disappointed. The immune system is designed to protect you from harm. Give it the support it needs, and it will serve you well.

Here is a concise prescription for the common cold:

GENERAL MEASURES

Rest (bed rest, better)

Drink large amount of fluids (preferably diluted vegetable juices, soups, and herb teas)

Limit simple sugar consumption (including fruit)

Use menthol preparations (such as Vicks VapoRub or White Flower Balm) on the upper chest at night to keep airways clear

NUTRITIONAL SUPPLEMENTS

Vitamin C, 500 to 1,000 milligrams every one to two hours (decrease if this produces excess gas or diarrhea)

Zinc lozenges, 1 lozenge containing 23 milligrams elemental zinc every two waking hours for one week

(*Note:* Prolonged zinc supplementation—more than one week—at this dose is not recommended, as it may lead to immunosuppression.)

BOTANICAL MEDICINES

Echinacea angustifolia (coneflower), *Hydrastis canadensis* (goldenseal), *Glycyrrhiza glabra* (licorice), or *Astragalus membranaceus* (astragalus) can be taken individually or in combination in the appropriate dosage.

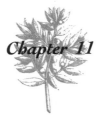

Chapter 11

CORTICOSTEROIDS

Corticosteroids are a group of drugs similar in structure and function to the natural corticosteroid hormones produced by the adrenal glands. Like the natural hormones, these drugs possess a wide range of activities. This chapter will focus on the use of oral preparations. Inhaled corticosteroids for asthma are discussed in Chapter 7, and topical corticosteroids in Chapter 12.

Corticosteroids can be prescribed as hormone-replacement therapy when the body fails to produce adequate amounts of corticosteroids due to Addison's disease or following surgical removal of the adrenal glands. However, the most common use of corticosteroids is in the treatment of a wide range of allergic and inflammatory conditions: asthma; rheumatoid arthritis and other autoimmune disorders like multiple sclerosis and lupus; Crohn's disease; ulcerative colitis; and serious cases of psoriasis and eczema. The drugs are also used to suppress the immune system in selected types of cancers and in preventing the rejection of a transplanted organ.

Prednisone

Prednisone is by far the most often prescribed oral corticosteroid. Other drugs in this category include prednisolone, methyl-prednisolone, dexamethasone, and betamethasone.

Used primarily in allergic and inflammatory conditions, prednisone blocks many key steps in the allergic and inflammatory response, including the production and secretion of the so-called inflammatory mediators such as histamine, prostaglandins, and leukotrienes by white blood cells.

This disruption of the normal defense functions of the white blood cells is great at stopping the inflammatory response, but essentially cripples the immune system.

Although prednisone is often of great benefit in the short-term management of many chronic inflammatory diseases, long-term use generally causes more problems than benefit. Long-term corticosteroid use has many significant side effects. It is for this reason that most physicians try to reserve the use of prednisone for acute conditions or exacerbations of a chronic inflammatory disease.

Because long-term treatment with artificial corticosteroids suppresses the natural production of corticosteroids by the adrenal gland, sudden withdrawal of the drugs may lead to collapse, coma, and death. Do not change your dosage of any corticosteroid without the supervision of a physician.

Side effects: The side effects of oral corticosteroids are a function of dosage levels and length of time with the medication. Most of the problems are not due to taking too much of the drug for a short period of time, but rather reflect long-term use. At lower doses (less than 10 milligrams per day), the most notable side effects are usually increased appetite, weight gain, retention of salt and water, and increased susceptibility to infection. These side effects are almost always expected with corticosteroids.

Common side effects of long-term corticosteroid use at higher dosage levels include: depression and other mental/emotional disturbances (up to 57 percent of patients being treated with high doses of prednisone for long periods of time[1]); high blood pressure; diabetes; peptic ulcers; acne; excessive facial hair in women; insomnia; muscle cramps and weakness; thinning and weakening of the skin; osteoporosis; and susceptibility to the formation of blood clots.

Dietary and Life-style Factors

Several conditions for which corticosteroids are often prescribed are discussed in detail in other parts of this book: Rheumatoid arthritis is discussed in Chapter 6; asthma in Chapter 7; eczema and psoriasis in Chapter 12. However, since corticosteroids are used for such a wide range of conditions, it is impossible to address the multitude of specific dietary and life-style factors for each disease that can be treated. Despite differences among the multitude of inflammatory and allergic conditions that are treated with corticosteroids, there are some common dietary and life-style factors involved.

In addition to adopting a healthful life-style, it is important for the individual with a condition currently being treated with corticosteroids to address the impact that food allergies, dietary fats, and dietary antioxidants may have on his or her health.

FOOD ALLERGIES

Virtually every condition treated with corticosteroids has responded to a diet that has eliminated food allergies.[2] The role of food allergies in rheumatoid arthritis, asthma, and eczema is discussed elsewhere. To further support the role of food allergies in chronic inflammatory disease, let's examine the role of diet in Crohn's disease and ulcerative colitis, the two major categories of inflammatory bowel disease (IBD). IBD is characterized by severe inflammation of the intestinal tract resulting in diarrhea, pain, fever, and weight loss.

Although food allergy has long been considered an important causative factor in the development of IBD, it is only recently that there have been studies utilizing a diet that eliminates foods that cause allergies in the treatment of both Crohn's disease and ulcerative colitis. For example, in a controlled trial of twenty patients with Crohn's disease, ten patients were put on a diet that excluded allergy-causing foods, and the other ten were placed on a high-fiber diet. At the end of six months, seven out of ten on the allergy-elimination diet remained symptom-free, compared with zero out of ten in the other group.[3]

In another study of patients with Crohn's disease, the allergy-elimination diet allowed fifty-one out of seventy-seven patients to remain on a diet alone without medications for periods up to fifty-one months.[4] Since Crohn's disease and ulcerative colitis are currently treated with corticosteroids, harsh drugs that impair the immune system, and since surgery is most often ineffective and produces numerous undesirable side effects, the results of these studies suggest that elimination of allergy-causing foods should be considered in the treatment of Crohn's disease and ulcerative colitis.

Guidelines on how to identify and eliminate food allergies are discussed in Chapter 22, "Designing a Healthful Diet."

DIETARY FATS

Fatty acids are important mediators of inflammation because of their ability to form either inflammatory or anti-inflammatory compounds known as prostaglandins. Manipulation of dietary-oil intake can significantly increase or decrease inflammation, depending on the type of oil being ingested.

Arachidonic acid is a fatty acid derived almost entirely from animal sources (meat, dairy products). It contributes greatly to the inflammatory process through its conversion to inflammatory prostaglandins and leukotrienes. In addition to arachidonic acid, animal foods tend to be high in saturated fats. Saturated fats can also increase the inflammatory response.

Vegetarian diets are often beneficial in the treatment of inflammatory conditions, presumably as a result of decreasing the availability of arachidonic acid for conversion to inflammatory prostaglandins and leukotrienes, while simultaneously supplying vegetable oils containing essential fatty acids like linoleic and linolenic acids. These fatty acids lead to the formation of prostaglandins, which actually inhibit inflammation.

Another important way of decreasing the inflammatory response is the consumption of cold-water fish such as mackerel, herring, sardines, and salmon. These fish are rich sources of eicosapentaenoic acid (EPA), which competes with arachidonic acid for prostaglandin and leukotriene production. The net effect of consumption of these fish or fish oil supplements is a significantly reduced inflammatory/allergic response. Several clinical studies have demonstrated a therapeutic effect when supplementing the diet with EPA in patients with chronic inflammatory diseases that are often treated with corticosteroids, including rheumatoid arthritis, asthma, lupus, multiple sclerosis, and ulcerative colitis.[5] However, supplementation may not be necessary if a serving of one of these cold-water fish is consumed at least once daily.

For vegetarians, flaxseed oil, canola oil, and evening primrose oil supplementation may provide similar benefit to EPA.[6,7] Nonetheless, it must be kept in mind that a vegetarian diet alone is therapeutic for many chronic inflammatory diseases.

To illustrate the power of dietary changes in fatty acids to improve a severe chronic degenerative disease, let's examine multiple sclerosis. Multiple sclerosis (MS) is a syndrome of progressive nervous system disturbances caused by destruction of a sheath of fatty material known as the myelin sheath, which surrounds nerves.

Dr. Roy Swank, professor of neurology, University of Oregon Medical School, has provided convincing evidence that a diet low in saturated fats, maintained over a long period of time (one study lasted more than thirty-four years), tends to halt the disease process.[8,9] Swank began successfully treating patients with his lowfat diet in 1948, a diet that recommends: (1) elimination of butter, hydrogenated oils (margarine and shortening), and an animal-fat intake of no more than 15 grams per day; (2) a daily intake of 40 to 50 grams or approximately three to four tablespoons of polyunsaturated vegetable oils; (3) at least 1 teaspoon of cod-liver oil daily; (4) a normal allowance of protein, mostly from vegetables, nuts, fish, white meat of turkey and chicken (skin removed), and lean meat; and (5) the consumption of fish three or more times a week.

The results of the thirty-four-year study of MS patients conducted by Dr. Swank from 1949 to 1984 are astounding.[9] Minimally disabled patients who followed his dietary recommendations experienced little disease progression, if at all. Only 5 percent failed to survive the thirty-four years of the study, whereas 80 percent who failed to follow the diet recommendations did not survive the study period. The moderately and severely disabled patients who followed the dietary recommendations also did far better than the group that didn't. In addition to dramatically reducing the death rate, the diet was shown to prevent worsening of the disease and greatly reduce fatigue.

Dr. Swank's results in MS treatment along with numerous other studies in other chronic degenerative diseases support the critical need to alter the production of prostaglandins and related compounds in these conditions by changing the source of dietary fatty acids. Dr. Swank's diet appears to be a good recommendation for virtually any chronic inflammatory or allergic condition. At the very least, such dietary manipulation will lessen the dosage of corticosteroids required.

DIETARY ANTIOXIDANTS

During inflammatory and allergic processes, there is a tremendous increase in the level of free radicals and pro-oxidants. These highly reactive molecules can bind to and destroy cellular components, which can overwhelm the body's defense mechanisms to produce significant tissue damage. It is a well-established fact that much of the damage and consequences of allergic and inflammatory conditions are the result of free radicals and pro-oxidants.

The cells of the body protect against free-radical and oxidative damage with the help of enzymes and their ability to incorporate from the diet valuable antioxidant compounds like beta-carotene, bioflavonoids, vitamins C and E, selenium, and sulfur-containing amino acids. It is, therefore, critically important that the diet of individuals be extremely high in plant foods to provide these substances. Furthermore, individuals with chronic inflammatory and allergic diseases usually require high-potency supplementation of antioxidant nutrients (see "Final Comments" for dosage levels). Several of these nutrients have shown clinical effects in chronic inflammatory conditions like rheumatoid arthritis.

Natural Alternatives to Corticosteroids

In addition to the measures discussed above—including supplementing the diet with essential fatty acids, fish oils, and antioxidants—there are other factors that have proven to be effective in several conditions often treated with corticosteroids. However, it is critical that these natural alternatives to corticosteroids be used along with all of the measures discussed above, especially the elimination of food allergies and dietary recommendations.

Pancreatin and Bromelain

Pancreatin refers to preparations of pancreatic enzymes isolated from fresh hog pancreas. Pancreatin preparations are often referred to as proteolytic enzymes, due to their protein-digesting activity. Pancreatin and bromelain, the protein-digesting enzyme of pineapple, have been

Table 11.1   Diseases That Pancreatin and Bromelain Can Improve

Autoimmune disorders
  Rheumatoid arthritis
  Lupus
  Scleroderma
Multiple sclerosis
Sports injuries and trauma
Herpes zoster (shingles)

shown to be effective anti-inflammatory agents in both clinical studies and experimental models.[10,11,12] Bromelain's anti-inflammatory actions are discussed on page 80. The major effect of these enzyme preparations is to lessen swelling and help the body reduce the level of circulating immune complexes.

Diseases associated with high levels of circulating immune complexes include rheumatoid arthritis, lupus erythematosus, periarteritis nodosa, scleroderma, ulcerative colitis, Crohn's disease, and multiple sclerosis. The presence of immune complexes is thought to contribute greatly to the disease process by activating the immune system against the body itself, which ultimately leads to tissue damage.

Experimental and clinical studies have shown that pancreatic enzyme preparations are extremely effective in reducing the levels of immune complex in the blood.[10,11] Furthermore, clinical improvements often correspond to decreases in immune complex levels.

Most studies have utilized the formulas marketed under the names Wobenzyme and Mulsal. However, it must be pointed out that these preparations are relatively weak in potency when compared with a number of enzyme preparations available in the United States. Presumably, by using higher-potency products, the impressive results demonstrated by Wobenzyme and Mulsal can be improved upon. It is preferable to use a full-strength undiluted pancreatic extract (8 to 10 times United States Pharmacopeia). Lower-potency pancreatin products are often diluted with salt, lactose, or galactose to achieve desired strength (e.g., 4 times or 1 time). For anti-inflammatory effects, the dosage recommendation for 10-times pancreatin is 500 to 1,000 milligrams three times a day, 10 to 20 minutes before meals.

The standard dosage of bromelain is based on its m.c.u. (milk clotting unit) activity. The most beneficial range of activity appears to be

1,800 to 2,000 m.c.u. The dosage for this range would be 400 to 600 milligrams three times daily, on an empty stomach.

Curcumin

Curcumin, the yellow pigment of turmeric (*Curcuma longa*) was briefly introduced in Chapter 6, "Arthritis Medications." In models of acute inflammation, curcumin is as effective as cortisone. However, while cortisone is associated with significant toxicity, curcumin displays virtually no toxicity.[13]

Sodium curcuminate, the most potent form of curcumin, can be produced by mixing turmeric with shaked lime. This mixture, applied as a poultice, is an ancient household remedy in India for sprains, muscular pain, and inflamed joints.

Used orally, curcumin exhibits many direct anti-inflammatory effects that, although weaker, are quite similar to cortisone's, including inhibiting leukotriene formation and inhibiting the response of white blood cells to various stimuli involved in the inflammatory process.[13]

In addition to these direct anti-inflammatory effects, curcumin must exert some indirect anti-inflammatory effects, because it is much less active in animals that have had their adrenal glands removed. Possible mechanisms of action include: (1) stimulation of the release of adrenal corticosteroids; (2) "sensitizing" or priming cortisone receptor sites, thereby potentiating cortisone action; and (3) preventing the breakdown of cortisol.

The clinical effect of curcumin in rheumatoid arthritis and inflammation is discussed on page 80. Although there is much research that still needs to be performed, the results of past studies indicate that curcumin may provide benefit in the treatment of inflammation. Furthermore, the safety of curcumin, compared with corticosteroids, is a major advantage.

Because studies in animals show that 40 to 85 percent of an oral dose of curcumin passes through the gastrointestinal tract unchanged, there remains a question on the absorption of orally administered curcumin.[14] To enhance absorption, curcumin is often formulated in conjunction with an equal amount of bromelain (a protein-digesting enzyme from pineapple). Bromelain has been shown to improve the absorption of other medications and it also has anti-inflammatory effects of its own. If a curcumin-bromelain combination is used, it is important to take it on an empty stomach twenty minutes before meals, or between meals.

Providing curcumin in a base of oil such as lecithin, fish oils, or essential fatty acids may also increase absorption. If this combination is used, taking it with meals is probably best.

The recommended dosage for curcumin in inflammation is 400 to 600 milligrams three times a day. To achieve a similar amount of curcumin using turmeric would require a dosage of 8,000 to 60,000 milligrams.

Final Comments

A concise prescription is in order in the treatment of a chronic inflammatory condition. After isolating and eliminating all allergens, it is essential to maintain a diet rich in plant foods (fruits, vegetables, whole grains, and legumes), and low in sugar, meat, refined carbohydrate, and saturated fat. Special foods and supplements for sufferers of chronic allergy and inflammation include: cold-water fish (mackerel, herring, sardines, and salmon) or their oils; cod-liver oil; flaxseed oil; onions and garlic; and flavonoid-rich berries or their extracts (cherries, hawthorn berries, blueberries, and blackberries).

A high intake of dietary antioxidants is critical to support normal protective mechanisms against tissue damage. In addition to eating a diet rich in fresh fruits and vegetables, supplementation is essential. With the exception of vitamin C, look for products that incorporate a broad spectrum of antioxidants in one pill. This will not only be more convenient, it will also reduce the cost. Several national manufacturers make excellent comprehensive antioxidant formulas, including Enzymatic Therapy, Twinlabs, Rainbow Light, and Source Naturals. Here are the levels of the individual antioxidant nutrients to take for the day:

Beta-carotene, 50,000 International Units

Vitamin C, 3 to 8 grams

Vitamin E, 800 to 1,200 International Units

Manganese, 15 milligrams

Selenium, 200 to 400 micrograms

Zinc, 30 to 45 milligrams

Other Supplements

EPA, 1.8 grams per day

Pancreatin (8 to 10X), 500 to 1,000 milligrams three times a day, 10 to 20 minutes before meals

Bromelain (800 to 2,000 m.c.u.), 400 to 600 milligrams three times daily, on an empty stomach

Curcumin, 400 to 600 milligrams three times a day

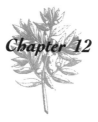

Chapter 12

C O R T I S O N E   C R E A M S ,

L O T I O N S ,   A N D   O I N T M E N T S

Cortisone-containing creams, lotions, and ointments are used for the temporary relief of a wide range of allergic and inflammatory conditions involving the skin. They are usually very effective in reducing the itching and inflammation that often accompany eczema, psoriasis, insect bites, poison oak or ivy, and minor skin rashes. The over-the-counter versions contain up to 0.5 percent hydrocortisone, while the prescription versions typically contain 1 or 2.5 percent hydrocortisone.

Side effects: In general, topical cortisone preparations are very safe. Local adverse reactions can include drying and thinning of the skin; allergic reactions; irritation; loss of pigmentation; excessive hair growth where they are applied; and acnelike eruptions.

The major risk when using cortisone preparations applied to the skin is the risk of infection. Cortisone suppresses the immune system and can mask the signs of skin infection. Therefore, an infection can develop and progress in severity without being noticed. Cortisone preparations should never be applied to skin that shows signs of infection—redness, heat, pus, and crusting—unless under strict medical supervision.

Since some of the cortisone is absorbed into the body through the skin, it can produce the same side effects as oral corticosteroids, especially when using the stronger prescription preparations over large areas of skin, or with the use of occlusive dressings, which do not allow the skin to breathe.

Dietary Factors

The occasional use of topical cortisone preparations for temporary relief of minor skin irritations is acceptable. However, for more chronic conditions like eczema and psoriasis, it is important to address the underlying cause.

Eczema (atopic dermatitis) is an intensely itchy, allergic disease of the skin. The area of skin affected is usually quite red, thick, and irritated. Eczema is commonly found on the face, wrists, and insides of elbows and knees.

Psoriasis is characterized by the appearance of a sharply bordered reddened rash or plaques composed of overlapping silvery scales. The rate at which skin cells divide in areas affected by psoriasis is roughly a thousand times greater than in normal skin. This is simply too fast for the cells to be shed, so they accumulate, resulting in a plaque formation. Psoriasis most often involves the scalp, the back side of wrists, elbows, knees, and ankles, and sites of repeated trauma.

Both eczema and psoriasis can be controlled quite well through diet. Basically, the same principles that apply to replacing oral corticosteroids (see previous chapter) with natural measures apply here as well: Eliminate food allergies and alter the intake of dietary oils.

ECZEMA

The role of food allergy as a major cause of eczema, especially in children, is well established. Control of eczema is dependent on finding and eliminating all, or at least most, of the food allergens. A recent study conducted at the Middlesex Hospital in London provides additional support on the role of food allergies as a cause of childhood eczema.[1] In this study, the researchers estimated that simply eliminating cow's milk, eggs, tomatoes, artificial colors, and food preservatives would help up to three quarters of children with moderate to severe eczema. If eliminating these foods fails to improve the condition, it is likely that another food is the culprit. An elimination diet (see page 267) can be used to identify food allergies.

In addition to food allergies, dietary oils are important in the presence of eczema. Specifically, patients with eczema appear to have an essential fatty acid deficiency. This deficiency results in decreased synthesis of the anti-inflammatory prostaglandins. Treatment with evening primrose oil has been shown both to normalize the essential fatty acid abnormalities and to relieve the symptoms of eczema in many patients.[2] Supplementation with other medicinal oils may provide similar benefits. It may be particularly important to increase the dietary intake of omega-3 oils, either by eating more coldwater fish (mackerel, herring, sardines, and salmon) or through consumption of nuts, seeds, flaxseed oil, or fish-oil supplements.

PSORIASIS

A number of dietary factors appear to be responsible for psoriasis, including incomplete protein digestion. If protein digestion is incomplete, or if there is inadequate intestinal absorption of amino acids, bacteria can break down the amino acids into many toxic compounds. A number of gut-derived toxins are implicated in the development of psoriasis. For example, a group of toxic amino acids known as polyamines (putrescine, spermidine, cadaverine) have been shown to be increased in individuals with psoriasis.[3] These compounds contribute greatly to the formation of skin plaques. Lowered skin and urinary levels of polyamines are associated with clinical improvement in psoriasis. The best way to prevent the excessive formation of polyamines is to keep protein intake, especially from animal foods, at moderate levels while simultaneously increasing the intake of dietary fiber.

Insufficient intake of dietary fiber is associated with increased levels of gut-derived toxins.[4] Dietary fiber is of critical importance in maintaining a healthy colon. Many fiber components are able to bind to bowel toxins and promote their excretion in the feces. It is therefore essential that the diet of an individual with psoriasis be rich in plant foods, especially whole grains, legumes, and vegetables.

Psoriatic patients have shown remarkable improvements while on a fasting and vegetarian treatment at a Swedish hospital where the effect of such diets on chronic inflammatory disease was being studied.[5] The improvement was probably due not only to decreased levels of gut-derived toxins and polyamines, but also to the changes in the intake of dietary oils.

Animal fats, particularly saturated fats and arachidonic acid, greatly increase the production of inflammatory compounds linked to stimulating the skin cells to divide too rapidly. It is best to eliminate consumption of meat (with the exception of fish) and other sources of saturated fats while increasing the consumption of polyunsaturated oils, especially omega-3 oils like flaxseed oil and fish oils. Several double-blind clinical studies have demonstrated that supplementing the diet with 10 to 12 grams of EPA oils results in significant improvement.[6,7] This would be equivalent to the amount of EPA in about a five-ounce serving of mackerel, salmon, sardines, or herring.

Patients with psoriasis must not drink alcohol. Alcohol consumption is known to worsen psoriasis considerably.[8] Alcohol's negative effects include the increased absorption of toxins from the gut, along with impaired liver function. The connection between the liver and psoriasis relates to one of the liver's basic tasks—filtering the blood. As mentioned above, psoriasis has been linked to several gut-derived toxins. If the liver is overwhelmed by an increased number of these toxins, or if there is a decrease in the liver's ability to filter them, the level of these compounds circulating in the blood will be increased, and the psoriasis will get much worse.

Natural Alternatives to Cortisone Creams

A number of botanical compounds have demonstrated an effect equal to or superior to cortisone when applied topically, but without side effects. Extracts of licorice and German chamomile are the most active. All natural creams/ointments containing one or both of these herbs offer an effective natural alternative to cortisone creams. Allantoin is another herbal substance that is often useful in treating mild skin disorders.

Licorice Extracts
Licorice (*Glycyrrhiza glabra*) contains a compound that, when applied to the skin, exerts an effect similar to that of cortisone in the treatment of eczema, contact and allergic dermatitis, and psoriasis.[9] The com-

pound, 18-beta-glycyrrhetinic acid, acts like cortisone, yet does not produce the negative side effects.[10] In several studies, glycyrrhetinic acid has been shown to be superior to topical cortisone, especially in chronic cases. For example, in one study of patients with eczema, 93 percent of the patients applying glycyrrhetinic acid demonstrated improvement, compared with 83 percent using cortisone.

The anti-inflammatory action of glycyrrhetinic acid is largely due to its ability to inhibit the formation and secretion of inflammatory compounds, an extremely important feature when the skin is irritated and inflamed as in psoriasis and eczema.[11]

Chamomile Extracts

Chamomile preparations are widely used in Europe for the treatment of a variety of common skin complaints, including eczema, psoriasis, and dry, flaky, irritated skin.[12] The flavonoid and essential-oil components of chamomile possess significant anti-inflammatory and antiallergy activity.

Allantoin

Allantoin is a compound isolated from comfrey root that has a long history of use in various skin-care products. Its effects on the skin are to soften, protect, and stimulate normal cell growth. Allantoin-containing preparations are useful in many skin complaints, especially those involving dry, scaly, or flaky skin such as eczema and psoriasis. Allantoin is extremely safe, nonallergenic, and nonirritating.

Final Comments

People with eczema and psoriasis usually need nutritional support. At the bare minimum, a zinc supplement providing a daily intake of 30 milligrams is indicated. For psoriasis, a special extract of milk thistle (*Silybum marianum*) known as "silymarin" has been reported to be of value.[13] Presumably this is a result of its ability to improve liver function, inhibit inflammation, and reduce excessive cellular proliferation. The standard dosage of silymarin is 70 to 210 milligrams three times daily.

If you have psoriasis, get a tan. Sunlight (ultraviolet light) and/or tanning beds often provide benefit to individuals with psoriasis. Sunlight is preferred to tanning beds because most tanning beds feature ultraviolet A (UVA), while sunlight provides both ultraviolet A and B (UVB). UVB exposure alone has been shown to be effective, with minimal side effects.

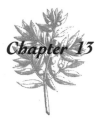

Chapter 13

DIABETES MEDICATIONS

Diabetes is a chronic disorder of carbohydrate, fat, and protein metabolism characterized by elevations of blood sugar (glucose) levels and a greatly increased risk of heart disease, stroke, kidney disease, blindness, and loss of nerve function. Diabetes can occur when the pancreas does not secrete enough insulin or if the cells of the body become resistant to insulin. Insulin is a hormone that promotes the uptake of blood sugar by the cells of the body. When there is not enough insulin or when there is a lack of sensitivity to insulin by the cells, the blood sugar cannot be absorbed by the body's cells. This can lead to serious complications.

Type I or Insulin-Dependent Diabetes Mellitus (IDDM) occurs most often in children and adolescents. It is associated with complete destruction of the beta cells of the pancreas, which manufacture the hormone insulin. These individuals will require lifelong insulin for the control of blood sugar levels. The Type I diabetic must learn how to manage his or her blood sugar levels on a day-by-day basis, modifying insulin types and dosage schedules as necessary, according to the results of regular blood sugar testing. About 10 percent of all diabetics are Type I.

Type II or Non–Insulin Dependent Diabetes Mellitus (NIDDM) usually has an onset after an individual is forty years of age. Up to 90 percent of all diabetics are Type II. Insulin levels may be low, normal, or elevated. Of greater importance in Type II diabetes is a lack of sensitivity to insulin by the cells of the body. Obesity is a major contributing factor to the loss of insulin sensitivity. Approximately 90 percent of individuals with Type II are obese.

In Type II diabetes, diet is of primary importance and must be tried diligently before a drug is used. Over 75 percent of Type II diabetes can be controlled by diet alone. Despite this high success rate, drugs or insulin are often used.

Diabetic Medications (Oral Hypoglycemic Drugs)

There is no question that a Type I diabetic requires insulin. This discussion of diabetes medications will be limited to oral blood sugar–lowering (hypoglycemic) drugs used in Type II diabetes. Oral hypoglycemic drugs are sulfa drugs (sulfonylureas) that appear to stimulate the secretion of additional insulin by the pancreas as well as enhance the sensitivity of body tissues to insulin. Some common examples of this class of drugs include (generic followed by some brand name):

Chlorpropamide (Diabinese)

Glipizide (Glucotrol)

Glyburide (DiaBeta, Micronase)

Tolazamide (Tolinase)

Tolbutamide (Orinase)

As a group, these drugs are not very effective. The rate of primary failure, an inability to control blood sugar levels after three months of continual treatment at an adequate dosage, is about 40 percent. Furthermore, these drugs generally lose their effectiveness over time. After an initial period of success, they will fail to produce a positive effect in about 30 percent of cases. The overall success rate of adequate control by long-term use of sulfonylureas is no more than 20 to 30 percent at best.

In addition to being of limited value, there is evidence to indicate that these drugs actually produce harmful long-term side effects. For example, in a landmark study conducted by the University Group Diabetes Program (UGDP) on the long-term effects of tolbutamide it was shown that the rate of death due to a heart attack or stroke was two and a half times greater than for the group controlling their Type II diabetes by diet alone.[1]

Due to the high risk of side effects, these drugs have to be used with extreme caution. They should not be used in the following situations:

Pregnancy
Known allergy to sulfa drugs
During infection, injury, or surgery
During long-term corticosteroid use

In addition, these drugs must be used with extreme caution in treating the very old, alcoholics, those taking multiple drugs, and those with impaired liver or kidney function.

Side effects: The major side effect of sulfonylureas is abnormally low blood sugar (hypoglycemia). Since blood sugar is the primary fuel for the brain, the symptoms of hypoglycemia usually affect mental function and include such problems as blurred vision, mental confusion, incoherent speech, bizarre behavior, convulsions, depression, other psychological disturbances, and irritability. One of the ways the body combats low blood sugar levels is by increasing epinephrine (adrenaline) secretion by the adrenal gland. Epinephrine secretion can result in accompanying symptoms of headache, sweating, weakness, hunger, heart palpitations, and "inward trembling." Drug-induced hypoglycemia is most likely to occur when fasting, after severe or prolonged exercise, or when alcohol is ingested.

Other possible side effects include allergic skin reactions, fatigue, indigestion, nausea and vomiting, and liver damage.

Dietary and Life-style Factors in Treating Diabetes

Diabetes, perhaps more than any other disease, is strongly associated with a Western diet rich in refined sugar, fat, and animal products.[2] Diabetes is quite rare in cultures consuming a more "primitive" diet rich in whole plant foods. However, as cultures switch from their native diets to more refined foods, their rate of diabetes increases, eventually reaching the same proportions seen in Western societies. The evidence indicting the Western diet and life-style as the ultimate causative factor in diabetes is overwhelming.[2,3]

Dietary modification and treatment is fundamental to the successful treatment of diabetes whether it be Type I or II. Although there are several commonly recommended diets in the management of diabetes, based on clinical research the best is not the one promoted by the American Diabetes Association (ADA), but rather one popularized by Dr. James Anderson.[4] The diet is high in cereal grains, legumes, and root vegetables, and restricts simple sugar and fat intake. It is called the high–complex carbohydrate, high-fiber diet, or HCF diet for short.

The HCF diet has substantial support and validation in the scientific literature as the diet of choice in the treatment of diabetes.[5] The positive effects of the HCF diet are many: reduced elevations in blood sugar levels after meals; increased tissue sensitivity to insulin; reduced cholesterol and triglyceride levels with increased HDL-cholesterol levels; and progressive weight reduction. If patients resume a conventional ADA diet, their insulin requirements return to prior levels. Obviously, the HCF is far superior to the one recommended by the American Diabetes Association.

Anderson basically promotes two HCF diets: one for the initial treatment of the hospitalized patient, and a home use, or maintenance, diet. In the hospitalized version, the caloric intake consists of 70 to 75 percent complex carbohydrates, 15 to 20 percent protein, only 5 to 10 percent fat; and the total fiber content is almost 100 grams per day. The caloric intake of the maintenance diet consists of 55 to 60 percent complex carbohydrates, 20 percent protein, 20 to 25 percent fat; and the total fiber content is still almost 100 grams per day.

On the maintenance HCF diet, available carbohydrate calories come from grain products (50 percent), fruits and vegetables (48 percent), and skim milk (2 percent). Protein is provided by fruits and vegetables (50 percent), grain products (36 percent), and skim milk and lean meat (14 percent). The fat is derived from grain products (60 percent), fruits and vegetables (20 percent), and skim milk and meat (12 percent). The dietary guidelines provided in Chapter 22, "Designing a Healthful Diet," will allow the diabetic to incorporate complex carbohydrates and fiber along with higher levels of legumes (peas and beans). In essence, an even healthier version of Anderson's HCF diet can be constructed. Consumption of legumes should be encouraged since a high-carbohydrate, legume-rich, high-fiber diet has been shown to improve all aspects of diabetic control.[6] The beneficial effects of legumes are primarily due to their water-soluble, gel-forming fiber components, which are similar to those of guar and pectin in producing a positive effect on blood sugar control.

Some individuals with diabetes will try to increase the fiber content of their diet through supplementation rather than through diet. Although fiber-supplemented diets are beneficial, they are not as effective as the HCF diet. Insulin dosages on fiber-supplemented diets can usually be reduced to one third of those used on control (ADA) diets, while the HCF diet has led to discontinuation of insulin therapy in approximately 60 percent of Type II patients, and significantly reduces doses in the other 40 percent.

THE IMPORTANCE OF IDEAL BODY WEIGHT

Body weight is a significant factor in blood sugar control. Even in nondiabetic individuals, significant weight gain results in carbohydrate intolerance, higher insulin levels, and insulin insensitivity in fat and muscle tissue.[7] The progressive development of insulin insensitivity is believed to be the underlying factor in the development of Type II diabetes. Weight loss corrects all of these abnormalities and significantly improves the metabolic disturbances of diabetes. In other words, since 90 percent of people with Type II diabetes are obese, the majority of Americans with diabetes could cure themselves simply by achieving their ideal body weight (see page 250).

EXERCISE

Exercise is critical in the treatment of diabetes, as it improves many aspects of blood sugar control. Physically fit diabetics experience many benefits: enhanced insulin sensitivity with a consequent diminished need for insulin injections; improved glucose tolerance; and reduced total serum cholesterol and triglycerides.

Natural Alternatives to Diabetes Medications

Proper treatment of diabetes requires much more than insulin, a drug, or a bottle of nutritional supplements. Foremost in the treatment of diabetes is diet. However, diet alone is not enough. Diabetics, especially Type I diabetics, have an increased need for many nutrients.[8] For example, since the transport of vitamin C into cells is facilitated by insulin, many diabetics do not have enough vitamin C inside the cells of the body. As a result, vitamin C deficiency exists in many diabetics despite an adequate dietary amount of vitamin C. The diabetic simply needs more vitamin C. A chronic, latent vitamin deficiency will lead to a number of problems for the diabetic, including an increased tendency to bleed (increased capillary permeability); poor wound healing; elevations in cholesterol levels; and a depressed immune system. Furthermore, vitamin C at high doses (for example, 2 grams per day) has been shown to reduce the accumulation of sorbitol within cells. Sorbitol is a sugar that is linked to many complications of diabetes, especially eye and nerve diseases. Other nutrients the diabetic needs more of include vitamins E and B, chromium, zinc, manganese, and magnesium. Supplementation is required to meet this increased demand.

Supplying the diabetic with certain key nutrients has been shown to improve blood sugar control, as well as help prevent or even improve many of the major diabetic complications, such as retinopathy (a disease of the retina, a portion of the eye), heart disease, kidney disease, diabetic cataracts, and nerve disease (neuropathy).[9] A good multiple vitamin and mineral formula should provide adequate levels of many key nutrients. Also, several nutritional-supplement manufacturers provide specific formulas to support an individual with diabetes.

In addition to nutritional supplements, certain medicinal plants are of value in diabetes. Many of these plants have been used since antiquity in the treatment of diabetes, and recent scientific investigation has confirmed that many are remarkably effective. Of necessity, the discussion in this chapter shall be limited to the three plants that appear most effective, are without side effects, and have substantial documentation of their benefits for diabetes.

Chromium

As a key constituent of the "glucose tolerance factor," chromium is a critical nutrient in diabetes. Supplementing the diet with chromium has been shown to decrease fasting glucose levels, improve glucose tolerance, lower insulin levels, and decrease total cholesterol and triglyceride levels, while increasing HDL-cholesterol levels.[10]

The best form of chromium may be chromium polynicotinate, a form composed of chromium bound to several niacin molecules. This is important as niacin administered along with chromium was shown to be more effective than chromium alone in improving blood sugar control.[11]

The diabetic should supplement his or her diet with 200 to 400 micrograms of chromium daily. In addition, it is important to exercise and to limit the intake of refined sugars and white flour products. Exercise increases tissue chromium concentrations,[12] while the consumption of sugar increases chromium excretion from the body.

Manganese

Manganese is an important cofactor in the key enzymes of glucose metabolism.[8] In guinea pigs, a deficiency of manganese results in diabetes and the frequent birth of offspring that develop pancreatic abnormalities or have no pancreas at all. Diabetics have been shown to have only one half the manganese of healthy individuals. A good daily dose of manganese for a diabetic is 30 milligrams.

Magnesium

Like manganese, magnesium is also involved in glucose metabolism. There is considerable evidence that diabetics should take supplemental magnesium. The reasons: magnesium deficiency is common in diabetics, and magnesium may prevent some of the complications of diabetes such as retinopathy and heart disease. Magnesium levels are usually low in diabetics and lowest in those with severe retinopathy.[13]

The recommended daily allowance (RDA) for magnesium is 350 milligrams for adult males and 300 milligrams for adult females. The diabetic may need twice that amount. Most of the magnesium should be derived from the diet. The average intake of magnesium by healthy adults in the United States ranges from 143 to 266 milligrams per day, far below the RDA. Food choices are the main reason. While magnesium occurs abundantly in whole foods, food processing refines out a very large portion of magnesium. The best dietary sources of magnesium are tofu, legumes, seeds, nuts, whole grains, and green leafy vegetables. Fish, meat, milk, and most commonly eaten fruit are quite low in magnesium. Most Americans consume a low-magnesium diet because their diets are high in refined foods, meat, and dairy products.

In addition to eating a diet rich in magnesium, diabetics should supplement their diets with 300 to 500 milligrams of magnesium. Also, they should take at least 50 milligrams of vitamin B_6 per day, as the level of vitamin B_6 inside the cells of the body appears to be intricately linked to the magnesium content of the cell. In other words, without vitamin B_6, magnesium will not get inside the cell and will, therefore, be useless.

Zinc

Zinc deficiency, like chromium deficiency, has been implicated in the development of diabetes.[8] Zinc is involved in virtually all aspects of insulin metabolism: synthesis, secretion, and utilization. Zinc also has a protective effect against beta-cell destruction and has well-known antiviral effects. Diabetics typically excrete too much zinc in the urine, and therefore require supplementation. Supplementation to diabetic mice has improved all aspects of glucose tolerance. Presumably zinc supplementation in humans may have similar effects. Diabetics should take at least 30 milligrams of zinc per day.

Biotin

This B vitamin has been shown to enhance insulin action and increase the activity of the enzyme glucokinase. This enzyme is responsible for the first step in glucose utilization by the liver. Glucokinase concentrations in diabetics are very low. Evidently, supplementing the diet with high doses of biotin improves glucokinase activity and glucose metabolism in diabetics. In one study, 16 milligrams of biotin per day resulted in significant improvements in blood glucose control in diabetics.[14]

Bitter Melon

Bitter melon (*Momordica charantia*), also known as balsam pear, is a tropical fruit widely cultivated in Asia, Africa, and South America. The unripe fruit is eaten as a vegetable. Bitter melon is a green cucumber-shaped fruit with gourdlike bumps all over it. It looks like an ugly cucumber. In addition to being eaten as a vegetable, unripe bitter melon has been used extensively in folk medicine as a remedy for diabetes.[15,16]

The blood sugar–lowering action of the fresh juice or extract of the unripe fruit has been clearly established.

Bitter melon contains several compounds with confirmed antidiabetic properties. Charantin, extracted by alcohol, is a hypoglycemic agent composed of mixed steroids, and is more potent than the oral hypoglycemic drug tolbutamide. Momordica also contains an insulinlike protein, polypeptide-P, which lowers blood sugar levels when injected under the skin into Type I diabetics.[17] Since it appears to have fewer side effects than insulin, it has been suggested as a replacement for some patients. The oral administration of two ounces of the juice has shown good results in clinical trials.[16,17]

Unripe bitter melon is available primarily at Asian grocery stores. Health-food stores may have bitter melon extracts, but the fresh juice is probably best to use, as it is the form used in the studies. Bitter melon juice is, in my opinion, very difficult to make palatable. As its name implies, it is quite bitter. If you desire the medicinal effects, it is best simply to plug your nose and take a two-ounce shot of the juice.

Onions and Garlic

Onions and garlic have significant blood sugar–lowering action.[16,17] The active principles are believed to be sulfur-containing compounds, allyl propyl disulphide (APDS) and diallyl disulphide oxide (allicin) respectively, although other constituents such as flavonoids may play a role as well.

Experimental and clinical evidence suggests that APDS lowers glucose levels by competing with insulin (also a disulphide) for insulin-inactivating sites in the liver, resulting in an increase of free insulin. ADPS administered in doses of 125 milligrams per kilogram of body weight to fasting humans causes a marked fall in blood glucose levels and an increase in serum insulin.[16] Allicin at doses of 100 milligrams per kilogram of body weight produces a similar effect.

Graded doses of onion extracts at levels sometimes found in the diet, that is, one to seven ounces of onion, reduce blood sugar levels during oral and intravenous glucose tolerance in a dose-dependent manner: The higher the dose, the greater the effect. The effects are similar in both raw and cooked onion extracts.[18]

The cardiovascular effects of garlic and onions—their cholesterol- and blood pressure–lowering actions—further substantiate the need for liberal intake of garlic and onions by the diabetic patient.

Gymnema Sylvestre

Gymnema sylvestre, a plant native to the tropical forests of India, has long been used as a treatment of diabetes. Recent scientific investigation has upheld its effectiveness in both Type I and Type II diabetes.

An extract of the leaves of *Gymnema sylvestre* given to twenty-seven patients with Type I diabetes on insulin therapy was shown to reduce insulin requirements and fasting blood sugar levels, and improve blood sugar control.[19] This study confirmed earlier work in animal studies. In Type I diabetes, gymnema appears to work by enhancing the action of insulin. Furthermore, there is some evidence that it may possibly regenerate or revitalize the beta cells of the pancreas.

Gymnema extract has also shown positive results in Type II diabetes.[20] In one study, twenty-two Type II diabetics were given gymnema extract along with their oral hypoglycemic drugs. All patients demonstrated improved blood sugar control. Twenty-one out of the twenty-two were able to reduce their drug dosage considerably, and five subjects were able to discontinue their medication and maintain blood sugar control with the gymnema extract alone.

The dosage for *Gymnema sylvestre* extract is 400 milligrams per day in both Type I and Type II diabetes. Gymnema extract is without side effect and exerts its blood sugar–lowering effects only in cases of diabetes. Given to healthy volunteers, it does not produce any blood sugar–lowering or hypoglycemic effects. This is in stark contrast to the oral hypoglycemic drugs.

Final Comments

The diabetic individual must be monitored carefully, particularly if he or she is on insulin or has relatively uncontrolled diabetes. Careful attention to symptoms, home glucose monitoring, and other blood tests are essential in monitoring the condition of the diabetic individual. As she or he employs some of the suggestions described in this chapter, drug dosages will have to be altered. A good working relationship with the prescribing doctor is critical.

As mentioned above, diabetics have an above average need for many nutrients. Supplementation is required to meet this increased demand.

In a nutshell, here are the key recommendations for daily supplementation:

Vitamin C, 3 to 8 grams
Vitamin E, 400 to 600 International Units
Vitamin B_6, 50 milligrams
Vitamin B_{12}, 1,000 micrograms
Biotin, 1,000 micrograms
Chromium, 200 to 400 micrograms
Magnesium, 300 to 500 milligrams
Manganese, 30 milligrams
Selenium, 200 micrograms
Zinc, 30 milligrams

A good multiple vitamin and mineral formula may provide adequate levels of most of these nutrients.

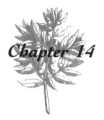

Chapter 14

GOUT MEDICATIONS

Gout is a common type of arthritis caused by an increased concentration of uric acid in biological fluids (such as blood, lymph, urine, and joint fluid). Uric acid is the final breakdown product of purine metabolism. Purines are made in the body and are also ingested in foods. In gout, uric acid crystals are deposited in joints, tendons, kidneys, and other tissues, where they cause considerable inflammation and damage.

The first attack of gout is characterized by intense pain, usually involving only one joint. The first joint of the big toe is affected in nearly half of the first attacks and is at some time involved in over 90 percent of individuals with gout. If the attack progresses, fever and chills will appear. The first attacks usually occur at night and often are preceded by a specific event such as dietary excess, alcohol ingestion, trauma, certain drugs, or surgery.

Gout is associated with affluence and is often called the "rich man's disease." Throughout history, the sufferer of gout has been depicted as a portly, middle-aged man sitting in a comfortable chair with one foot resting painfully on a soft cushion as he consumes great quantities of meat and wine. In fact, the traditional picture does have some basis in reality, as meats, particularly organ meats, are high-purine foods, while alcohol inhibits uric acid secretion by the kidneys. Furthermore, even today, gout is primarily a disease of adult men; over 95 percent of sufferers of gout are men over the age of thirty. The incidence of gout is approximately three adults in one thousand, although as many as 10 to 20 percent of the adult population have elevated uric acid levels in the blood.[1]

Basic Gout Medications

There are basically two types of gout medication: drugs used to treat acute attacks of gout and drugs that reduce the level of uric acid in the body. In the treatment of acute attacks, colchicine or nonsteroidal anti-inflammatory drugs (NSAIDs) such as indomethacin, phenylbutazone, naproxen, and fenoprofen are used. Colchicine is the drug of choice when the diagnosis of gout is in question; however, NSAIDs are now preferred over colchicine in acute attacks when a firm diagnosis of gout has been made. Since NSAIDs are discussed fully elsewhere (see page 67), they will not be discussed here.

In the treatment of chronic gout, physicians often measure the amount of uric acid in a twenty-four-hour collection of urine to identify whether a gout sufferer is an overproducer of uric acid (greater than 800 milligrams) or an underexcretor (less than 800 milligrams). The overproducer is usually prescribed allopurinol, while the underexcretor is given probenecid or sulfinpyrazone.

Colchicine

Colchicine is an anti-inflammatory drug that was originally isolated from the plant *Colchicum autumnale* (autumn crocus, meadow saffron). Colchicine has no effect on uric acid levels. Rather, it stops the inflammatory process by lowering the acidity of the joint tissues, thereby increasing the solubility of uric acid and dissolving uric acid crystals. Colchicine also inhibits the migration of white blood cells into areas of inflammation.

The reason colchicine is still the preferred drug when the diagnosis of gout is in question is that if it is gout, colchicine will bring about almost immediate relief. If it isn't gout, colchicine will not affect whatever illness the patient may have. It is somewhat diagnostic in initial attacks, as over 90 percent of patients with gout show dramatic improvement in symptoms within the first twelve hours after receiving colchicine. However, as many as 80 percent of patients are unable to tolerate an optimal dose because of gastrointestinal side effects such as severe nausea, abdominal cramps, vomiting and/or diarrhea, which may precede or coincide with clinical improvement.[2]

Low doses of colchicine are often incorporated with probenecid (see below) in an effort to prevent recurrent gout attacks. Examples of this combination include the brands Colabid, ColBENEMID, and Proben-C.

Side effects: Colchicine is an extremely powerful drug that has significant side effects. Side effects are typically a function of dosage; that is, the greater the dosage, the more likely it is that side effects will appear. As mentioned above, most patients will experience significant gastrointestinal discomfort. Other possible side effects include: allergic reactions; loss of hair; suppression of bone marrow resulting in low white blood cell counts; anemia; fatigue; abnormal bleeding and bruising; peripheral nerve inflammation characterized by numbness; "pins and needles" sensations; pain; weakness in the hands and/or feet; liver damage; and inflammation of the colon resulting in bloody diarrhea.

Allopurinol

Allopurinol works to lower uric acid levels by inhibiting its formation. It also inhibits the activity of xanthine oxidase, the enzyme responsible for the final conversion of purines into uric acid. Allopurinol is best used in gout patients who overproduce, as opposed to underexcrete, uric acid.

Side effects: In general, allopurinol is well tolerated. The most common side effect is the development of a skin rash. Because these skin reactions can be quite severe and indicate more serious problems, if a rash develops, discontinue use and consult your physician immediately. Other possible side effects include headache, dizziness, fatigue, loss of hair, and liver damage.

Probenecid and Sulfinpyrazone

These two drugs increase the excretion of uric acid. They are used primarily in the long-term management of gout in patients who have elevated blood and tissue uric acid levels due to an inability to excrete uric acid.

Side effects: Because probenecid and sulfinpyrazone increase the excretion of uric acid, they increase the risk of developing kidney stones. Patients with a history of kidney stones or kidney disease should not take either drug.

Other than kidney stones, the most common side effects of probenecid and sulfinpyrazone are gastrointestinal irritation (nausea, vomiting, gastric pain), headache, and mild skin rashes. Other possible side effects include reduced appetite, sore gums, liver damage, bone-marrow suppression, and kidney damage.

Dietary Factors in Treating Gout

It is a well-accepted fact that most cases of gout can be treated effectively with diet alone. However, with the advent of potent drugs like allopurinol, many physicians do not even stress the value of diet therapy to their patients. The dietary treatment of gout involves the following guidelines, each of which will be briefly summarized below:

Elimination of alcohol intake

Low purine diet

Achievement of ideal body weight

Liberal consumption of complex carbohydrates

Low fat intake

Low protein intake

Liberal fluid intake

ALCOHOL

Alcohol increases uric acid production and reduces uric acid excretion by increasing lactate production (a result of the breakdown of alcohol), which impairs kidney function. The net effect is a significant increase in serum uric acid levels. Alcohol consumption is often a precipitating factor in acute attacks of gout. Elimination of alcohol is all that is needed to reduce uric acid levels and prevent gout in many individuals.[1]

LOW-PURINE DIET

A low-purine diet has been the mainstay of the dietary therapy of gout for many years. Foods with high purine levels should be entirely omitted. These include organ meats, red meats, shellfish, yeast (brewer's and baker's), herring, sardines, mackerel, and anchovies.

WEIGHT REDUCTION

Individuals with gout are typically obese, prone to high blood pressure and diabetes, and are at a greater risk for cardiovascular disease. Weight reduction in obese individuals significantly reduces serum uric acid levels. Achieving ideal body weight may be the most important dietary goal in gout.

CARBOHYDRATES, FATS, AND PROTEINS

Refined carbohydrates (particularly sugar and white flour products) and saturated fats should be kept to a minimum, as the former increase uric acid production while the latter decrease uric acid excretion. Protein intake should not be excessive as it has been shown that uric acid synthesis may be accelerated in both normal and gouty patients by a high protein intake.

FLUID INTAKE

Liberal fluid intake keeps the urine diluted and promotes the excretion of uric acid. Furthermore, dilution of the urine reduces the risk of kidney stones.

Natural Alternatives to Gout Medications

Although diet alone is effective in most cases of gout, there are several natural compounds that can help. In addition to recommendations given in Chapter 6, "Arthritis Medications," all of which are also effective for gout, here are some specific suggestions for gout.

Flavonoids

Consuming the equivalent of one-half pound of fresh cherries per day has been shown to be very effective in lowering uric acid levels and preventing attacks of gout.[2] Cherries, hawthorn berries, blueberries, and other dark red-blue berries are rich sources of anthocyanidins and proanthocyanidins. They are available year-round in fresh, frozen, or extract form. These flavonoid compounds are what give these fruits their deep red-blue color. They are also the compounds that make these fruits remarkable in their ability to prevent destruction of joint structures.

Other types of flavonoids may be of benefit to individuals with gout. For example, the flavonoid quercetin has demonstrated several beneficial effects in experimental studies. Quercetin may offer significant protection by inhibiting uric acid production in a fashion similar to the drug allopurinol, as well as inhibiting the manufacture and release of inflammatory compounds.[3,4] Quercetin is widely found in fruits and vegetables. For best results, 200 to 400 milligrams of quercetin should be taken with bromelain (see page 80) between meals, as bromelain is believed to enhance the absorption of quercetin and other medications.

Folic Acid

Folic acid has been shown to inhibit xanthine oxidase, the enzyme responsible for producing uric acid.[5] In fact, research has demonstrated that folic acid is an even greater inhibitor of xanthine oxidase than allopurinol, suggesting that folic acid at pharmacological doses may be an effective treatment in gout. Positive results in the treatment of gout have been reported, but the data are incomplete and uncontrolled.[6] The dosage of folic acid required is in the range of 10 to 40 milligrams per day.

Final Comments

A secondary type of gout, sometimes called saturnine gout, can result from lead toxicity.[7] Historically, saturnine gout was due to the consumption of alcoholic beverages stored in vessels containing lead (such as leaded crystal). While these are still a concern, nowadays lead contamination from the environment (water, air, food) is a bigger problem. In the United States alone, emissions from industrial sources and leaded gasoline put more than six hundred thousand tons of lead into the atmosphere to be inhaled or—after being deposited on food crops, in fresh water, and soil—to be ingested. Hair mineral analysis is a good screening test for lead toxicity. I recommend it be performed in any patient suffering from gout.

If lead is the source of the problem, special foods and nutrients that help "get the lead out" include: artichokes, beets, carrots, dandelion, cabbage-family vegetables, whole grains, legumes, vitamin C, zinc, choline, methionine, cysteine, and flavonoids.

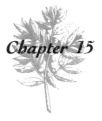

Chapter 15

HEADACHE MEDICATIONS

Headaches rank ninth among the most common causes of visits to physicians. The pain of a headache comes from outside the brain, because the brain tissue itself does not have sensory nerves. Pain arises from the outer lining of the brain (the meninges) and from the scalp and its blood vessels and muscles when these structures are stretched or tensed.

Although a headache may be associated with a serious medical condition, most headaches are not serious. Headaches can be caused by a wide variety of factors, but the overwhelming majority requiring medical attention are either tension or migraine headaches. A quick way to differentiate between the two is the nature of the pain. Tension headaches usually have a steady, constant, dull pain that starts at the back of the head or in the forehead and spreads over the entire head, giving the sensation of pressure or a vise grip applied to the skull. In contrast, migraine headaches are vascular headaches characterized by a throbbing or pounding sharp pain in the head.

A tension headache is usually caused by tightening in the muscles of the face, neck, or scalp as a result of stress or poor posture. The tightening of the muscles results in pinching of a nerve or its blood supply, which results in the sensation of pain and pressure. Relaxation of the muscle usually brings about immediate relief.

Migraine headaches are caused by excessive dilation (expansion) of a blood vessel in the head. Migraines are a surprisingly common disorder, affecting 15 to 20 percent of men and 25 to 30 percent of women. More than half of migraine sufferers have a family history of the illness.

Although many migraines come without warning, other migraine sufferers do have warning symptoms (auras) before the onset of pain. Typical auras last a few minutes and include: blurring or bright spots in the vision; anxiety; fatigue; disturbed thinking; and numbness or tingling on one side of the body.

Common Headache Medications

Tension headaches are treated with mild pain-relieving medicines (analgesics) like aspirin, acetaminophen (Tylenol), or ibuprofen (Advil, Motrin). Since aspirin and ibuprofen have been discussed elsewhere (page 67), only acetaminophen will be discussed below. An acute migraine headache is most often treated with ergotamine. For prevention, many doctors prescribe either ergotamine, beta-blockers, calcium channel blockers, or nonsteroidal anti-inflammatory drugs. Only ergotamine will be discussed below, as these other drugs were reviewed earlier (page 106).

Acetaminophen (Tylenol, Datril, Panadol, Anacin-3)
Acetaminophen, like aspirin and ibuprofen, can reduce pain and fever, but, unlike aspirin, it doesn't have an anti-inflammatory effect, and therefore, is not used in inflammatory conditions such as arthritis. But it is recommended by many physicians for conditions of minor pain, like most tension headaches, because it is gentler to the stomach than aspirin or ibuprofen. However, acetaminophen does have problems of its own. Most important, it can cause liver and kidney damage. While this is usually not a problem for the occasional user unless taking a massive dose (10 grams), the regular user is at risk.

Side effects: Acetaminophen is usually well tolerated if it is taken as directed and on an occasional basis. Skin rashes and other allergic reactions are the most common side effects. At high dosages (10 to 15 grams), severe liver damage can occur. This damage can even be fatal. Long-term use of acetaminophen, as well as of ibuprofen and aspirin, is associated with an increased risk for kidney disease.

Ergotamine

Ergotamine is usually given as ergotamine tartrate, with or without caffeine, belladonna, or barbiturates. It is the most widely used medical drug in the treatment of migraine. Ergotamine works by constricting the blood vessels of the head, thereby preventing or relieving the excessive dilation of the blood vessels that causes the pain of migraine headaches.

Although ergotamine is definitely effective when administered intramuscularly—by inhalation or by suppository—oral ergotamine (which is poorly absorbed by the gastrointestinal tract) is no more effective than a placebo in an acute migraine.

Side effects: Early recognition of the common signs and symptoms of acute and chronic toxicity of ergotamine is important. Symptoms of acute poisoning include: vomiting; diarrhea; dizziness; rise or fall of blood pressure; slow, weak pulse; shortness of breath; convulsions; and loss of consciousness. Symptoms of chronic poisoning include two types of manifestations: those resulting from blood vessel contraction and reduced circulation—numbness and coldness of the extremities, tingling, pain in the chest, heart-valve lesions, hair loss, decreased urination, and gangrene of the fingers and toes; and those resulting from nervous system disturbances—vomiting, diarrhea, headache, tremors, contractions of the facial muscles, and convulsions.

Dietary and Life-style Factors in Treating Headaches

There is little doubt that food allergy/intolerance is the major cause of migraine headaches. These same factors may also play a role in tension headaches. Many carefully designed studies have shown that the detection and removal of allergic/intolerant foods will eliminate or greatly reduce migraine symptoms in the majority of sufferers.[1-6] The most common allergens are milk, wheat, chocolate, food additives, artificial sweeteners like aspartame (Nutrasweet), tomatoes, and fish.

Foods such as chocolate, cheese, beer, and wine, as well as aspartame, precipitate migraine attacks in many people not only due to aller-

Table 15.1   Precipitating Factors in Migraine and Tension Headaches

Foods, e.g., allergens, chocolate, cheese, cured meats
Alcohol, especially red wine
Nitrates, monosodium glutamate, nitroglycerin
Emotional changes, especially let-down after stress and intense
     emotions such as anger
Hormonal changes, e.g., menstruation, ovulation, effects of birth-
     control pills
Too little or too much sleep
Exhaustion
Poor posture
Muscle tension
Weather changes, e.g., barometric pressure changes, exposure to sun
Glare
Withdrawal from caffeine or other drugs that constrict blood vessels

gies, but also because these foods contain compounds known as "vasoactive amines," which can trigger migraines in sensitive individuals by causing blood vessels to expand. Many migraine sufferers have been found to have significantly lower levels of a platelet enzyme that normally breaks down these dietary amines. Since red wine contains substances that are potent inhibitors of this enzyme, it often triggers migraines in these individuals, especially if consumed along with high vasoactive amine foods like cheese.[7]

Natural Alternatives to Headache Medications

One of my favorite instructors while I was going to medical school was Dr. Bill Mitchell. He said something during a lecture that I have always remembered: "You don't get a headache for lack of aspirin." Dr. Mitchell's philosophy is to get at the cause of an illness and then address that cause with as natural a treatment as possible. In the treatment of headache, this usually means eliminating a precipitating factor.

Usually, simply identifying and eliminating the cause is all that is needed. However, if additional support is required, here are two very useful natural alternatives to consider—magnesium, and the herb feverfew.

Magnesium

Several researchers have provided substantial links between low magnesium levels and both migraine and tension headaches, based on both theory and clinical observations. A magnesium deficiency is known to set the stage for the events that can cause a migraine attack as well as a tension headache.[8] Low brain and tissue magnesium concentrations have been found in patients with migraines, indicating a need for supplementation, since one of magnesium's key functions is to maintain the tone of the blood vessels.[9]

Another possible benefit of magnesium for migraine sufferers may be its ability to improve mitral valve prolapse. Mitral valve prolapse refers to a loss of tone or slight deformity of the mitral valve of the heart, which causes leakage of the valve and produces a heart murmur that can be heard by a stethoscope. A prolapse of the mitral valve is linked to migraines because it leads to changes in blood platelets that makes them release substances that ultimately cause the blood vessels in the head to expand. Since research has shown that 85 percent of patients with mitral valve prolapse have chronic magnesium deficiency, magnesium supplementation is indicated. This recommendation is further supported by several studies showing oral magnesium supplementation improves mitral valve prolapse.[10,11]

For best results, use a highly absorbable form of magnesium like magnesium aspartate or citrate at a dose of 350 to 500 milligrams per day.

Feverfew (Tanacetum parthenium)

Feverfew has been used for centuries to relieve fever, migraines, and arthritis. Physician John Hill, in his book *The Family Herbal* (1772), noted, "In the worst headache this herb exceeds whatever else is known." Recently, there has been tremendously increased interest in feverfew in the treatment of headaches. This renewed interest began in the 1970s in Britain, and increased public awareness led to scientific investigation. A 1983 survey found that 70 percent of 270 migraine sufferers who had eaten feverfew daily for prolonged periods claimed that the herb decreased the frequency and/or intensity of their attacks.[12]

Many of these patients had been unresponsive to orthodox medicines. This improvement prompted two clinical investigations of the therapeutic and preventive effects of feverfew in migraine treatment.

The first double-blind study was done at the London Migraine Clinic, using patients who reported being helped by feverfew.[12] Those patients who received the placebo (and as a result stopped using feverfew) had a significant increase in the frequency and severity of headaches, nausea, and vomiting during the six months of the study, while patients taking feverfew showed no change in the frequency or severity of their symptoms. Two patients in the placebo group who had been in complete remission during self-treatment with feverfew leaves developed recurrence of incapacitating migraine and had to withdraw from the study. The resumption of self-treatment led to renewed remission of symptoms in both patients.

The second double-blind study was performed at the University of Nottingham.[13] The results of the study clearly demonstrated that feverfew was effective in reducing the number and severity of migraine attacks.

Follow-up studies to clinical results have shown feverfew works in the treatment and prevention of migraine headaches by inhibiting the release of blood vessel–dilating substances from platelets, inhibiting the production of inflammatory substances, and reestablishing proper blood vessel tone.[14]

The effectiveness of feverfew is dependent upon adequate levels of parthenolide, the active ingredient. The preparations used in the clinical trials had a parthenolide content of 0.2 percent. The dosage of feverfew used in the London Migraine Clinic study was one capsule containing 25 milligrams of the freeze-dried pulverized leaves twice daily. In the Nottingham study, it was one capsule containing 82 milligrams of dried powdered leaves once daily. While these low dosages may be effective in preventing an attack, a higher dose (1 to 2 grams) is necessary during an acute attack. Feverfew is extremely well tolerated and no serious side effects have been reported. However, chewing the leaves can result in small ulcerations in the mouth and swelling of the lips and tongue. This condition occurs in about 10 percent of users.

Final Comments

If you suffer from chronic migraine or tension headaches, I would strongly recommend that you see a chiropractor or an acupuncturist. Both chiropractic manipulation and acupuncture have been shown to be effective in providing relief from headaches. Some other natural or noninvasive methods to consider include biofeedback, transcutaneous electrical nerve stimulation (TENS), massage, and relaxation techniques.

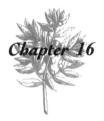

LAXATIVES

Laxatives are used to relieve constipation, a condition that affects over four million people in the United States.[1] This high rate of constipation translates to over four hundred million dollars in annual sales of laxatives in this country. There are many causes of constipation, most of which are listed in Table 16.1. In general, inappropriate diet, inadequate exercise, and laxative/enema abuse are the most common causes.

Since the frequency of defecation and the consistency and volume of stools vary so greatly from individual to individual, it is difficult to determine what is normal. Nonetheless, most nutritionally oriented physicians consider two to three bowel movements per day as ideal. This is the number that is typically found in healthy people eating a high-fiber diet and getting adequate exercise.

Common Laxatives

While constipation will usually respond to a high-fiber diet, plentiful fluid consumption, and exercise, this appears to be too much to ask of many sufferers of chronic constipation. Instead of following this natural approach, many people are content to become dependent upon laxatives. The three most popular types of laxatives currently in use are bulking agents, stimulant laxatives, and stool softeners.

Table 16.1 Causes of Constipation

Dietary: highly refined and low-fiber foods, inadequate fluid intake

Physical inactivity: inadequate exercise, prolonged bed rest

Pregnancy: can cause change in bowel activity

Advanced age: can cause change in bowel activity

Drugs: anesthetics, antacids (aluminum and calcium salts); anticholinergics (bethanechol, carbachol, pilocarpine, physostigmine, ambenonium); anticonvulsants, antidepressants (tricyclics, monoamine oxidase inhibitors); antihypertensives, antiparkinsonism drugs, antipsychotics (phenothiazines); beta-adrenergic blocking agents (propanolol); bismuth salts, diuretics, iron salts, laxatives and cathartics (chronic use); muscle relaxants, opiates, toxic metals (arsenic, lead, mercury)

Metabolic abnormalities: low potassium stores, diabetes, kidney disease

Endocrine abnormalities: low thyroid function, elevated calcium levels, pituitary disorders

Structural abnormalities: abnormalities in the structure or anatomy of the bowel

Bowel diseases: diverticulosis, irritable bowel syndrome (alternating diarrhea and constipation), tumor

Neurogenic abnormalities: nerve disorders of the bowel (aganglionosis, autonomic neuropathy); spinal cord disorders (trauma, multiple sclerosis, tabes dorsalis); disorders of the splanchnic nerves (tumors, trauma); cerebral disorders (strokes, parkinsonism, neoplasm)

Enemas: (chronic use)

BULKING AGENTS

Bulking agents are laxatives that approximate most closely the natural mechanism that promotes a bowel movement and are, therefore, the recommended choice as initial therapy for constipation. They can be composed of natural plant fibers derived from psyllium seed, kelp, agar, pectin, and plant gums like karaya and guar. Or, they can be purified semisynthetic polysaccharides like methyl-cellulose and carboxymethyl cellulose sodium. Psyllium-containing laxatives are the most popular and usually the most effective.

Side effects: Bulking agents are extremely safe, as long as sufficient fluids are consumed with them. Failure to consume sufficient fluid could cause the formation of a very hard stool that is difficult to pass. Bulking agents must not be used if there is evidence of bowel obstruction (severe abdominal pain and absence of intestinal noises). Please consult a physician before taking a bulk laxative if you have severe abdominal pain.

STIMULANT LAXATIVES

Stimulant laxatives act on the large intestine by increasing peristalsis (the muscular activity of the colon). The most common stimulant laxatives are derived from either cascara sagrada (Rhamnus purshiana) or senna (*Cassia senna*). Both plants have long been used as laxatives. It is best to use commercial over-the-counter sources rather than the crude plant, however, because the former contain standardized concentrates of the laxative components. Although extremely effective in promoting bowel movements, use of stimulant laxatives should be avoided. They should never be used as an initial treatment of constipation, nor should they ever be used for more than one week of treatment.

Side effects: Stimulant laxatives can produce severe cramping, electrolyte and fluid deficiencies, and malabsorption of nutrients. Since the laxative components of senna and cascara are absorbed into breast milk, it may cause diarrhea in breast-fed infants. Stimulant laxatives should not be used if symptoms of appendicitis are present (abdominal pain, nausea, and vomiting). Long-term use of stimulant laxatives can lead to a poorly functioning colon and dependence on the laxative for relief.

STOOL SOFTENERS

Docusate calcium and docusate potassium are the most popular stool softeners. Docusate softens the stool by promoting the mixing of water and fatty substances in the stool. Many over-the-counter preparations contain stimulant laxatives with a stool softener because docusate is not very effective in relieving chronic constipation on its own. Like stimulant laxatives, stool softeners should only be used for short-term therapy of less than one week.

Side effects: Since stool softeners are inert substances that are not absorbed, they are safe. However, because they can increase the absorption of other compounds that are potentially harmful, they must be used with care. Consequently, the FDA requires the following warning statement on docusate-containing formulas: "Do not take this product if you are taking a prescription drug or mineral oil."

Dietary Factors in Treating Constipation

A low-fiber diet is probably the greatest contributor to chronic constipation. A high level of dietary fiber increases both the frequency and quantity of bowel movements, decreases the transit time of stools, decreases the absorption of toxins from the stool, and appears to be a preventive factor in several diseases.

Particularly effective in relieving constipation are bran and prunes. The typical recommendation for bran is one-half cup of bran cereal per day, increasing to one-and-a-half cups over several weeks. Corn bran is more effective than wheat bran, while oat bran is less irritating and a better absorber of fats. For best results, adequate amounts of fluids must also be consumed (at least thirty-two ounces per day). Whole prunes as well as prune juice possess good laxative effects. Eight ounces is usually an effective dose.

Natural Alternatives to Laxatives

Many laxatives are natural products, so the real natural alternative to laxatives is to "retrain" the bowels. If constipation has been a chronic problem and laxatives have been used frequently, bowels will need to be retrained to produce regular bowel movements. Listed below are recommended rules for reestablishing bowel regularity. The recommended procedure will take four to six weeks.

Table 16.2   Rules for Bowel Retraining

Find and eliminate known causes of constipation
Never repress an urge to defecate
Eat a high-fiber diet, particularly fruits and vegetables
Drink six to eight glasses of fluid (water and/or fresh juices) per day
Sit on the toilet at the same time every day (even when the urge to
    defecate is not present), preferably, immediately after breakfast or
    exercise
Exercise at least twenty minutes, three times per week
Stop using laxatives (except as discussed below to reestablish bowel
    activity) and enemas

Week one: Every night before bed, take a stimulant laxative
containing either cascara or senna. Take the lowest amount necessary
to ensure a reliable bowel movement every morning.

Weekly thereafter: Each week, decrease dosage by one half. If
constipation recurs, go back to the previous week's dosage. Decrease
dosage if diarrhea occurs.

Final Comments

A frequent cause of constipation is the so-called irritable bowel syndrome (IBS), a very common condition in which the large intestine (colon) fails to function properly. In addition to constipation, IBS can include a combination of any of the following symptoms: abdominal pain and distension; more frequent bowel movements with pain, or relief of pain with bowel movements; diarrhea; excessive production of mucus in the colon; symptoms of indigestion such as flatulence, nausea, or loss of appetite; and varying degrees of anxiety or depression.

IBS can be treated in most circumstances simply by increasing the intake of dietary fiber and eliminating food allergies. If additional support is needed, look for a special peppermint oil product in health-food stores—Peppermint Plus is an enteric-coated peppermint oil capsule made by Enzymatic Therapy.

Peppermint oil has been shown to inhibit intestinal spasm and relieve gas.[2] A special procedure of coating a capsule containing peppermint oil prevents the oil from being released in the stomach. Without the special coating, peppermint oil tends to produce heartburn.

Enteric-coated peppermint oil has been used in treating the irritable bowel syndrome in Europe for many years.[3,4] In one double-blind cross-over study, it was shown to significantly reduce the abdominal symptoms of the irritable bowel syndrome.[4] The study concluded that "Peppermint oil in enteric-coated capsules appears to be an effective and safe preparation for symptomatic treatment of the irritable bowel syndrome." Many sufferers of the irritable bowel syndrome are told that it is a condition they will just have to live with. Before giving up hope, they should try enteric-coated peppermint oil. The recommended dosage for Peppermint Plus is one or two capsules between meals three times a day.

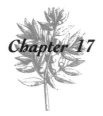

PEPTIC ULCER MEDICATIONS

An ulcer usually refers to a peptic ulcer. The most common locations for peptic ulcer formation are in the stomach (gastric ulcer) and the first portion of the small intestine (duodenal ulcer). Although duodenal and gastric ulcers occur at different locations, they appear to be the result of similar events. Specifically, the development of a duodenal or gastric ulcer is a result of the acidic secretions of the stomach damaging the lining of the duodenum or stomach.

The acid secreted by the stomach is strong enough to burn your skin and produce an ulcer. So how do the stomach and duodenum protect against ulcer formation? There are actually several important ways, including: the production of a mucus that lines the stomach and intestinal walls and protects against ulcer formation; the constant renewing of intestinal cells; and the secretion of substances that neutralize the acid when it comes in contact with the stomach and intestinal linings.

Under normal circumstances, there are enough protective factors to prevent ulcer formation. However, when there is a decrease in the integrity of these protective factors, an ulcer can occur. A loss of integrity can be a result of alcohol, drugs (particularly drugs used in arthritis), nutrient deficiency, stress, and many other factors.

Although symptoms of a peptic ulcer may be absent or quite vague, most peptic ulcers are associated with abdominal discomfort noted forty-five to sixty minutes after meals, or during the night. In a typical case, the pain is described as gnawing, burning, cramplike, or aching, or as "heartburn." Eating or using antacids usually results in great relief.

Individuals with any symptoms of a peptic ulcer need competent medical care. Peptic ulcer complications such as hemorrhage, perforation, and obstruction represent medical emergencies that require immediate hospitalization. Individuals with peptic ulcer should be monitored by a physician, even if following the natural approaches discussed below.

Common Peptic Ulcer Medications

Current medical treatment of peptic ulcers focuses on reducing gastric acidity with antacids and drugs that block stomach acid secretion. Though effective, these treatments can be expensive, carry some risk of toxicity, disrupt normal digestive processes, and alter the structure and function of the cells that line the digestive tract. The latter factor is just one of the reasons why peptic ulcers will develop again if medications are discontinued.

Antacids

Although antacids are widely used to relieve ulcer symptoms, their use dose pose certain risks. In fact, many popular antacids should not be used by individuals with peptic ulcers. The calcium carbonate antacids (Tums, Alka-2) actually produce a "rebound" effect on gastric acid secretion and may cause kidney stones, while the sodium bicarbonate antacids (Rolaids, Alka-Seltzer, Bromo-Seltzer) have a tendency to induce systemic alkalosis and interfere with heart and kidney function. The antacids typically used in the treatment of peptic ulcers are aluminum-magnesium compounds (Maalox, Mylanta, Digel), which may cause calcium and phosphorus depletion. They may also cause aluminum toxicity or the accumulation of aluminum in the brain. Antacids are more fully discussed in Chapter 5.

H2-receptor Antagonists

These drugs work to block the action of histamine on the secretion of stomach acid. Histamine normally acts on the acid-secreting cells of the stomach in a manner that results in the secretion of stomach acid. By blocking this effect of histamine, stomach acid output is greatly reduced, resulting in immediate relief in most instances. H2-receptor antagonists differ from the antihistamines used in allergy medications, which are

H1-receptor antagonists. Each drug class acts on a different type of histamine receptor.

Examples of H2-receptor antagonists include cimetidine (Tagamet), ranitidine (Zantac), famotidine (Pepcid), and nizatidine (Axid). These drugs are among the most popular and biggest-selling. In fact, Zantac is the biggest-selling drug in the history of the pharmaceutical industry. In 1992, its sales were over three billion dollars. Tagamet's 1992 sales were over one billion dollars.

There are two very good reasons why these drugs are such big moneymakers: (1) They are very expensive (typically, more than one hundred dollars per month); and (2) because they do not address the underlying cause, approximately 70 to 90 percent of patients who take H2-receptor antagonists and then discontinue them will have a relapse within a year.

The H2-receptor antagonists are good examples of why many people speculate that drug companies work together to reap big profits. Tagamet was introduced in 1977 and had a virtual lock on the antiulcer market until 1983, when Zantac was introduced. Citing improved tolerance and fewer side effects, Glaxo, the manufacturer, charged a premium for Zantac. Rather than lower the price for Tagamet in an attempt to compete against Zantac, Smith Kline, the manufacturer of Tagamet, actually increased its price. Since then, the price of both drugs has increased in a parallel fashion. When Merck and Eli Lilly entered this drug class with Pepcid (1986) and Axid (1988), respectively, they also charged a premium for their drugs rather than try to compete on the basis of price. The obvious question is: Do drug companies work together to raise prices rather than compete on a price basis? In my opinion, there is little doubt that the answer is yes.

Side effects: As a class, these drugs are associated with numerous side effects, but are for some reason generally regarded as safe. In fact, there is a big push by the manufacturers to make them available as over-the-counter drugs. However, this does not seem wise, as these drugs not only have side effects, but are associated with adverse interactions when combined with many other drugs.

Because H2-receptor antagonists block a vital bodily function involved in digestion, digestive disturbances are quite common and can include nausea, constipation, and diarrhea. Nutrient deficiencies may result because of impaired digestion. Other possible side effects include liver damage, allergic reactions, headaches, breast enlargement in men, hair loss, osteoporosis, dizziness, depression, insomnia, or impotence.

Bismuth Preparations

Recently a bacterium, *Helicobacter pylori* (HP for short), has been thought to play a role in the development of peptic ulcers.[1] Whether HP is a direct cause or simply a contributor to ulcer formation has not yet been determined. What is known is that HP can be found in 70 to 75 percent of gastric ulcers and 90 to 100 percent of duodenal ulcers. HP burrows itself into the junction between the intestinal cells and then secretes an enzyme that breaks down the mucus, which protects the intestinal lining. Indigestion, inflammation, and ulceration can follow.

Preliminary results indicate that killing HP may prove to be an effective treatment of peptic ulcers.[1] The most encouraging studies have utilized bismuth preparations. Bismuth is a naturally occurring mineral that can act as an antacid. The best-known and most widely used bismuth preparation is bismuth subsalicylate (Pepto-Bismol). However, bismuth subcitrate has produced the best results in peptic ulcers. Unfortunately, this form is currently not available in the United States.

Side effects: Bismuth is extremely safe when taken at prescribed dosages. It may cause a temporary and harmless darkening of the tongue and/or stool. Bismuth subsalicylate should not be taken by children recovering from the flu, chicken pox, or other viral infection, as it may mask the nausea and vomiting associated with Reye's syndrome, a rare but serious illness.

Dietary and Life-style Factors in Treating Peptic Ulcers

A healthful diet and life-style go a long way in preventing peptic ulcers. Important dietary and life-style factors to consider include dietary fiber, food allergies, smoking, alcohol intake, and stress.

FIBER

A diet rich in fiber is both preventive and therapeutic.[2] This effect is probably a result of fiber's ability to promote a healthy protective layer of mucin in the stomach and intestines as well as act as a buffering agent. Although several fibers (pectin, guar gum, psyllium) often used to supplement the diet have been shown to produce beneficial effects,[3,4] it is best simply to eat a diet rich in plant foods (see Chapter 22, "Designing a Healthful Diet").

FOOD ALLERGIES

Strange as it may seem, there is much evidence pointing to food allergy as a prime causative factor in peptic ulcers.[5] In addition, a diet eliminating food allergies has been used with great success in treating and preventing recurrent ulcers.[6] Food allergy may explain the high recurrence rate of peptic ulcers. If food allergy is the cause, the ulcer will continue to recur until the food has been eliminated from the diet.

It is ironic that many people with peptic ulcers soothe themselves by consuming milk, a highly allergenic food. Milk should be avoided on the basis of allergy alone. There is additional evidence suggesting that milk should be avoided in patients with peptic ulcers. Population studies show that higher milk consumption creates a greater likelihood of ulcers, as milk significantly increases stomach acid production.[7]

SMOKING

A factor strongly linked to peptic ulcers is smoking. Increased frequency, decreased response to peptic ulcer therapy, and an increased mortality due to peptic ulcer are all related to smoking. Three postulated mechanisms for this association are: decreased pancreatic bicarbonate secretion (an important neutralizer of gastric acid); increased reflux of bile salts into the stomach; and acceleration of gastric contents emptying into the duodenum.

Bile salts are extremely irritating to the stomach and initial portions of the duodenum, and bile salt reflux induced by smoking appears to be the most likely factor responsible for the increased peptic ulcer rate in smokers. The psychological aspects of smoking are also important, since the chronic anxiety and psychological stress associated with smoking appear to worsen ulcer activity.

STRESS AND EMOTIONAL FACTORS

While stress is widely believed to be an important factor in the development of peptic ulcers, this theory is not based on clinical evidence. In the medical literature, the role of stress in the development of peptic ulcer is controversial.

Although several studies have shown that the number of stressful life events is not significantly different in peptic ulcer patients as compared with carefully selected ulcer-free controls, this really doesn't hold much significance because it is not simply the amount of stress that is important to consider. What is more important is an individual's response to stress. Two people can experience the same stressful situation, yet handle it in completely different ways. Ulcer patients have been characterized as tending to repress emotions rather than express what they feel. Learning to deal with stress and to express emotion is critical to long-term health.

Natural Alternatives to Peptic Ulcer Medications

The natural approach to treating peptic ulcers is first to identify, and then eliminate or reduce all factors that can contribute to the development of peptic ulcers: food allergy, low-fiber diet, cigarette smoking, stress, alcohol consumption, and drugs (especially aspirin and other nonsteroidal anti-inflammatory drugs). Once the causative factors have been controlled or eliminated, the focus is directed at healing the ulcers and promoting tissue resistance.

Selected Nutrients
Numerous individual nutrients have been shown to be important to the health of the stomach and intestinal lining. Most important are vitamins A, C, and E, and zinc.[8] They have been shown to inhibit the development

of ulcers in laboratory animals, and several clinical studies have shown a positive therapeutic effect as well. Rather than take each of these nutrients separately, it may be best to simply take a good multiple vitamin-mineral preparation (see Chapter 24, "A Quick Guide to Nutritional Supplements").

Cabbage Juice

Cabbage juice was shown to be extremely effective in the treatment of peptic ulcers by Dr. Garnett Cheney at Stanford University's School of Medicine, as well as by other researchers in the 1950s.[9,10] Cheney believed that cabbage juice contained a substance he called "vitamin U" (the U stood for ulcer). Although this factor was never clearly identified, Cheney demonstrated that fresh cabbage juice is extremely effective in the treatment of peptic ulcers, usually within seven days. Here was one of Dr. Cheney's favorite juice recipe recommendations:

½ head or 2 cups of green cabbage
4 ribs of celery
2 carrots

Green cabbages are best, but red cabbages are also beneficial. Cut the cabbage into long wedges and feed through the juicer, followed by the celery and carrots.

DEGLYCYRRHIZINATED LICORICE (DGL)

A special licorice extract known as "deglycyrrhizinated licorice," or DGL for short, is a remarkable antiulcer agent.[11,12] DGL's mode of action is different from the current medications used for the treatment of peptic ulcers. Rather than inhibit the release of acid, licorice stimulates the normal defense mechanisms that prevent ulcer formation. Specifically, DGL improves both the quality and quantity of the protective substances that line the stomach and intestinal tract; increases the life span of the intestinal cell; and improves blood supply to the intestinal lining.

Numerous studies over the years have found DGL to be an effective antiulcer compound. In several head-to-head comparison studies, DGL has been shown to be more effective than Tagamet, Zantac, or antacids in both short-term treatment and maintenance therapy of peptic ulcers.[13,14] As noted earlier, while these drugs are associated with significant side effects, DGL is extremely safe and costs only a fraction of what the drugs cost. For example, while Tagamet and Zantac typically cost over a hundred dollars for a month's supply, DGL is available in health-food stores at fifteen dollars for a month's supply.

DGL in Gastric Ulcers

In a study of DGL in gastric ulcers, thirty-three gastric ulcer patients were treated with either DGL (760 milligrams, three times a day) or a placebo for one month.[15] There was a significantly greater reduction in ulcer size in the DGL group (78 percent) than in the placebo group (34 percent). Complete healing occurred in 44 percent of those receiving DGL, but in only 6 percent of the placebo group.

Gastric ulcers are often a result of the use of alcohol, aspirin or other nonsteroidal anti-inflammatory drugs, caffeine, and other factors that decrease the integrity of the gastric lining. As DGL has been shown to reduce the gastric bleeding caused by aspirin, DGL is strongly indicated for the prevention of gastric ulcers in patients requiring long-term treatment with ulcerogenic drugs, such as aspirin, nonsteroidal anti-inflammatory agents, and corticosteroids.[16]

DGL in Duodenal Ulcers

DGL is also effective in treating duodenal ulcers. In one study, forty patients with chronic duodenal ulcers of four to twelve years' duration and more than six relapses during the previous year were treated with DGL.[12] All of the patients had been referred for surgery because of relentless pain, sometimes with frequent vomiting, despite treatment with bed rest, antacids, and anticholinergic drugs. Half of the patients received 3 grams of DGL daily for eight weeks; the other half received 4.5 grams per day for sixteen weeks. All forty patients showed substantial improvement, usually within five to seven days, and none required surgery during the one year follow-up. Although both dosages were effective, the higher dose was significantly more effective than the lower dose.

In another, more recent study, the therapeutic effect of DGL was compared with that of antacids or cimetidine in 874 patients with confirmed chronic duodenal ulcers.[14] Ninety-one percent of all ulcers healed within twelve weeks; there was no significant difference in healing rate among the groups. However, there were fewer relapses in the DGL group (8.2 percent) than in those receiving cimetidine (12.9 percent) or antacids (16.4 percent). These results, coupled with DGL protective effects, suggest that DGL is a superior treatment for duodenal ulcers.

Dosage Instructions for DGL: In order to be effective in healing peptic ulcers, it appears that DGL must mix with saliva. DGL may promote the release of salivary compounds that stimulate the growth and regeneration of stomach and intestinal cells. The standard dose for DGL is two to four 380-milligram chewable tablets either between or twenty minutes before meals. Dosage should be continued for eight to sixteen weeks, depending on the response. DGL is available at health-food stores.

Final Comments

The natural approach to treating peptic ulcers is clearly superior to the current medical treatment, because it addresses the cause of most people's ulcers—a lack of factors that protect against ulcer development. Here are six concise recommendations that I give to my patients with ulcers:

1. Eliminate sugar and refined carbohydrates like white flour from your diet.
2. Eliminate milk and eggs.
3. Increase your consumption of whole grains, legumes, and vegetables.
4. Get a juicer and drink sixteen to twenty-four ounces of vegetable juice per day, including the regular consumption of cabbage juice.
5. Take a high-potency multiple vitamin-mineral formula with meals.
6. Take two tablets of DGL twenty minutes before meals.

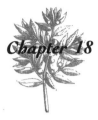

PROSTATE MEDICATIONS

The prostate is a single, doughnut-shaped gland about the size of a chestnut that lies below the male bladder and surrounds the urethra. The prostate secretes fluids that lubricate the urethra to prevent infection and to increase sperm motility. The prostatic secretions account for 30 percent of the volume of semen.

Enlargement of the prostate (benign prostatic hyperplasia, or BPH) is an extremely common condition that affects more than half of men over forty years of age in the United States. Because the enlarged prostate will pinch off the flow of urine, BPH is characterized by symptoms of bladder obstruction such as increased urinary frequency, nighttime awakening to empty bladder, and reduced force and caliber of urination.

Note: BPH can only be diagnosed by a physician. Do not self-diagnose. If you are experiencing any symptoms associated with BPH, see your physician immediately for proper diagnosis.

If left untreated, BPH will eventually obstruct the bladder outlet, resulting in the retention of urine in the blood (uremia). As this is a potentially life-threatening condition, proper treatment is crucial. In the past, medical treatment involved a procedure known as a TURP (transurethral resection of the prostate). Because this surgery is associated with complications and will often make matters worse, it should be avoided unless absolutely necessary.

Common Prostate Medication

Finesteride (Proscar) is currently the only approved drug in the treatment of BPH. It works by inhibiting the activity of an enzyme, 5-alpha-reductase, involved in male sex hormone (testosterone) metabolism. Finesteride blocks the transformation of testosterone to dihydrotestosterone, a very potent hormone derived from testosterone, within the prostate. Dihydrotestosterone is responsible for the overproduction of prostate cells, which ultimately results in prostatic enlargement.

Although Proscar has received much attention, based on the results of the clinical trials, it is much less effective than the extract of *Serenoa repens* (discussed below). Less than 50 percent of patients on Proscar will experience clinical improvement after taking the drug for one year, and it must be taken for at least six months before any improvement can be expected. Proscar costs about seventy-five dollars a month. Merck has predicted sales will soon reach one billion dollars annually. However, men with prostate enlargement would receive far better results from the natural alternatives discussed below.

Side effects: In general, finesteride appears to be well tolerated. Decreased libido, ejaculatory disorders, and impotence are the most common side effects reported, but occur in no more than 5 percent of patients. Finesteride may suppress the levels of prostatic-specific antigen, the marker for prostate cancer.

Dietary Factors in Treating BPH

Diet appears to play a critical role in preventing as well as treating BPH. It's particularly important to avoid pesticides, increase the intake of zinc and essential fatty acids, and keep cholesterol levels below 220 milligrams per deciliter.

AVOID PESTICIDES

In trying to treat or prevent BPH, the diet should be as free as possible from pesticides and other contaminants, since many of these compounds (dioxin, polyhalogenated biphenyls, hexachlorobenzene, dibenzofurans) can ultimately lead to BPH.[1] Synthetic hormones fed to animals to fatten them up before slaughter have been shown to produce changes in rat prostates similar to BPH.[1]

The tremendous increase in the occurrence of BPH in the last few decades may reflect the ever-increasing effect that toxic chemicals have on our health. BPH is perhaps just one of many health problems that may be due to these toxic substances. A diet rich in natural whole foods (preferably organically grown) may offer some protection due to the presence, in particular, of minerals (calcium, magnesium, zinc, selenium, germanium), vitamins, plant pigments (flavonoids, carotenes, chlorophyll), fiber (especially gel-forming and mucilaginous types), and sulfur-containing compounds, all of which have activity that helps the body deal with toxic chemicals and heavy metals.

ZINC AND ESSENTIAL FATTY ACIDS

Paramount to an effective BPH prevention and treatment plan is adequate zinc intake and absorption. Zinc supplementation has been shown to reduce the size of the prostate—as determined by rectal examination, X ray, and endoscopy—and to reduce symptoms in the majority of patients.[2] The clinical efficacy of zinc is probably due to its critical involvement in many aspects of hormonal metabolism.

Foods rich in zinc include nuts and seeds. These foods also provide an excellent source of essential fatty acids which, like zinc, have shown positive results in the treatment of BPH. In one study, the administration of a mixture of essential fatty acids to nineteen subjects with BPH showed a reduction in the amount of residual urine in the bladder.[3] In twelve of the nineteen, there was no residual urine by the end of several weeks of treatment. These effects appear to be due to the correction of an underlying essential fatty acid deficiency, since the prostatic and seminal lipid levels and ratios are often abnormal in persons with BPH.[4,5] Based on this evidence alone, increasing the intake of nuts and seeds or supplementation with zinc and/or essential fatty acids appears indicated.

An old folk remedy for BPH is to eat one-quarter to one-half cup of pumpkin seeds each day. This appears to be a very sound recommendation due to the high zinc and essential fatty acid content of pumpkin seeds. Flaxseed oil, sunflower oil, evening primrose oil, and soy oil are all appropriate vegetable oils to add to the diet to ensure the essential fatty acid requirement is being met. One tablespoon per day is usually a sufficient amount.

CHOLESTEROL

Breakdown products of cholesterol have been shown to accumulate in the prostate tissue affected with either BPH or cancer. These metabolites of cholesterol initiate degeneration of prostatic cells, which can promote prostatic enlargement. Drugs that lower cholesterol levels have been shown to have a favorable influence on BPH, preventing the accumulation of cholesterol in the prostatic cells and limiting subsequent formation of damaging cholesterol metabolites.[1] Every effort should be made to keep the total cholesterol level below 200 milligrams per deciliter.

AVOID BEER

It is important to avoid beer, as it has been linked to BPH. A suggested reason is that beer increases the release by the pituitary gland of the hormone prolactin.[6] Prolactin increases the uptake of testosterone and its conversion to dihydrotestosterone within the prostate. Drugs that reduce prolactin levels, like bromocryptine, reduce many of the symptoms of BPH. However, these drugs have severe side effects and are therefore not widely used. It appears that the trace mineral zinc and vitamin B_6 can reduce prolactin levels as well, yet produce no side effects at prescribed doses.[7,8]

Natural Alternatives to Prostate Medications

In many cases, the dietary recommendations above will bring about clinical improvement. If additional treatment is necessary, there are several natural products to choose from, but the best is the fat-soluble extract of saw palmetto berries.

Saw Palmetto Berry Extract

Saw palmetto (*Serenoa repens*) is a small scrubby palm tree native to the West Indies and the Atlantic Coast of North America from South Carolina to Florida. It bears berries that have a long history of use in folk medicine as an aphrodisiac and sexual rejuvenator. These berries have also been used for centuries in treating conditions of the prostate. In recent clinical studies, the therapeutic effect of the fat-soluble extract of saw palmetto berries has been shown to greatly improve the signs and symptoms of an enlarged prostate.[9-12] The purified fat-soluble extract is a well-defined medicinal plant extract containing between 85 and 95 percent fatty acids and sterols.

Like Proscar, the therapeutic effect of the saw palmetto extract appears to be due to its inhibition of dihydrotestosterone, the compound that causes prostate cells to multiply excessively. However, the saw palmetto extract goes well beyond Proscar in that it not only inhibits the formation of dihydrotestosterone, but also inhibits its binding at cellular binding sites. Since Proscar has no effect on blocking the binding of dihydrotestosterone, saw palmetto has much greater antagonizing effects on dihydrotestosterone in the prostate than does Proscar. These effects are translated into very positive clinical results.[13-25]

Table 18.1   Clinical Studies Demonstrating the Efficacy of Saw Palmetto (*Serenoa Repens*)* in BPH

Authors	Type of Study	# Patients	Length of Study	Results
Boccafoschi, et al.	Double-blind	22	60 days	Significant difference for: volume voided, maximum flow, mean flow, dysuria, nocturia

Authors	Type of Study	# Patients	Length of Study	Results
Cirillo, et al.	Open	47	4 months	Significant difference for: dysuria, nocturia, urine flow
Tripodi, et al.	Open	40	30–90 days	Significant difference for: dysuria, nocturia, volume of prostate, voiding rate, residual urine
Emili, et al.	Double-blind	30	30 days	Significant difference for: number of voidings, strangury, maximum and mean urine flow, residual urine
Greca, et al.	Open	14	1–2 months	Significant difference for: dysuria, perineal heaviness, nocturia, volume of urine per voiding, interval between two diurnal voidings, sensation of incomplete voiding
Duvia, et al.	Controlled trial vs Pygeum africanum	30	30 days	Significant difference for: voiding rate
Tasca, et al.	Double-blind	30	31–90 days	Significant difference for: frequency, urine flow measurement
Cukier, et al.	Double-blind	168	60–90 days	Significant difference for: dysuria, frequency, residual urine

Authors	Type of Study	# Patients	Length of Study	Results
Crimi, et al.	Open	32	4 weeks	Significant difference for: dysuria, nocturia, volume of prostate, voiding rate
Champault, et al.	Double-blind	110	28 days	Significant difference for: dysuria, nocturia, flow measurement, residual urine
Mattei, et al.	Double-blind	40	3 months	Significant difference for: dysuria, nocturia, residual urine

*dose = 320 milligrams per day

Saw Palmetto Versus Proscar

Numerous studies on the saw palmetto extract have shown it to be effective in nearly 90 percent of patients (see Table 18.1), usually in a period of four to six weeks. In contrast, Proscar is effective in reducing the symptoms in less than 50 percent of patients after taking the drug for one year. To illustrate saw palmetto extract's superiority over Proscar, let's look at the effect of both on the maximum urine flow rate, a good indicator of bladder neck obstruction due to an enlarged prostate. The following data are based on pooled information on saw palmetto extract from studies listed in Table 18.1 and pooled data on Proscar found in the *Physicians' Desk Reference*.

Table 18.2   Saw Palmetto Versus Proscar on Urine Flow Rate (milliliters per second)

	Saw Palmetto Extract	Proscar
Initial measurement	9.53 ml/sec	9.6 ml/sec
3 months	13.15 ml/sec*	10.4 ml/sec
12 months	**	11.2 ml/sec

	Saw Palmetto Extract	*Proscar*
% increase	38% in 3 months	16% in 12 months

*Many studies on the saw palmetto extract were less than 90 days; final measurements were calculated as 90-day measurements.

**There are no long-term studies on saw palmetto extract, yet the effect at 3 months (or less) is obviously superior to that of Proscar.

Clearly, the saw palmetto extract is superior to Proscar; it is also significantly less expensive, as it is at least one fourth the price compared with Proscar. Unfortunately, most men with BPH will never hear about the saw palmetto berry extract. Merck has the FDA to thank for that. Despite saw palmetto extract's clear superiority over Proscar, in 1990 the FDA rejected an application to have saw palmetto approved in the treatment of BPH. The result is that even though saw palmetto extract is more effective, less expensive, and much safer than Proscar, manufacturers and distributors of the extract cannot make any claims for their product. In Europe, *Serenoa repens* extracts are widely prescribed by physicians as medicines. In the United States, *Serenoa repens* extracts identical to those used in Europe are available in health-food stores as "food supplements," and no health claims can be made. As a result, very few men know about this natural alternative.

Dosage instructions for saw palmetto: The dosage of fat-soluble saw palmetto extract standardized to contain 85 to 95 percent fatty acids and sterols is 160 milligrams twice daily. If you want the best results, make sure you are using the right extract at the right dosage. Saw palmetto extract is completely safe—no significant side effects have ever been reported in the clinical trials of the extract or with saw palmetto berry ingestion. Detailed toxicology studies on the extract have been carried out on mice, rats, and dogs and indicate that the extract has no toxic effects.

Pygeum africanum

Pygeum africanum is a large evergreen tree native to Africa, where it has been used for a variety of health complaints. The purified fat-soluble extract of the bark of *Pygeum africanum* has demonstrated clinical efficacy similar to the extract of saw palmetto.[9,10,25] However, in a head-to-head comparison study, the saw palmetto extract exhibited greater efficacy and tolerability.[18] The mechanism of action of the pygeum extract is not as well defined as that of saw palmetto, but appears to work via its inhibition of cholesterol uptake by the prostate, antagonizing testosterone, and reducing prostatic inflammation. The standard dosage is 100 milligrams twice daily.

Flower Pollen

The flower pollen extract known as cernilton has been used to treat prostatitis and BPH in Europe for more than twenty-five years.[11] It has been shown to be quite effective in several double-blind clinical studies in the treatment of prostatitis due to inflammation or infection.[12,26] The extract has been shown to exert some anti-inflammatory action and produce a contractile effect on the bladder while simultaneously relaxing the urethra. Cernilton and similar products are available in health-food stores. They are perhaps better suited for prostatitis than BPH. The standard dosage for cernilton or similar products is two tablets of 500 milligrams each three times daily.

Amino Acids

The combination of glycine, alanine, and glutamic acid (in the form of two 360-milligram capsules administered three times daily for two weeks, and one capsule three times daily thereafter) has been shown in several studies to relieve many of the symptoms of BPH. In a controlled study of forty-five men, nighttime urination was relieved or reduced in 95 percent of the group, urgency reduced in 81 percent, frequency reduced in 73 percent, and delayed urination alleviated in 70 percent.[27]

These results have also been reported in other controlled studies.[28] The mechanism of action is unknown, but may be due to glycine's role as an inhibitory neurotransmitter in the central nervous system. Amino acid therapy is probably only palliative and not curative.

Final Comments

Benign prostatic hyperplasia represents a major medical problem in the United States. Prevention is the best measure. Six factors of critical importance in a prevention plan are:

1. Maintain an adequate zinc intake.
2. Maintain an adequate vitamin B_6 intake.
3. Eliminate or reduce the amount of beer and other alcohol consumed.
4. Maintain serum cholesterol below 200 milligrams per deciliter.
5. Establish an adequate intake of essential fatty acids by eating a handful of nuts or seeds each day or using flaxseed oil as a salad dressing.
6. Limit dietary and environmental exposure to pesticides and other environmental contaminants.

In addition to these general factors, if an individual is already experiencing symptoms of prostatic enlargement, he should take the following:

Zinc, 30 to 45 milligrams daily

Saw Palmetto (*Serenoa repens*) (liposterolic extract), 160 milligrams twice daily in extract standardized to contain 85 to 95 percent fatty acids and sterols

An additional recommendation is to take a hot sitz bath (a partial-immersion bath of the pelvic region). Although a sitz bath is more easily taken in a specially constructed tub, it may also be effective in a regular bathtub. Heat the water to 105 to 115 degrees Fahrenheit, and immerse the pelvis in the water for three to ten minutes, followed by cool sponging of the pelvic area. The primary effect of the sitz bath is relaxation and opening of the urinary passageway. Hot sitz baths are not indicated in cases of acute inflammation or infection of the prostate.

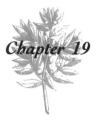

SEDATIVE MEDICATIONS

Over the course of a year, more than one half of the population of the United States will have difficulty falling asleep. About 33 percent of Americans experience insomnia on a regular basis. Many use over-the-counter sedative medications to combat insomnia, while others seek stronger drugs. Each year, up to ten million people in this country receive prescriptions for drugs to help them go to sleep.

Insomnia can have many causes, but the most common reasons are depression, anxiety, and tension. If psychological factors do not seem to be the cause, various foods, drinks, and medications may be responsible. There are numerous compounds in food and drink and well over three hundred drugs that can interfere with normal sleep.

Common Sedative Medications

The two primary classes of drugs used in the treatment of insomnia are antihistamines and benzodiazepines. Antihistamines are available in over-the-counter sleeping pills, contain either diphenhydramine or doxylamine, and act to prevent the manufacture of histamine in the brain. This produces drowsiness and sleep. Antihistamines are discussed in Chapter 7.

Table 19.1 Common Causes of Insomnia

Anxiety or tension
Depression
Environmental change
Emotional arousal
Fear of insomnia
Fear of sleep
Hypoglycemia
Disruptive environment
Pain or discomfort
Caffeine
Drugs
Alcohol

Table 19.2 Over-the-Counter Sedatives

Diphenhydramine	*Doxylamine*
Benadryl	Doxysom
Compoz	Ultra Sleep
Nervine	Unisom
Nytol	
Sleep-Eze 3	
Sleepinal	
Sominex	
Twilite	

Benzodiazepines

The benzodiazepine drugs such as triazolam (Halcion), diazepam (Valium), and chlordiazepoxide (Librium) have become the primary drugs prescribed for anxiety and insomnia. Other drugs in this category include: lorazepam (Ativan), prazepam (Centrax), flurazepam (Dalmane), clonazepam (Clonopin), halazepam (Paxipam), temazepam (Restoril), oxazepam (Serax), clorazepate (Tranxene), and alprazolam (Xanax).

The benzodiazepines act to induce sleep by enhancing the action of the nerve transmitter gamma-aminobutyric acid (GABA), which in turn blocks the arousal of brain centers. Benzodiazepines are not designed for long-term use, as they are addictive, associated with numerous side effects, and cause abnormal sleep patterns. The latter factor is responsible for the development of a vicious cycle. The patient takes the drug to induce sleep which, in turn, causes further disruption of normal sleep by suppressing REM (rapid eye movement) sleep. During REM sleep, the body is more physiologically active, meaning repair and rejuvenative processes take place during REM. We also dream during REM sleep. Because the patient does not experience adequate REM sleep while on a benzodiazepine, he or she will typically wake up with a "hangover" and often will feel more tired than when going to sleep. Patients may then turn to a stimulant, such as coffee, to get them going again. There is more. When a patient tries to withdraw from long-term use of benzodiazepines, REM sleep is increased, leading to nightmares and further sleep disturbances, among other withdrawal symptoms.

Benzodiazepines, especially Halcion, have been receiving a lot of negative attention in the media over the past few years. More people are "waking up" to the fact that these drugs can be quite dangerous if used more often than occasionally. But if you have taken a benzodiazepine for more than four weeks, do not suddenly stop taking the drug. It is important to work with your physician to taper off the drug gradually to avoid potentially dangerous withdrawal symptoms. Symptoms of withdrawal can include: anxiety, irritability, sensations of panic, insomnia, nausea, headache, impaired concentration, memory loss, depression, extreme sensitivity to the environment, seizures, hallucinations, and paranoia.

Side effects: Benzodiazepines can produce many side effects, such as dizziness, drowsiness, and impaired coordination, so it is important not to drive or engage in any potentially dangerous activity while on these drugs. Alcohol should never be consumed with benzodiazepines.

Benzodiazepines will often produce a morning "hangover" feeling. Other possible side effects include allergic reactions, headache, blurred vision, nausea, indigestion, diarrhea or constipation, and lethargy.

The most serious side effects of the benzodiazepines relate to their effects on memory and behavior. Because the drugs act on brain chemistry, significant changes in brain function and behavior can occur. Severe amnesia or memory impairment of events while on the drug, nervousness, confusion, hallucinations, bizarre behavior, and extreme irritability and aggressiveness may result. Benzodiazepines have also been shown to increase feelings of depression, including suicidal thinking.

Dietary and Life-style Factors in Treating Insomnia

There are several dietary and life-style factors to consider in relieving insomnia. They include eliminating the food and drink compounds that impair sleep processes, avoiding nocturnal hypoglycemia, learning to relax, and exercising. Each of these factors is discussed below.

ELIMINATING INHIBITORS OF SLEEP

It is essential that the diet be free of natural stimulants such as caffeine and related compounds. Coffee, as well as less obvious caffeine sources such as soft drinks, chocolate, coffee-flavored ice cream, hot cocoa, and tea must all be eliminated.

The sensitivity to the stimulant effects of caffeine is extremely variable from one person to the next.[1] What determines sensitivity to caffeine's stimulatory effects is largely a reflection of how quickly the body can eliminate caffeine. In other words, some people are more sensitive to the effects of caffeine than other people are, due to a slower elimination of these substances from the body. Even small amounts of caffeine, such as those found in decaffeinated coffee or chocolate, may be enough to cause insomnia in some people.

Another substance that must be eliminated is alcohol, which produces a number of effects that impair sleep. In addition to causing the release of adrenaline, alcohol impairs the transport of the amino acid tryptophan into the brain, where it is converted to serotonin, a natural sleep-promoting substance.

AVOIDING NOCTURNAL HYPOGLYCEMIA

Nocturnal hypoglycemia (low nighttime blood-glucose level) is an important cause of sleep-maintenance insomnia. When there is a drop in the blood glucose level, it causes the release of hormones like adrenaline, glucagon, cortisol, and growth hormone, which regulate glucose levels. These compounds stimulate the brain and are a natural signal that it is time to eat.

Many people in the United States suffer from faulty glucose metabolism, either hypoglycemia or diabetes, because of overeating refined carbohydrates. The dietary guidelines given in Chapter 13, "Diabetes Medications," as well as in Chapter 22, "Designing a Healthful Diet," are important to follow to prevent nocturnal hypoglycemia.

Good snacks to eat thirty to forty-five minutes before bedtime to keep blood sugar levels steady throughout the night are oatmeal and other whole grain cereals, whole grain breads and muffins, and other complex carbohydrates. These foods will not only help maintain proper blood sugar levels, they actually can help promote sleep by increasing the level of the natural sleep-promoting substance, serotonin, within the brain. Avoid snacks high in refined sugars at or near bedtime.

LEARNING TO RELAX

Many people never learn how to really relax. Although an individual may relax by simply sleeping, watching television, or reading a book, these activities may not produce a body response known as the "relaxation response." Relaxation techniques seek to counteract the results of stress by inducing its opposite reaction—relaxation.

The physiological effects of the relaxation response are opposite to those seen with stress. With the stress response, the sympathetic nervous system dominates. The sympathetic nervous system is designed to protect us against immediate danger and therefore keeps us awake and alert. With the relaxation response, the parasympathetic nervous system dominates. The parasympathetic nervous system controls bodily functions such as digestion, breathing, and heart rate during periods of rest, relaxation, visualization, meditation, and sleep.

One of the most popular techniques for turning on the parasympathetic nervous system and producing the relaxation response in the treatment of insomnia and anxiety is called progressive relaxation. The technique is based on a very simple procedure of comparing tension against relaxation. Many people are not aware of the sensation of relaxation. In progressive relaxation, an individual is educated on what it feels like to relax by comparing relaxation to muscle tension.

The individual will first be asked to contract a muscle forcefully for a period of one to two seconds and then give way to a feeling of relaxation. Since the procedure goes progressively through all the muscles of the body, eventually a deep state of relaxation results. The procedure begins by contracting the muscles of the face and neck, holding the contraction for a period of at least one to two seconds, and then relaxing those muscles. Next the upper arms, chest, and back are contracted, then relaxed, followed by the lower arms and hands. The process is repeated down the body, that is, the abdomen, the buttocks, the thighs, the calves, and the feet. In the treatment of insomnia, this whole practice is repeated two or three times or until it produces sleep.

EXERCISING

Regular physical exercise is known to improve general well-being as well as promote improvement in sleep quality. Exercise should be performed in the morning or early evening, not before bedtime, and should be of moderate intensity. Usually twenty minutes of aerobic exercise at a heart rate between 60 and 75 percent of maximum (the maximum pulse rate is approximately 220, minus age in years) is sufficient. See Chapter 23 for additional information on how to design an exercise program.

Natural Alternatives to Sedative Medications

Foremost in the natural approach to treating insomnia is the elimination of those factors known to disrupt normal sleep patterns, such as sources of caffeine, alcohol, and drugs. Since insomnia is largely due to psychological factors, these should be considered and handled before simply inducing sleep pharmacologically. Counseling and/or stress-reduction techniques such as progressive relaxation and exercise are often very effective. If these general measures produce no improvement, there are several natural alternatives to sedative medications that can be used, but the best available is the use of the herb valerian. Once a normal sleep pattern has been established, valerian use should be slowly decreased.

Valerian

Valerian (*Valeriana officinalis*) has been widely used in folk medicine as a sedative. Recent scientific studies have substantiated valerian's ability to improve sleep quality and relieve insomnia.[2,3,4] In a large double-blind study involving 128 subjects, it was shown that an aqueous extract of valerian root improved the subjective ratings for sleep quality and sleep latency (the time required to get to sleep), but left no "hangover" the next morning.[2]

In a follow-up study, valerian extract was shown to reduce sleep latency significantly, and improve sleep quality in sufferers of insomnia under laboratory conditions. Valerian was suggested to be as effective in reducing sleep latency as small doses of benzodiazepines.[3] The difference, however, arises in the fact that synthetic compounds also result in increased morning sleepiness. Valerian on the other hand, actually reduces morning sleepiness.

As a mild sedative, valerian may be taken in the following doses thirty to forty-five minutes before bedtime:

Dried root (or as tea), 1 to 2 grams

Tincture (1:5), 4 to 6 milligrams (1 to 1.5 teaspoons)

Fluid extract (1:1), 1 to 2 milligrams (0.5 to 1 teaspoon)

Valerian extract (0.8 percent valeric acid), 150 to 300 milligrams

If morning sleepiness does occur, reduce dosage. If dosage was not effective, be sure to eliminate those factors that disrupt sleep, such as caffeine and alcohol, before increasing dosage.

Tryptophan

Since the synthesis of serotonin within the brain is dependent on the availability of the amino acid tryptophan, supplementing the diet with tryptophan produces very good results in relieving insomnia. Tryptophan administration at a dose of 1 to 3 grams has been shown to reduce the time required to go to sleep as well to as decrease awakenings in numerous double-blind clinical studies.[5,6,7]

Unfortunately, at the time of this writing, tryptophan is no longer available to American consumers. For several decades, L-tryptophan was used by hundreds of thousands of people in the United States safely and effectively for insomnia and depression. But in October 1989, some people taking tryptophan started reporting strange symptoms to physicians—severe muscle and joint pain, high fever, weakness, swelling of the arms and legs, and shortness of breath. The syndrome was dubbed EMS (eosinophilia-myalgia syndrome). This led to the removal of all products containing more than 100 milligrams of L-tryptophan from the market on November 17, 1989. As of May 1992, the number of reported EMS cases was 1,541, including 38 deaths.

All cases of tryptophan-induced EMS could be traced to one manufacturer, Showa Denko. Of the six Japanese companies that supplied tryptophan to the United States, Showa Denko was the largest in that it supplied 50 to 60 percent of all the tryptophan being used in this country. Due to a change in manufacturing procedures, the tryptophan produced by Showa Denko from October 1988 to June 1989 became contaminated with a substance now linked to EMS.[8]

Tryptophan has remained off the market despite the fact that, before the Showa Denko incident, it had been used safely for decades. There are numerous examples of contaminated foods and medicines causing health problems and even death. Yet in most industries, once the problem of contamination is solved, manufacturers are again allowed to market their products, whether contaminated grapes, Perrier, or hamburgers from Jack in the Box. But, for some reason, tryptophan has not been allowed back on the marketplace, even though the contamination issue is resolved. We can hope that tryptophan will become available again in the very near future. It is interesting to note that one of the best treatments of EMS is noncontaminated tryptophan.[9]

Final Comments

The restless-legs syndrome is another significant cause of insomnia. This syndrome is characterized by an irresistible urge to move the legs while trying to sleep and while awake. Although the restless-legs syndrome is most often found in people consuming too much caffeine, some patients with restless-legs syndrome respond well to extremely high doses of folic acid (35 to 60 milligrams daily).[10] This syndrome is believed to be a result of a folic acid deficiency or perhaps an increased need for folic acid in some individuals.

Almost all patients with restless-legs syndrome have nocturnal myoclonus, a nerve and muscle disorder characterized by repeated contractions of one or more muscle groups, typically of the leg, during sleep. Each muscle jerk usually lasts less than ten seconds. The person with nocturnal myoclonus is normally unaware of the disorder and only complains of either frequent nocturnal awakenings or excessive daytime sleepiness. But questioning the sleep partner often reveals the myoclonus. Vitamin E has been used successfully in nocturnal myoclonus. Take at least 400 IUs per day.

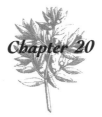

Chapter 20

WEIGHT-LOSS AIDS

Weight loss is perhaps the most challenging health goal for many Americans. Few people want to be overweight, yet only 5 percent of people who need to lose twenty pounds or more and only 66 percent of people just a few pounds overweight are able to attain and maintain "normal" body weight.

Dieters are constantly bombarded with new reports of "wonder" diets to follow. There are literally hundreds of diets, diet programs, and weight-loss aids that claim to be the answer to the problem of obesity. The basic equation for losing weight never changes. In order for an individual to lose weight, caloric intake must be less than the amount of calories burned. The most sensible approach to weight loss is to decrease caloric intake and increase exercise simultaneously.

Common Weight-Loss Aids

The only approved substances available without a prescription as weight-loss aids are phenylpropanolamine (PPA) and benzocaine. While prescription amphetamines can also promote weight loss, these effects are only short-lived, as the body develops a tolerance to such drugs. Furthermore, because amphetamines have a tremendous potential for abuse, dependence, and side effects, they are rarely prescribed for weight loss anymore.

Phenylpropanolamine (PPA)

PPA is an amphetaminelike substance with milder stimulant effects. PPA is thought to promote weight loss by reducing the appetite, but this effect is debatable. The American Medical Association's Drug Evaluations states that PPA-containing products are only "minimally effective," and many standard pharmacology texts state that PPA is ineffective as an appetite suppressant.

How PPA was ever approved as a weight-loss aid has been the subject of much interest. The FDA Advisory Review Panel admitted that the studies they used as a basis for their decision were flawed— and they were also unpublished. The panel's approval of PPA has been severely criticized by many medical experts who feel that the use of PPA poses a danger to the public. While the panel recommended a daily dosage of 150 milligrams, the maximum dosage that the FDA would sanction was 75 milligrams.

Side effects: Side effects with PPA are common, especially if the recommended dosage is exceeded. Nervousness, restlessness, insomnia, headache, nausea, and elevations of blood pressure are some of PPA's adverse effects. People taking PPA should monitor their blood pressure, as PPA can produce severe elevations, even in people with normal blood pressure. People with high blood pressure, diabetes, thyroid disease, and depression should not take PPA unless under the supervision of a physician.

Benzocaine

Benzocaine is a widely used anesthetic that is incorporated into chewing gum, lozenge, or candy as a weight-loss aid. Benzocaine acts to reduce appetite by numbing the taste receptors on the tongue. Since one of the reasons we eat is because we like the taste of food, the belief is that chewing gum or eating candy containing benzocaine will lead to less food consumption. Although this sounds reasonable, benzocaine as an appetite suppressant has even less scientific support than PPA.

Side effects: Benzocaine is generally regarded as safe. Although side effects have been reported, they are rare. Fatal allergic reactions have occurred, suggesting that long-term use should be avoided.

Dietary and Life-style Factors in Weight-Loss Success

Successful permanent weight loss must incorporate a healthful diet, adequate exercise, and a positive mental attitude. All the components are critical and interrelated; no single component is more important than another. Improvement in one facet may be enough to result in some positive changes, but impacting all three yields the best results.

The ultimate goal for anyone trying to lose weight is to retrain one's attitude and body into accepting a lower body weight. Research has found that each person has a natural "set point" weight that is determined primarily by the size or amount of fat stored in the individual fat cells throughout the body. The set point is a problem when trying to lose weight because, when the fat cell becomes smaller, it sends a message to the brain to eat. Since the obese individual often has both more and larger fat cells, the result is an overpowering urge to eat.

Most diets don't work because the obese individual can only fight off the impulse to eat for a time, and eventually, the signal becomes too strong to ignore. The result is rebound overeating, with individuals often exceeding their previous weight. In addition, their set point is now set at a higher level, making it even more difficult to lose weight. This is known as the "yo-yo" or "ratchet" effect.

The set point seems to be tied to the sensitivity of fat cells to the hormone insulin. Insulin is a hormone that is secreted by the pancreas. Its primary function is to help regulate blood sugar levels by promoting the uptake of blood glucose by cells of the body. Obesity leads to insulin insensitivity and vice versa. When cells become insensitive to insulin, blood sugar reaches higher than normal levels and may ultimately lead to diabetes.

The key to overcoming the fat cell's set point appears to be increasing the sensitivity of the fat cells to insulin. The set-point theory suggests that a weight-loss plan that does not improve insulin sensitivity will most likely fail to provide long-term results. Fortunately, insulin sensitivity can be improved and the set point lowered through exercise and diet.

INCREASING SELF-ESTEEM

The first step in a successful weight-loss program is to employ measures to increase self-esteem, to which, typically, the obese individual has experienced much psychological trauma. Fashion trends, insurance programs, college placements, employment opportunities—all discriminate against the obese person. Consequently, obese people learn many self-defeating and self-degrading attitudes. They are led to believe that fat is "bad," which often results in a vicious cycle of low self-esteem, depression, overeating for consolation, increased fatness, social rejection, and further lowering of self-esteem. Counseling is often necessary to change attitudes about being obese and to aid in the improvement of self-esteem. If this problem is not dealt with, even the most perfect diet and exercise plan will fail. Improving the way overweight people feel about themselves assists them in changing their eating behaviors.

Increasing self-esteem and promoting a positive mental attitude are critical factors in a successful weight-loss program. In order to achieve these goals, it is necessary to exercise or condition the attitude in a way that is similar to the conditioning of the body. Chapter 21, "Developing a Positive Mental Attitude," contains exercises designed to help people achieve the kind of permanent weight-loss results they really want.

DIET AND WEIGHT LOSS

In order to lose one pound of fat by diet alone in one week, an individual needs to have a negative caloric intake of 500 calories per day or 3,500 calories per week. To lose two pounds of fat each week, there must be a negative caloric balance of 1,000 calories a day. This can be achieved by decreasing the amount of calories ingested and/or by exercise. To reduce one's caloric intake by 1,000 calories is often difficult, as is burning an additional 1,000 calories per day by exercise (a person would need to jog for ninety minutes, play tennis for two hours, or take a brisk walk for two and a half hours). The most sensible approach to weight loss is to decrease caloric intake *and* to increase exercise. The figure and tables in Chapter 22, "Designing a Healthful Diet," can help you determine your ideal body weight and caloric needs, as well as provide guidelines to construct a healthful diet.

Perhaps the most important recommendation for individuals trying to lose weight is to eat more. That's right, eat more. One of the biggest mistakes people make when trying to lose weight is trying to starve themselves to achieve their goal. It is critical to provide the body with the high-quality nutrition it needs during weight loss. If the body is not fed, it feels that it is starving. The result: metabolism will slow down, and less fat will be burned. It is clear that you must eat to lose weight. But instead of choosing high-calorie foods, you must eat high-fiber, low-calorie foods. These foods can reset the set point and help you achieve long-term, permanent results. Here are ten weight-loss tips that really work.

1. Avoid snacking. Eat regular, planned meals. If you feel a need for a snack, drink a glass of fresh vegetable juice, eat a piece of fruit, have a salad, or eat carrot or celery sticks.

2. Reduce intake of fatty foods, spreads, salad dressings, butter, and other sources of fats. Keep fat intake to a minimum.

3. At lunch and dinner, eat large quantities of fresh vegetables and salads to fill you up.

4. Eat high-fiber whole grain breads and cereals instead of white bread and refined cereals.

5. Eliminate high-calorie desserts and sweets by substituting fresh fruits.

6. Avoid alcohol and soft drinks.

7. Drink a glass of fresh fruit juice thirty to forty-five minutes before your main meal. The fructose (fruit sugar) in the fresh juice will dampen your appetite, resulting in fewer calories being consumed.

8. When eating out, choose restaurants that offer lowfat choices. Avoid fast-food restaurants.

9. Learn to eat slowly. Enjoy your meals; allow your body time to realize it has been fed.

10. Avoid eating late at night, as the calories tend to be stored rather than burned for energy.

EXERCISE AND OBESITY

Physical inactivity may be the major cause of obesity in the United States. Childhood obesity seems to be associated more with inactivity than overeating, and strong evidence suggests that 80 to 86 percent of adult obesity begins in childhood. In the adult population, obese adults are less active than their leaner counterparts. Regular exercise is a necessary component of a weight-loss program due to the following factors:

1. When weight loss is achieved by dieting without exercise, a substantial portion of the total weight loss comes from the lean tissue—primarily as water loss.

2. When exercise is included in a weight-loss program, there is usually an improvement in body composition, due to a gain in lean body weight because of an increase in muscle mass and a decrease in body fat.

3. Exercise helps counter the reduction in basal metabolic rate (BMR) that usually accompanies dieting alone.

4. Exercise increases the BMR for an extended period of time following the exercise session.

5. Moderate to intense exercise allows your body to eat more healthful portions without overeating.

6. Those who exercise during and after weight reduction are better able to maintain the weight loss than those who do not.

Guidelines for designing an exercise program are given in Chapter 23, "The Importance of Exercise."

Natural Alternatives to Weight-Loss Aids

There are no "magic bullets" that will melt away fat, but there are some natural substances that can help. The most effective natural weight-loss aids are fiber supplements and so-called thermogenic formulas, which contain herbs to speed up fat metabolism.

FIBER SUPPLEMENTS

A fiber-deficient diet is an important factor in the development of obesity. Dietary fiber plays a role in preventing obesity by: (1) slowing the eating process; (2) increasing excretion of calories in the feces; (3) improving glucose tolerance; and (4) suppressing the appetite by stimulating release of appetite-suppressing hormones like cholecystokinin and its intestinal bulking action.

Perhaps the prime effects of fiber on obesity are related to improving glucose metabolism. Blood sugar problems (hypoglycemia and diabetes) appear to be one of the problems most clearly related to inadequate dietary fiber intake.[1] Numerous clinical trials have demonstrated the beneficial effects on blood sugar control of supplementing the diet with fiber (see Chapter 13, "Diabetes Medications"). These data suggest that in addition to eating a high-fiber diet, supplementing the diet with more fiber may provide increased benefit in weight loss as well.

Fiber has been shown to reduce feelings of hunger and consequently reduce the intake of food.[1,2] Several clinical trials have demonstrated that a daily supplement of 5 grams of fiber is of great value in the treatment of obesity.[3,4,5] Fiber's main action appears to be reducing caloric consumption by increasing the feeling of fullness and decreasing the feeling of hunger.

The best fiber sources are psyllium, guar gum, glucomannan, gum karaya, and pectin, because they are rich in water-soluble fibers. Be sure to drink adequate amounts of water when taking any fiber supplement, especially if it is in tablet form. If you have a disorder of the esophagus, do not take fiber supplements in pill form, as they may expand in the esophagus and lead to blockage of the esophagus, a very serious disorder.[6]

THERMOGENIC FORMULAS

Have you ever wondered why some people can eat all the food they want and still stay thin, while other people seem to put on weight easily? The common answer is that it comes down to metabolism. Many individuals are predisposed to obesity because they have a very efficient ability to lay down fat in tissue, while others have a very efficient ability to burn fat.

A certain amount of the food we consume is converted immediately to heat. This process is known as diet-induced thermogenesis (heat production). The activity of diet-induced thermogenesis is what determines whether an individual is likely to be obese. In lean individuals, a meal may stimulate up to a 40-percent increase in heat production. In contrast, obese individuals often display only a 10-percent or less increase in heat production. The food energy is stored rather than converted to heat.

The reason for the decreased thermogenesis in obese individuals is impaired sympathetic nervous system activity. This portion of the nervous system controls many body functions, including metabolism. In other words, the reason why many obese individuals have a "slow metabolism" is that there is a lack of stimulation by the sympathetic nervous system. Several plant stimulants can activate the sympathetic nervous system, thereby increasing the metabolic rate and thermogenesis. By addressing the underlying defect in metabolism, weight loss is the result.

Plant Stimulants

Various plants have a long history of use by the majority of cultures worldwide to increase energy levels and help cope with rough environments. Although many stimulants, like coffee, are routinely abused in our current society, natural stimulants offer significant benefit if used when indicated at an appropriate level. Weight loss is a prime example of proper indication for use.

In addition to individual plant compounds exhibiting stimulatory effects, combinations of herbs have been shown to accentuate each individual plant's action. Another way of saying this: The plants exert synergistic effects (1 + 1 = 3). For example, the weight-loss-promoting action of ephedrine is amplified considerably by caffeine-containing herbs like green tea (*Camellia sinensis*) or cola nut (*Cola nitida*), as well as coffee.

Ephedrine and Caffeine Combinations in Weight Loss

Ephedrine has been shown to promote weight loss in experimental and clinical studies.[7,8] It appears to promote weight loss primarily by increasing the metabolic rate of fat tissue and decreasing appetite. In other words, ephedrine simultaneously speeds up metabolism and reduces caloric intake. Its action, however, can be greatly enhanced when it is used in combination with caffeine.

The potentiating effect of caffeine on ephedrine's action has been observed in numerous weight-loss studies in animals and humans. For example, in one animal study, when ephedrine was used alone it resulted in losses of 14 percent in body weight and 42 percent in body fat. However, when it was used in combination with caffeine or theophylline, there was a loss of 25 percent in body weight and 75 percent in body fat.[9] In contrast, when either caffeine or theophylline was used alone, there was no significant loss in body weight. The reason for the decrease in body weight is an increased metabolic rate and fat-cell breakdown promoted by ephedrine and enhanced by caffeine and theophylline.

Studies on human subjects have also demonstrated that ephedrine combined with caffeine and theophylline is at least twice as effective as ephedrine alone in increasing the metabolic rate of the obese individual.[10,11] Significant weight loss can result when such combinations are used, because the mixture effectively normalizes the impaired thermogenic response to food in obese subjects and raises overall metabolic rate by an average of nearly 10 percent.

Plant stimulants are not for everyone. However, they do appear to be quite useful in weight-loss programs. The dosage used in the human studies of the plant stimulants in their purified form was 22 milligrams ephedrine and 80 milligrams caffeine per day. As a point of reference, a cup of coffee typically has 150 milligrams of caffeine and would produce about the same degree of stimulant effect. However, the stimulant effect is not what is the most important in weight loss. Ultimately, the most important aspect is the effect on the fat cells.

In order to produce the desired weight-loss benefit, herbal products containing ephedrine and caffeine must contain properly combined formulas. Using herbal extracts standardized for their stimulant levels may offer additional benefits over herbal products or stimulant-containing beverages, which do not specify the level of ephedrine or caffeine. Although these latter forms may produce a stimulant effect, in terms of promoting weight loss through thermogenesis, it is best to use well-defined formulas. These formulas ensure the proper ratio of ephedrine to caffeine. This ratio, as well as the amounts of its components, is critical to the overall effectiveness of the product. The dosage of the particular formula used should be consistent with the clinical studies on the pure compounds. In other words, calculate the dosage of the herbal product necessary to provide 22 milligrams of ephedrine and 80 milligrams of caffeine per day.

Even though the dosage of the stimulants required for increasing thermogenesis is relatively low, some people are more sensitive to the effects of caffeine and ephedrine than other people, due to a slower elimination of these substances from the body.[12] It is best to take the product early in the day and eliminate all other sources of stimulants (for example, coffee, black tea, colas) while taking a thermogenic aid. If you have high blood pressure, heart disease, or are using antidepressant medication, you must consult with your doctor before taking a thermogenic formula that contains ephedrine.

Final Comments

Permanent results require permanent changes in choosing what foods to eat and when to eat them. Nonetheless, some people find that meal-replacement formulas can be used effectively to achieve ideal body weight. Meal-replacement formulas are mixed with water, juice, or milk to produce a drink that is then used to replace a meal. While these formulas can provide short-term benefit, in the long run, a successful program must incorporate healthier food choices. There are numerous meal-replacement formulas on the market. Here are five guidelines for choosing a healthful version:

1. Look for a product that contains high-quality protein from grains and legumes, whey, or hydrolyzed lactalbumin. Avoid casein-based formulas. Casein, a milk protein, is often difficult for people to digest. Many people are allergic to it, and it has been shown to raise blood cholesterol levels. Casein is used not only in many meal-replacement formulas—it is also used in glues, molded plastics, and paints.

2. The formula should contain at least 5 grams of a combination of soluble and insoluble dietary fibers per serving.

3. Look for balanced high-quality nutrition with enhanced levels of nutrients critical to weight loss, such as chromium.

4. The formula should have a low total fat content, but supply some essential fatty acids.

5. The formula should not contain sweeteners, artificial flavors, or other artificial food additives. Refined sugar leads to loss of blood sugar control, diabetes, and obesity. Sucrose (white table sugar) is often the first ingredient of many meal-replacement formulas.

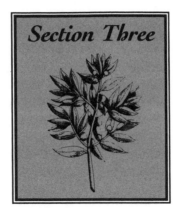

Section Three

Staying Healthy

Health is a term that is difficult to define; a definition somehow tends to place unnecessary boundaries on its meaning. The World Health Organization defines health as "a state of complete physical, mental, and social well-being, not merely the absence of disease or infirmity." This definition provides a positive range of health well beyond the absence of sickness.

The presence of health or disease often comes down to individual responsibility. In this context, responsibility means choosing a healthful alternative over a less healthful one. If you want to be healthy, simply make healthful choices.

Many of our health practices and life-style factors are based on both habit and marketing hype. The health practices and life-style of our parents usually become intricately woven into the fabric of our own life-styles. Meanwhile, a great deal of time, energy, and money is spent on trying to influence diet and life-style choices. There is a constant bombardment in the mass media of fast-food restaurant commercials, cigarette advertisements, sporting events sponsored by beer companies, and other messages that seek to influence our lives.

The first step in achieving and maintaining health is taking personal responsibility. The second step is taking the appropriate action to achieve the results you desire.

Achieving and maintaining good health is usually quite easy if an individual follows the basic principles: positive mental attitude, a healthful diet, and exercise. The importance of these three essential components of a healthful life-style is discussed in this section. Along with another category, supplemental measures, they provide guidelines for attaining good health.

Trying to "sell" people on health is often difficult. In order to be healthy, one needs commitment. The reward is not easily seen or felt. It is usually not until the body fails us in some manner that we realize we haven't taken care of it. Ralph Waldo Emerson said, "The first wealth is health."

The reward for most people who maintain a positive mental attitude, eat a healthful diet, and exercise regularly is a healthy life filled with very high levels of energy, joy, vitality, and a tremendous passion for living.

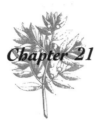

Chapter 21

BUILDING A POSITIVE
MENTAL ATTITUDE

More and more evidence is accumulating demonstrating that what we think and feel has a tremendous effect on the way our body functions. The most important factor in maintaining or attaining good health is a consistent positive mental attitude. Researchers in the medical and psychological fields are concluding that our level of optimism is a major determining factor in our level of wellness. Optimists view the misfortunes of life as temporary setbacks, challenges, or opportunities for growth. Research shows optimists are healthier and may even live longer than pessimists.[1,2]

According to Martin Seligman, Ph.D., a leading authority on optimism, we are, by nature, optimists, and optimism is a necessary step toward achieving our goals in life.[3] The first step in building an optimistic or positive mental attitude is taking personal responsibility for your own positive mental state, your life, your current situation, and your health. The next step is taking action to make the changes you desire.

Conditioning Your Attitude

In order to achieve a positive attitude or high self-esteem, you need to exercise or condition your attitude in a manner similar to the way you condition your body. I have developed an exercise designed to help you achieve the kind of permanent results you really want by conditioning you for success. You will need to get a notebook, which will become your personal journal. A journal is a powerful tool to help you stay in touch with your feelings, thoughts, and emotions. This exercise, designed to help you learn how to adopt healthier attitudes, will provide the foundation. Your daily personal journal will build upon this foundation.

EXERCISE ONE—CREATING A POSITIVE GOAL STATEMENT

Learning to set goals in a way that results in a positive experience is critical to your success. The following guidelines can be used to set any goal, including your desired weight. You can use goal-setting to create a "success cycle." Achieving goals helps you feel better about yourself and the better you feel, the more likely you will be to achieve your goals.

- In your notebook, state your goal in positive terms; do not use any negative words in your goal statement. For example, it is better to say and write, "I enjoy eating heathful, low-calorie, nutritious foods," rather than "I will not eat sugar, candy, ice cream, and other fattening foods."

- Make your goal attainable and realistic. Again, goals can be used to create a success cycle and positive self-image. Little things add up to make a major difference in the way you feel about yourself.

- Be specific. The more clearly your goal is defined, the more likely you are to reach it. For example, if you want to lose weight, what is the weight you desire? What are the measurements or body fat percentage you desire?

- State your goal in present tense, not future tense. In order to reach your goal, you have to believe you have already attained it. "You'll see it when you believe it." You must program yourself to achieve the goal. See and feel yourself having already achieved the goal.

Goal Statement

Use the guidelines above to construct a positive goal statement. Example: "My body is strong and beautiful. I have 23-percent body fat and I weigh 125 pounds. I feel good about myself and my body. I am

losing two pounds a week by making healthful food choices, and I feel
fantastic!!"

Short-term Goals

Any voyage begins with one step and is followed by many other steps.
Short-term goals can be used to help you achieve those long-term results
described in your positive goal statement. Get in the habit of asking
yourself the following question each morning and evening: What must
I do today to achieve my long-term goal?

Final Comments

For most people, a positive attitude doesn't happen all at once. It
happens by degrees, subtle changes accumulating one by one. Would
you be in good physical condition if you only exercised once? It takes
conditioning. The same is true for your attitude.

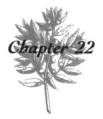

Chapter 22

DESIGNING A
HEALTHFUL DIET

There is little debate that a healthful diet must be rich in whole "natural" and unprocessed foods. Of particular importance are plant foods, such as fruits, vegetables, grains, beans, seeds, and nuts. These foods contain not only valuable nutrients, but also dietary fiber and other food compounds that have remarkable health-promoting properties. A diet rich in plant foods offers significant protection against the development of chronic degenerative conditions like heart disease, cancer, diabetes, strokes, and arthritis.[1,2,3]

The Government and Nutrition Education

Throughout the years, various governmental organizations have published dietary guidelines, but it has been the recommendations of the United States Department of Agriculture (USDA) that have become the most widely known. In 1956, the USDA published "Food for Fitness—A Daily Food Guide." This became popularly known as the Basic Four Food Groups:

1. The Milk Group included milk, cheese, ice cream, and other milk-based foods.
2. The Meat Group included meat, fish, poultry, and eggs, with dried legumes and nuts as alternatives.

3. The Fruit and Vegetable Group included all varieties.

4. The Breads and Cereals Group included all varieties.

One of the major problems with the Basic Four Food Groups model was that it graphically suggested that the food groups were equal in health value. The result has been overconsumption of animal products, dietary fat, refined carbohydrates—and insufficient consumption of fiber-rich foods like fruits, vegetables, and legumes. Following such a diet has caused many premature deaths, chronic diseases, and increased health-care costs. According to a recent U.S. Surgeon General's Report on Nutrition and Health, diet-related diseases account for 68 percent of all deaths in this country.

Table 22.1   Diseases Associated with a Diet Low in Plant Foods

Metabolic: Obesity, diabetes, kidney stones, gallstones, gout
Cardiovascular: Hypertension, cerebrovascular disease, ischemic heart disease, varicose veins, deep-vein thrombosis, pulmonary embolism
Gastrointestinal: Constipation, appendicitis, diverticulitis, diverticulosis, hemorrhoids, colon cancer, irritable bowel syndrome, ulcerative colitis, Crohn's disease
Other: Dental caries, autoimmune disorders, multiple sclerosis, thyrotoxicosis, many skin conditions

In an attempt to create a new model in nutrition education, the USDA developed the "Eating Right Food Pyramid." (See page 248). The pyramid has not changed the food groups per se. Instead, it stresses the importance of making fresh fruits, vegetables, and whole grains the basis of a healthful diet by placing them at the widest parts of the pyramid structure.

How to Design a Healthful Diet

Most people give very little thought to the design of their diet. They are motivated to eat foods based on sensual needs rather than on what their body

Figure 22.1   Eating Right Food Pyramid

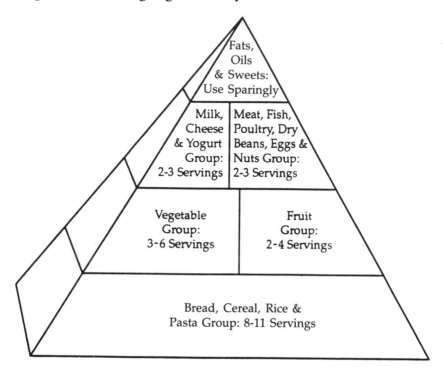

requires. Health is largely a conscious decision. Awareness of what to eat, in what quantities, and of healthful ways to prepare food is critical.

The American Dietetic Association (ADA), in conjunction with the American Diabetes Association and other groups, has developed the Exchange System, a convenient tool for the rapid estimation of the calorie, protein, fat, and carbohydrate content of a diet. Originally created for use in designing dietary recommendations for diabetics, the exchange method is now used in the calculation and design of virtually all therapeutic diets. Unfortunately, the ADA exchange plan does not place a strong enough focus on the quality of food choices.

The Healthy Exchange System presented here is a more beneficial version, because it emphasizes healthier food choices and focuses on unprocessed, whole foods. The diet is prescribed by allotting the number of exchanges (servings) allowed per food group for one day. There are seven exchange groups (lists); however, the milk and meat lists should be considered optional.

THE HEALTHY EXCHANGE SYSTEM

List 1—vegetables
List 2—fruits
List 3—breads, cereals, and starchy vegetables
List 4—legumes (beans)
List 5—fats, oils, nuts, and seeds
List 6—milk
List 7—meats, fish, cheese, and eggs

Because all food portions within each exchange list provide approximately the same calories, proteins, fats, and carbohydrates per serving, it is easy to construct a diet with the following components:

Carbohydrates: 65 to 75 percent of total calories
Fats: 15 to 25 percent of total calories
Protein: 10 to 15 percent of total calories
Dietary fiber: at least 50 grams

Of the carbohydrates ingested, 90 percent should be complex carbohydrates or naturally occurring sugars. Refined carbohydrate and concentrated sugars (including honey, pasteurized fruit juices, and dried fruit, as well as sugar and white flour) should be limited to less than 10 percent of the total calorie intake.

Constructing a diet that meets these recommendations is simple when using the exchange lists. In addition, the recommendations ensure a high intake of vital whole foods, particularly vegetables, rich in nutritional value.

The table below shows the fat, carbohydrate, and protein composition per serving for each exchange list.

Table 22.2 Macro-Nutrient Composition per Serving

List	Protein grams	Fat grams	Carbohydrate grams	Fiber grams	Calories Kilocalories (Kcal)
Vegetables	3	0	11	1–3	50
Fruits	0	0	20	1–3	80
Breads, etc.	2	0	15	1–4	70
Legumes	7	0.5	15	6–7	90
Fats	0	5	0	0	45
Milk (skim)	8	0	12	0	80
Meats, etc.	7	3	0	0	55

HOW MANY CALORIES DO YOU NEED?

In determining caloric needs, first it is necessary to determine ideal body weight and frame size. The most popular height and weight charts are the tables of "desirable weight" provided by the Metropolitan Life Insurance Company. The most recent edition of these tables, published in 1983, follows. It gives weight ranges for men and women at one-inch increments of height for three body-frame sizes. ("Determining Frame Size" follows table.)

Table 22.3 1983 Metropolitan Life Height and Weight Table

Weights for adults twenty-five to fifty-nine years of age based on lowest mortality. Weight in pounds according to frame size in indoor clothing (five pounds for men, three pounds for women), wearing shoes with one-inch heels.

Height	Small Frame	Medium Frame	Large Frame
Men			
5'2"	128–134	131–141	138–150
5'3"	130–136	133–143	140–153
5'4"	132–138	135–145	142–156
5'5"	134–140	137–148	144–160

Men (cont.)

5'6"	136–142	139–151	146–164
5'7"	138–145	142–154	149–168
5'8"	140–148	145–157	152–172
5'9"	142–151	148–160	155–176
5'10"	144–154	151–163	158–180
5'11"	146–157	154–166	161–184
6'0"	149–160	157–170	164–188
6'1"	152–164	160–174	168–192
6'2"	155–168	164–178	172–197
6'3"	158–172	167–182	176–202
6'4"	162–176	171–187	181–207

Women

4'10"	102–111	109–121	118–131
4'11"	103–113	111–123	120–134
5'0"	104–115	113–126	122–137
5'1"	106–118	115–129	125–140
5'2"	108–121	118–132	128–143
5'3"	111–124	121–135	131–147
5'4"	114–127	124–138	134–151
5'5"	117–130	127–141	137–155
5'6"	120–133	130–144	140–159
5'7"	123–136	133–147	143–163
5'8"	126–139	136–150	146–167
5'9"	129–142	139–153	149–170
5'10"	132–145	142–156	152–173
5'11"	135–148	145–159	155–176
6'0"	138–151	148–162	158–179

Determining Frame Size

To make a simple determination of your frame size: Extend your arm and bend the forearm upward at a 90-degree angle. Keep the fingers straight and turn the inside of your wrist away from your body. Place the thumb and index finger of your other hand on the two prominent bones on either side of your elbow. Measure the space between your fingers with a tape measure. Compare your measurement with the following measurements for medium-framed individuals. A lower reading indicates a small frame; higher readings, a large frame.

Table 22.4   Medium-Frame Measurements

Men
Height in 1" heels   *Elbow breadth*
5'2" to 5'3"   2½" to 2⅞"
5'4" to 5'7"   2⅝" to 2⅞"
5'8" to 5'11"   2¾" to 3"
6'0" to 6'3"   2¾" to 3⅛"
6'4"   2⅞" to 3¼"

Women
Height in 1" heels   *Elbow breadth*
4'10" to 5'3"   2¼" to 2½"
5'4" to 5'11"   2⅜" to 2⅝"
6'0"   2½" to 2¾"

After determining your desirable weight in pounds, convert it to kilograms by dividing it by 2.2. Next, take that number and multiply it by the following calories, depending upon activity level:

Little physical activity: 30 calories
Light physical activity: 35 calories
Moderate physical activity: 40 calories
Heavy physical activity: 45 calories

Weight (in kilograms) × Activity Level = Approximate Calorie Requirements: ——— × ——— = ———

For example, I weigh 195 pounds divided by two equals 88 kilograms. I would rate my physical activity level as moderate. Even though I exercise at least five days a week for a minimum of one hour, during most of the day I am sedentary. Therefore, my equation would look like this:

88 × 40 = 3,520 calories

EXAMPLES OF EXCHANGE RECOMMENDATIONS
(SEE HEALTHY EXCHANGE LISTS, PAGE 257)

1,500-CALORIE VEGAN DIET DAILY INTAKE

List 1—vegetables: 5 servings

List 2—fruits: 2 servings

List 3—breads, cereals, and starchy vegetables: 9 servings

List 4—legumes (beans): 2.5 servings

List 5—fats, oils, nuts, and seeds: 4 servings

Percentage of calories as carbohydrates: 67 percent

Percentage of calories as fats: 18 percent

Percentage of calories as protein: 15 percent

Protein content: 55 grams (all from plant sources)

Dietary fiber content: 31 to 74.5 grams

To review the material above, this recommendation would result in an intake of approximately 1,500 calories, of which 67 percent are derived from complex carbohydrates and naturally occurring sugars, 18 percent from fat, and 15 percent from protein. The protein intake is entirely from plant sources but still provides approximately 55 grams, an amount well above the recommended daily allowance of protein intake for someone requiring 1,500 calories. At least one half of the fat servings should be from nuts, seeds, and other whole foods from List 5: Fats, Oils, Nuts, and Seeds. The dietary fiber intake would be approximately 31 to 74.5 grams.

1,500-CALORIE OMNIVORE DIET DAILY INTAKE

List 1—vegetables: 5 servings

List 2—fruits: 2.5 servings

List 3—breads, cereals, and starchy vegetables: 6 servings

List 4—legumes (beans): 1 serving

List 5—fats, oils, nuts, and seeds: 5 servings

List 6—milk: 1 serving

List 7—meats, fish, cheese, and eggs: 2 servings

Percentage of calories as carbohydrates: 67 percent
Percentage of calories as fats: 18 percent
Percentage of calories as protein: 15 percent
Protein content: 61 grams (75 percent from plant sources)
Dietary fiber content: 19.5 to 53.5 grams

2,000-CALORIE VEGAN DIET DAILY INTAKE

List 1—vegetables: 5.5 servings
List 2—fruits: 2 servings
List 3—breads, cereals, and starchy vegetables: 11 servings
List 4—legumes (beans): 5 servings
List 5—fats, oils, nuts, and seeds: 8 servings

Percentage of calories as carbohydrates: 67 percent
Percentage of calories as fats: 18 percent
Percentage of calories as protein: 15 percent
Protein content: 79 grams (all from plant sources)
Dietary fiber content: 48.5 to 101.5 grams

2,000-CALORIE OMNIVORE DIET DAILY INTAKE

List 1—vegetables: 5 servings
List 2—fruits: 2.5 servings
List 3—breads, cereals, and starchy vegetables: 13 servings
List 4—legumes (beans): 2 servings
List 5—fats, oils, nuts, and seeds: 7 servings
List 6—milk: 1 serving
List 7—meats, fish, cheese, and eggs: 2 servings

Percentage of calories as carbohydrates: 66 percent
Percentage of calories as fats: 19 percent
Percentage of calories as protein: 15 percent
Protein content: 78 grams (72 percent from plant sources)
Dietary fiber content: 32.5 to 88.5 grams

2,500-CALORIE VEGAN DIET DAILY INTAKE

List 1—vegetables: 8 servings
List 2—fruits: 3 servings
List 3—breads, cereals, and starchy vegetables: 17 servings
List 4—legumes (beans): 5 servings
List 5—fats, oils, nuts, and seeds: 8 servings

Percentage of calories as carbohydrates: 69 percent
Percentage of calories as fats: 15 percent
Percentage of calories as protein: 16 percent
Protein content: 101 grams (all from plant sources)
Dietary fiber content: 33 to 121 grams

2,500-CALORIE OMNIVORE DIET DAILY INTAKE

List 1—vegetables: 8 servings
List 2—fruits: 3.5 servings
List 3—breads, cereals, and starchy vegetables: 17 servings
List 4—legumes (beans): 2 servings
List 5—fats, oils, nuts, and seeds: 8 servings
List 6—milk: 1 serving
List 7—meats, fish, cheese, and eggs: 3 servings

Percentage of calories as carbohydrates: 66 percent
Percentage of calories as fats: 18 percent
Percentage of calories as protein: 16 percent
Protein content: 102 grams (80 percent from plant sources)
Dietary fiber content: 40.5 to 116.5 grams

3,000-CALORIE VEGAN DIET DAILY INTAKE

List 1—vegetables: 10 servings
List 2—fruits: 4 servings
List 3—breads, cereals, and starchy vegetables: 17 servings

List 4—legumes (beans): 6 servings

List 5—fats, oils, nuts, and seeds: 10 servings

Percentage of calories as carbohydrates: 70 percent

Percentage of calories as fats: 16 percent

Percentage of calories as protein: 14 percent

Protein content: 116 grams (all from plant sources)

Dietary fiber content: 50 to 84 grams

3,000-CALORIE OMNIVORE DIET DAILY INTAKE

List 1—vegetables: 10 servings

List 2—fruits: 3 servings

List 3—breads, cereals, and starchy vegetables: 20 servings

List 4—legumes (beans): 2 servings

List 5—fats, oils, nuts, and seeds: 10 servings

List 6—milk: 1 serving

List 7—meats, fish, cheese, and eggs: 3 servings

Percentage of calories as carbohydrates: 67 percent

Percentage of calories as fats: 18 percent

Percentage of calories as protein: 15 percent

Protein content: 116 grams (81 percent from plant sources)

Dietary fiber content: 45 to 133 grams

Note: Use above recommendations as the basis for calculating other calorie diets. For example, for a 4,000-calorie diet, add the 2,500 to the 1,500 or double the 2,000-calorie diet. For a 1,000-calorie diet, divide the 2,000-calorie diet in half.

The Healthy Exchange Lists

LIST 1—VEGETABLES

Vegetables are excellent sources of vitamins, minerals, and health-promoting fiber compounds. Vegetables are fantastic "diet" foods because they are very high in nutritional value, but low in calories. (Please notice that starchy vegetables like potatoes and yams are included in List 3—Breads, Cereals, and Starchy Vegetables. Legumes are found in List 4.) In addition to eating vegetables whole, you can consume vegetables as fresh juice. There is also a list of "free" vegetables on page 258. These vegetables are termed "free foods" and can be eaten in any desired amount because the calories they contain are offset by the number of calories your body burns in the process of digestion. These foods are especially valuable diet foods, as they help to keep you feeling satisfied between meals.

As the recommendations for vegetables in the Healthy Exchange System is quite high, many individuals may find it necessary to juice their fresh, raw vegetables. Juicing allows for easy absorption of the health-giving properties of fresh fruits and vegetables in larger amounts.

This list shows the vegetables to use for one vegetable exchange. One cup cooked vegetables or fresh vegetable juice, or two cups raw vegetables equals one exchange.

Artichoke (1 medium)

Asparagus

Bean sprouts

Beets

Broccoli

Brussels sprouts

Carrots

Cauliflower

Eggplant

Greens

   Beet

continued

Chard
Collard
Dandelion
Kale
Mustard
Spinach (cooked)
Turnip
Mushrooms
Okra
Onions
Rhubarb
Rutabaga
Sauerkraut
String beans, green or yellow
Summer squash
Tomatoes, tomato juice, vegetable juice cocktail
Zucchini

The following "free" vegetables may be eaten in any quantity desired, especially in their raw form.

Alfalfa sprouts
Bell peppers
Bok choy
Cabbage (all varieties)
Celery
Chicory
Chinese cabbage
Cucumber
Endive
Escarole
Lettuce (all varieties)

Parsley
Radishes
Spinach (raw)
Turnips
Watercress

LIST 2—FRUITS

Fruits make excellent snacks, as they contain fructose or fruit sugar. This sugar is absorbed slowly into the bloodstream, thereby allowing the body time to utilize it. Fruits are also excellent sources of vitamins and minerals as well as health-promoting fiber compounds. However, fruits are not as nutrient-dense as vegetables because they are typically higher in calories. That is why vegetables are favored over fruits in weight-loss plans and overall health-giving diets.

Each of the following equals one exchange:

Fresh Juice, 1 cup (8 ounces)
Pasteurized juice, ⅔ cup
Apple, 1 large
Applesauce (unsweetened), 1 cup
Apricots (dried), 8 halves
Apricots (fresh), 4 medium
Banana, 1 medium
Berries
　　Blackberries, 1 cup
　　Blueberries, 1 cup
　　Cranberries, 1 cup
　　Raspberries, 1 cup
　　Strawberries, 1½ cups
Cherries, 20 large
Dates, 4
Figs (dried), 2

Figs (fresh), 2

Grapefruit, 1

Grapes, 20 large

Mango, 1 small

Melons

    Cantaloupe, ½ small

    Honeydew, ¼ medium

    Watermelon, 2 cups

Nectarine, 2 small

Orange, 1 large

Papaya, 1½ cups

Peach, 2 medium

Persimmon (native), 2 medium

Pineapple, 1 cup

Plums, 4 medium

Prune juice, ½ cup

Prunes, 4 medium

Raisins, 4 tablespoons

Tangerine, 2 medium

Additional fruit exchanges (no more than one per day):

Honey, 1 tablespoon

Jams, jellies, preserves, 1 tablespoon

Sugar, 1 tablespoon

LIST 3—BREADS, CEREALS, AND STARCHY VEGETABLES

Breads, cereals, and starchy vegetables are classified as complex carbohydrates. Chemically, complex carbohydrates are made up of long chains of simple carbohydrates or sugars. The body has to digest or break down the large sugar chains into simple sugars. Therefore, the sugar from complex carbohydrates enters the bloodstream more slowly. As a result, blood sugar levels and appetite are better controlled.

Complex carbohydrate foods like whole grain breads, cereals, and starchy vegetables are higher in fiber and nutrients but lower in calories than foods high in simple sugars like cakes and candies. One of the following equals one exchange:

Breads
 Bagel (small), ½
 Dinner roll, 1
 Dried bread crumbs, 3 tablespoons
 English muffin (small), ½
 Tortilla (6-inch), 1
 Whole wheat, rye, or pumpernickel, 1 slice

Cereals
 Bran flakes, ½ cup
 Cereal (cooked), ½ cup
 Cornmeal (dry), 2 tablespoons
 Flour, 2½ tablespoons
 Grits (cooked), ½ cup
 Pasta (cooked), ½ cup
 Puffed cereal (unsweetened), 1 cup
 Rice or barley (cooked), ½ cup
 Wheat germ, ¼ cup
 Other unsweetened cereal, ¾ cup

Crackers
 Arrowroot, 3
 Graham (2½"-square), 2
 Matzo (4" × 6"), ½
 Rye wafers (2" × 3½"), 3
 Saltines, 6

Starchy vegetables
 Corn, ⅓ cup

continued

Corn on cob, 1 small

Parsnips, ⅔ cup

Potato (mashed), ½ cup

Potato (white), 1 small

Squash (winter, acorn, or butternut), ½ cup

Yam or sweet potato, ¼ cup

Prepared foods

Biscuit, 2″ diameter (omit 1 fat exchange), 1

Corn bread, 2″ × 2″ × 1″ (omit 1 fat exchange), 1

French fries, 2–3″ long (omit 1 fat exchange), 8

Muffin, small (omit 1 fat exchange), 1

Pancake, 5″ × ½″ (omit 1 fat exchange), 1

Potato or corn chips (omit 2 fat exchanges), 15

Waffle, 5″ × ½″ (omit 1 fat exchange), 1

LIST 4—LEGUMES (BEANS)

Legumes are fantastic foods as they are rich in important nutrients and health-promoting compounds. Legumes help improve liver function, lower cholesterol levels, and are extremely effective in improving blood sugar control. Since obesity and diabetes have been linked to loss of blood sugar control (insulin insensitivity), legumes appear to be extremely important in weight-loss plans and in the dietary management of diabetes.

One-half cup of the following cooked or sprouted beans equals one exchange:

Black-eyed peas

Chick peas

Garbanzo beans

Kidney beans

Lentils

Lima beans

Pinto beans

Soybeans, including tofu (omit 1 fat exchange)

Split peas

Other dried beans and peas

LIST 5—FATS, OILS, NUTS, AND SEEDS

As stated earlier, animal fats are typically solid at room temperature and are referred to as saturated fats, while vegetable fats are liquid at room temperature and are referred to as unsaturated fats or oils. Vegetable oils provide the greatest source of the essential fatty acids linoleic acid and linolenic acid. These fatty acids function in our bodies as components of nerve cells, cellular membranes, and hormonelike substances. Fats also provide the body with energy.

While fats are important to human health, too much fat in the diet, especially saturated fat, is linked to numerous cancers, heart disease, and strokes. It is strongly recommended by most nutritional experts that the total fat intake be kept below 30 percent of the total calories. It is also recommended that at least twice as much unsaturated fat be consumed as saturated fat.

Each of the following equals one exchange:

Polyunsaturated

Vegetable Oils, 1 teaspoon

   Canola

   Corn

   Flaxseed

   Safflower

   Soy

   Sunflower

Almonds, 10 whole

Avocado (4″ diameter), ⅛

Peanut butter, 2 tablespoons

Peanuts
    Spanish, 20 whole
    Virginia, 10 whole
Pecans, 2 large
Seeds, 1 tablespoon
    Flax
    Pumpkin
    Sesame
    Sunflower
Walnuts, 6 small
Monounsaturated
Olive oil, 1 teaspoon
Olives, 5 small
Saturated (use sparingly)
Bacon, 1 slice
Butter, 1 teaspoon
Cream (heavy), 1 tablespoon
Cream (light or sour), 2 tablespoons
Cream cheese, 1 tablespoon
Mayonnaise, 1 teaspoon
Salad dressings, 2 teaspoons

LIST 6—MILK

Is milk for everybody? Definitely not. Many people are allergic to milk or lack necessary enzymes to digest it. The drinking of cow's milk is a relatively new dietary practice for humans. Its recent introduction into the human diet may be the reason so many people have difficulty with it. Certainly, milk consumption should be limited to no more than two servings per day.

One cup equals one exchange:

Nonfat milk or yogurt

2% milk (omit one fat exchange)

Lowfat yogurt (omit one fat exchange)

Whole milk (omit two fat exchanges)

Yogurt (omit two fat exchanges)

LIST 7—MEATS, FISH, CHEESE, AND EGGS

When choosing from this list, it is important to choose primarily from the lowfat group, and remove the skin of poultry. This will keep the amount of saturated fat low. Although many people advocate vegetarianism, the exchange list below provides high concentrations of certain nutrients difficult to get in an entirely vegetarian diet, such as the full range of amino acids, vitamin B_{12}, and iron. The most important recommendation may be to use these foods in small amounts as "condiments" in the diets, rather than as mainstays.

Each of the following equals one exchange:

Low fat (less than 15 percent fat content)

Beef: Baby beef, chipped beef, chuck, steak (flank, plate), round (bottom, top), tenderloin plate ribs, all cuts rump, spare ribs, tripe, 1 ounce

Cottage cheese (lowfat), ¼ cup

Fish, 1 ounce

Lamb: Leg, loin (roast and chops), rib, shank, shoulder, sirloin, 1 ounce

Poultry: Light meat of chicken or turkey without skin, 1 ounce

Veal: Cutlet, leg, loin, rib, shank, shoulder, 1 ounce

Medium fat (for each omit ½ fat exchange)

Beef: Ground (15 percent fat), canned corned beef, rib eye, round (ground commercial), 1 ounce

Cheese (e.g., mozzarella, ricotta, farmer's, Parmesan), 1 ounce

Eggs, 1

Organ meats, 1 ounce

Pork: Boston butt, Canadian bacon, loin (all tenderloin), picnic and boiled ham, shoulder, 1 ounce

High fat (for each exchange omit 1 fat exchange)
Beef: Brisket, corned beef, ground beef (more than 20 percent fat), hamburger, roasts (rib), steaks (club and rib), 1 ounce

Cheese (e.g., cheddar, blue cheese, brie), 1 ounce

Duck or goose, 1 ounce

Lamb: Breast, 1 ounce

Pork: Country-style ham, deviled ham, ground pork, loin, spareribs, 1 ounce

Finding and Controlling Food Allergies

In addition to following the guidelines of the Healthy Exchange System, people with food allergies need to consider some other recommendations. A food allergy occurs when there is an adverse reaction to the ingestion of a food. The reaction may or may not be mediated by the immune system. The reaction may be caused by a food protein, starch, or other food component, or by a contaminant found in the food (colorings, preservatives, etc.). A classic food allergy occurs when an ingested food molecule acts as an antigen, which is defined as a substance that can be bound by an antibody, and is bound by allergic antibodies known as immunoglobulin E (IgE). IgE then binds to specialized white blood cells known as mast cells and basophils. This binding brings about the release of substances like histamine, which causes swelling and inflammation.

Other words often used to refer to a food allergy include: food hypersensitivity, food anaphylaxis, food idiosyncrasy, food intolerance, pharmacologic (druglike) reaction to food, metabolic reaction to food, and food sensitivity.

The number of people suffering from food allergies has increased dramatically during the last fifteen years. Some physicians claim that food allergies are the leading cause of most undiagnosed symptoms, and that at least 60 percent of the American population suffers from symptoms associated with food reactions. Theories of why the incidence has increased include: increased stresses on the immune system (such as greater chemical pollution in the air, water, and food); earlier weaning and earlier introduction of solid foods to infants; genetic manipulation of plants, resulting in food components with greater allergenic tendencies; and increased ingestion of fewer foods. Probably all of these and more have contributed to the increased frequency and severity of symptoms.

Signs and Symptoms of Food Allergies

Food allergies have been implicated as a causative factor in a wide range of conditions.[4,5] The actual symptoms produced during an allergic response depend on the location of the immune system activation, the mediators of inflammation involved, and the sensitivity of the tissues to specific mediators.

Identifying Food Allergies

Although there are laboratory tests that identify food allergies, many physicians believe that oral food challenge is the best way of diagnosing adverse reactions to foods. The most popular challenge method involves using an elimination diet. The patient is placed on a limited diet; commonly eaten foods are eliminated and replaced with either hypoallergenic foods and foods rarely eaten, or special hypoallergenic meal replacement formulas. The standard elimination diet (also known as an oligoantigenic diet) consists of lamb, chicken, potatoes, rice, banana, apple, and a cabbage-family vegetable (cabbage, Brussels sprouts, broccoli). There are variations of the elimination diet that are suitable. The important thing is that no allergenic foods be consumed.

The individual stays on this limited diet for at least one week and up to one month. If the symptoms are related to food allergy or sensitiv-

Table 22.5   Symptoms and Diseases Commonly Associated with Food Allergy

System	Symptoms and Dieases
Gastrointestinal	Canker sores, celiac disease, chronic diarrhea, gas, gastritis, irritable colon, malabsorption, stomach ulcer, ulcerative colitis
Genitourinary	Bed-wetting, chronic bladder infections, kidney disease
Immune	Chronic infections, frequent ear infections
Brain	Anxiety, depression, hyperactivity, inability to concentrate, insomnia, irritability, mental confusion, personality change, seizures
Musculoskeletal	Bursitis, joint pain, low back pain
Respiratory	Asthma, chronic bronchitis, wheezing
Skin	Acne, eczema, hives, itching, skin rash
Miscellaneous	Arrthymia, edema, fainting, fatique, headache, hypoglycemia, itchy nose or throat, migraines, sinusitis

ity, they will typically disappear by the fifth or sixth day of the diet. If the symptoms do not disappear, it is possible that a reaction to a food in the elimination diet is responsible, in which case an even more restricted diet must be utilized.

After one week, individual foods are reintroduced according to some plan where a particular food is reintroduced every two days. Methods range from reintroducing only a single food every two days, to one every one or two meals. Usually after the one-week "cleansing" period, the patient will have developed an increased sensitivity to offending foods.

Reintroduction of sensitive foods will typically produce a more severe or recognizable symptom than before. A carefully detailed record must be maintained describing when foods were reintroduced and what symptoms appeared upon reintroduction. It can be very useful to track the wrist pulse during reintroduction, as pulse changes may occur when an allergic food is consumed.

Dealing with Food Allergies

Once a food allergy has been determined, the simplest and most effective method of dealing with it is through avoidance. Avoidance means not only avoiding the food in its most identifiable state (for example, eggs in an omelet), but also in its hidden state (eggs in bread). Closely related foods with similar components may also need to be eliminated (rice and millet in patients with severe wheat allergy).

It is also important to eliminate food additives. Food additives are used to prevent spoiling or enhance flavor, and include such substances as preservatives, artificial colors, artificial flavorings, and acidifiers. The FDA has approved the use of over twenty-eight hundred different food additives. Although the government has banned many synthetic food additives, it should not be assumed that all those currently used in our food supply are safe. There are still numerous synthetic food additives in use that are being linked to allergies and such diseases as depression, asthma, hyperactivity or learning disabilities in children, and migraine headaches.[4]

If a person has multiple food allergies, the so-called rotary diversified diet is the best method to follow. This diet is made up of a highly varied selection of foods that are eaten in a definite rotation or order to prevent the formation of new allergies and to control preexisting ones. Tolerated foods are eaten at regularly spaced intervals of four to seven days. For example, if a person has wheat on Monday, he or she will have to wait until Friday to have anything with wheat in it again. This approach is based on the principle that infrequent consumption of tolerated foods is not likely to induce new allergies or increase any mild allergies, even in highly sensitized and immunocompromised individuals. As tolerance for eliminated foods returns, in some cases they may be added back into the rotation schedule without reactivation of the allergy.

It is not simply a matter of rotating tolerated foods; food families must also be rotated. Foods, whether animal or vegetable, come in families. The reason it is important to rotate food families is that foods in one family can "cross-react" with allergy-inducing foods. Steady consumption of foods that are members of the same family can lead to allergies. Food families need not be as strictly rotated as individual foods. It is usually recommended to avoid eating members of the same food family two days in a row. Table 22.6 lists family classifications for edible plants and animals, while a simplified four-day rotation diet plan is provided in Table 22.7.

Table 22.6   Edible Plant and Animal Kingdom Taxonomic List

Vegetables

Legumes	*Mustard*	*Parsley*	*Potato*	*Grass*	*Lily*
Beans	Broccoli	Anise	Chili	Barley	Asparagus
Cocoa bean	Brussels sprout	Caraway	Eggplant	Corn	Chives
Lentil	Cabbage	Carrot	Peppers	Oat	Garlic
Licorice	Cauliflower	Celery	Potatoes	Rice	Leek
Peanut	Mustard	Coriander	Tobacco	Rye	Onions
Peas	Radish	Cumin	Tomato	Wheat	
Soybean	Turnip	Parsley			
Tamarind	Watercress				
Laurel	*Sunflower*	*Beet*	*Buckweat*		
Avocado	Artichoke	Beet	Buckwheat		
Camphor	Lettuce	Chard	Rhubarb		
Cinnamon	Sunflower	Spinach			
Gourds	*Plums*	*Citrus*	*Cashew*	*Nuts*	*Beech*
Cantaloupe	Almond	Grapefruit	Cashew	Brazil nut	Beechnut
Cucumber	Apricot	Lemon	Mango	Pecan	Chestnut
Honeydew	Cherry	Lime	Pistachio	Walnut	Chinquapin
Melons	Peach	Mandarin			nut
Pumpkin	Persimmon	Orange			
Squash	Plum	Tangerine			
Zucchini					
Banana	*Palm*	*Grape*	*Pineapple*	*Rose*	*Birch*
Arrowroot	Coconut	Grape	Pineapple	Blackberry	Filbert
Banana	Date	Raisin		Loganberry	Hazelnut
Plantain	Date sugar			Raspberry	
				Rose hips	
				Strawberry	

Apple	*Blueberry*	*Pawpaw*				
Apple	Blueberry	Papaya				
Pear	Cranberry	Pawpaw				
Quince	Huckleberry					

Mammals *(Meat/Milk)*	*Birds* *(Meat/Egg)*	*Fish*		*Crustaceans*	*Mollusks*
Cow	Chicken	Catfish	Salmon	Crab	Abalone
Goat	Duck	Cod	Sardine	Crayfish	Clams
Pig	Goose	Flounder	Snapper	Lobster	Mussels
Rabbit	Hen	Halibut	Trout	Prawn	Oysters
Sheep	Turkey	Mackerel	Tuna	Shrimp	Scallops

Table 22.7 Four-day Rotation Diet

Food Family	*Food*
Day 1	
Citrus	Lemon, orange, grapefruit, lime, tangerine, kumquat, citron
Banana	Banana, plantain, arrowroot (musa)
Palm	Coconut, date, date sugar
Parsley	Carrots, parsnips, celery, celery seed, celeriac, anise, dill, fennel, cumin, parsley, coriander, caraway
Spices	Black and white pepper, peppercorn, nutmeg, mace
Subucaya	Brazil nut
Bird	All fowl and game birds, including chicken, turkey, duck, goose, guinea, pigeon, quail, pheasant, eggs
Juices	Juice (preferably fresh) may be made and used from any fruits and vegetables listed above, in any combination desired, without adding sweeteners.

Food Family	Food
Day 2	
Grape	All varieties of grapes, raisins
Pineapple	Juice-pack, water-pack, or fresh
Rose	Strawberry, raspberry, blackberry, loganberry, rose hips
Gourd	Watermelon, cucumber, cantaloupe, pumpkin, squash, other melons, zucchini, pumpkin or sqash seeds
Beet	Beet, spinach, chard
Legume	Pea, black-eyed pea, dry beans, green beans, carob, soybeans, lentils, licorice, peanut, alfalfa
Cashew	Cashew, pistacho, mango
Birch	Filbert, hazelnut
Flaxseed	Flaxseed
Swine	All pork products
Mollusks	Abalone, snail, squid, clam, mussel, oyster, scallop
Crustaceans	Cray, crayfish, lobster, prawn, shrimp
Juices	Juice (preferably fresh) may be made and used without added sweeteners from any fruits, berries, or vegetables listed above, in any combination desired, including fresh alfalfa and some legumes.
Day 3	
Apple	Apple, pear, quince
Gooseberry	Currant, gooseberry
Buckwheat	Buckwheat, rhubarb
Aster	Lettuce, chicory, endive, escarole, globe artichoke, dandelion, sunflower seeds, tarragon
Potato	Potato, tomato, eggplant, peppers (red and green), chili pepper, paprika, cayenne, ground cherries
Lily (onion)	Onion, garlic, aspargus, chives, leeks
Spurge	Tapioca
Herb	Basil, savory, sage, oregano, horehound, catnip, spearmint, peppermint, thyme, marjoram, lemon balm

Day 3 (continued)
Food Family   *Food*

Walnut	English walnut, black walnut, pecan, hickory nut, butternut
Pedalium	Sesame
Beech	Chestnut
Saltwater fish	Herring, anchovy, cod, sea bass, sea trout, mackerel, tuna, swordfish, flounder, sole
Freshwater fish	Sturgeon, salmon, whitefish, bass, perch
Juices	Juice (preferably fresh) may be made and used without added sweeteners from any fruits and vegetables listed above, in any combination

Day 4

Plum	Plum, cherry, peach, apricot, nectarine, almond, wild cherry
Blueberry	Blueberry, huckleberry, cranberry, wintergreen
Pawpaw	Pawpaw, papaya, papain
Mustard	Mustard, turnip, radish, horseradish, watercress, cabbage, Chinese cabbage, broccoli, cauliflower, Brussels sprouts, kale, kohlrabi, rutabaga
Laurel	Avacado, cinnamon, bay leaf, sassafras, cassia buds or bark
Grass	Wheat, corn, rice, oats, barley, rye, wild rice, cane, millet, sorghum, bamboo sprouts
Orchid	Vanilla
Protea	Macadamia nut
Conifer	Pine nut
Fungus	Mushrooms and yeast (brewer's yeast, etc.)
Bovid	Milk products—butter, cheese, yogurt, beef and milk products, oleomargarine, lamb
Juices	Juice (preferably fresh) may be made and used without added sweeteners from any fruits and vegetables listed above, in any combination desired.

Final Comments

I firmly believe that the quality of one's life is directly related to the quality of the foods one routinely ingests. The human body is the most remarkable machine in the world, but most Americans are not feeding the body the high-quality fuel it deserves. When a machine does not receive the proper fuel or maintenance, how long can it be expected to run in an efficient manner? If your body is not fed the full range of nutrients it needs, how can it be expected to stay in a state of good health?

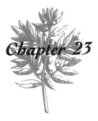

Chapter 23

THE IMPORTANCE

OF EXERCISE

The health benefits of regular exercise cannot be overstated. The immediate effect of exercise is stress on the body; however, with a regular exercise program, the body adapts. The body's response to this regular stress is that it becomes stronger, functions more efficiently, and has greater endurance. Exercise is a vital component of health.

Physical Benefits of Exercise

The entire body benefits from regular exercise largely as a result of improved cardiovascular and respiratory function. Simply stated, exercise enhances the transport of oxygen and nutrients into cells. At the same time, exercise enhances the transport of carbon dioxide and waste products from the tissues of the body to the blood stream, and ultimately, to eliminative organs.

Regular exercise is particularly important in reducing the risk of heart disease. It does this by lowering cholesterol levels, improving blood and oxygen supply to the heart, increasing the functional capacity of the heart, reducing blood pressure, reducing obesity, and exerting a favorable effect on blood clotting.[1]

Psychological and Social Benefits of Exercise

Regular exercise makes people not only look better, but also feel better. Tension, depression, feelings of inadequacy, and worries diminish greatly with regular exercise. Exercise alone has been demonstrated to have a tremendous impact on improving mood and the ability to handle stressful life situations.

In a recent study published in the *American Journal of Epidemiology*, it was found that increased participation in exercise, sports, and physical activities is strongly associated with decreased symptoms of depression (feelings that life is not worthwhile, low spirits); anxiety (restlessness, tension); and malaise (rundown feeling, insomnia).[2]

Overall Health Benefits of Exercise

- Improved cardiovascular function is achieved, as noted by a decreased heart rate, improved heart contraction, reduced blood pressure, and decreased blood cholesterol levels.
- Reduced secretions of adrenaline and noradrenaline result in response to psychological stress.
- Improved oxygen and nutrient utilization occurs in all tissues.
- Improved self-esteem, mood, and frame of mind are felt.
- Increased endurance and energy levels are experienced.

How to Start an Exercise Program

The first thing to do is to make sure you are fit enough to start an exercise program. If you have been mostly inactive for a number of years or have a previously diagnosed illness, see your physician first.

If you are fit enough to begin, the next thing to do is select an activity that you feel you would enjoy. The best exercises are the kind that get your heart moving. Aerobic activities such as walking briskly, jogging, bicycling, cross-country skiing, swimming, aerobic dance, and racquet sports are good examples. Brisk walking (five miles an hour) for approximately thirty minutes may be the very best form of exercise for weight loss. Walking can be done anywhere. It doesn't require any expensive equipment, just comfortable clothing and well-fitted shoes, and the risk for injury is extremely low.

Exercise draws from all of the fat stores of the body, not just from local deposits of the body parts being used. While aerobic exercise generally enhances weight-loss programs, weight-training programs can also substantially alter body composition, by increasing lean body weight and decreasing body fat.[3] Thus, weight training may be just as, or more, effective than aerobic exercise in maintaining or increasing lean body weight.[4]

INTENSITY OF EXERCISE

Exercise intensity is determined by measuring your heart rate (the number of times your heart beats per minute). This determination can be quickly done by placing your index and middle finger of one hand on the side of the neck just below the angle of the jaw, or on the opposite wrist. Beginning with zero, count the number of heartbeats for six seconds. Simply add a zero to this number and you have your pulse. For example, if you counted fourteen beats, your heart rate would be 140. Would this be a good number? It depends upon your "training zone."

A quick and easy way to determine your maximum training heart rate is simply to subtract your age from 185. For example, if you are 40 years old, your maximum heart rate would be 145. To determine the bottom of the training zone, simply subtract 20 from this number. In the case of a 40-year-old, this would be 125. So, the training range would be a heartbeat between 125 and 145 beats per minute. For maximum health benefits, you must stay in this range and never exceed it.

DURATION AND FREQUENCY

A minimum of fifteen to twenty minutes of exercising at your training heart rate at least three times a week is necessary to gain any significant benefits from exercise. It is better to exercise at the lower end of your training zone for longer periods of time than it is to exercise at a higher intensity for a shorter period of time. It is also better if you can make exercise a part of your daily routine.

Final Comments

The key to getting the maximum benefit from exercise is to make it enjoyable. Choose an activity that you enjoy and have fun with. If you can find enjoyment in exercise, you are much more likely to exercise regularly. You don't get in good physical condition by exercising once. It must be performed on a regular basis. So, make it fun.

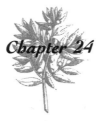

Chapter 24

A QUICK GUIDE TO

NUTRITIONAL SUPPLEMENTS

In the last few years, more Americans than ever are taking nutritional supplements. Despite the fact that there is tremendous scientific evidence to support the beneficial effects of nutritional supplementation, medical experts have not overwhelmingly endorsed nutritional supplementation. Some say diet alone can provide all the essential nutrition necessary, while many others tout the health benefits of vitamins and minerals. The consumer is left in the middle trying to figure out which side is right.

First of all, to an extent, both sides are right. What it boils down to is the criterion of "optimum" nutrition being used. If an expert believes optimum nutrition simply means no obvious signs of nutrient deficiency, his or her answer to whether supplementation is necessary is going to be different from that of an expert who thinks of optimum nutrition as the level of nutrition that will allow a person to function at the highest degree possible with vitality, energy, and enthusiasm for living. What it comes down to then is an argument of philosophy.

Do you believe that good health is simply a matter of not being sick? Or, do you believe that good health is much more than that? It is the goal of optimal health that drives people to take nutritional supplements.

Who Takes Vitamins?

Taking vitamin and mineral supplements has become a way of life for most Americans. Data from the first and second United States Health and Nutrition Examination Survey (HANES I and II) conducted in the 1970s indicated that almost 35 percent of the American population between eighteen and seventy-four years of age took vitamin/mineral supplements regularly.[1] During the 1980s and early 1990s, it is estimated, that number has nearly doubled, so that now, over 60 percent of Americans take vitamin or mineral supplements.

The HANES data demonstrated some interesting facts about supplement users.[1] Perhaps the most interesting finding was that persons with the highest dietary nutrient intakes are the most likely to take a multiple vitamin-mineral supplement. This fact is extremely significant, as it says a great deal about how these individuals view "optimum" nutrition. They are not using nutritional supplements to improve a nutrient-poor diet. Instead, they are using supplements truly as they are intended: that is, to supplement a good, healthful diet.

Other interesting findings included: College-educated individuals are much more likely to take a multiple supplement than those with less education; more women take supplements than men; supplement use is highest in the West and lowest in the South; individuals of normal weight or lighter are more likely to take supplements than heavier individuals; and individuals who exercise regularly are more likely to take supplements than those who do not exercise regularly.

The Need for Nutritional Supplementation

Many Americans, even those who are obese, consume a diet inadequate in nutritional value, yet not to a point where obvious nutrient deficiencies are apparent. The term *subclinical* or *marginal deficiency* is often used to describe this concept. A subclinical deficiency indicates a deficiency of a particular vitamin or mineral that is not severe enough to produce a classic deficiency sign or symptom. Complicating the matter is the fact that in many instances, the only clue to a subclinical nutrient deficiency may be fatigue, lethargy, difficulty in concentration, a lack of well-being, or some other vague symptom. Diagnosis of subclinical deficiencies is an extremely difficult process that involves detailed dietary or laboratory analysis.

Is there evidence to support the contention that subclinical vitamin and mineral deficiencies are common? Definitely yes. During recent years, the United States government has sponsored a number of comprehensive studies (HANES I and II, Ten-State Nutrition Survey, USDA nationwide food-consumption studies) to determine the average nutritional status of the population's diet. These studies have revealed that marginal nutrient deficiencies exist in a substantial portion of the American population (approximately 50 percent), and that for some selected nutrients in certain age groups more than 80 percent of the group consumed less than the recommended dietary allowance (RDA).[2]

These studies indicate that the chances of consuming a daily diet meeting the RDA for all nutrients is extremely unlikely for most Americans. In other words, while it is theoretically possible that healthy individuals can get all the nutrition they need from foods, the fact is that most Americans do not even come close to meeting all their nutritional needs through diet alone. In an effort to increase their intake of essential nutrients, many Americans look to vitamin and mineral supplements.

Is the RDA Enough?

Recommended Dietary Allowances for vitamins and minerals have been prepared by the Food and Nutrition Board of the National Research Council since 1941.[3] These guidelines were originally developed to reduce the rates of severe nutritional deficiency diseases such as scurvy (deficiency of vitamin C), pellagra (deficiency of niacin), and beriberi (deficiency of vitamin B_1). Another critical point is that the RDAs were designed to serve as the basis for evaluating the adequacy of diets of groups of people, not individuals. Individuals simply vary too widely in their nutritional requirements. As stated by the Food and Nutrition Board, "Individuals with special nutritional needs are not covered by the RDAs."

A tremendous amount of scientific research indicates that the "optimal" level for many nutrients, especially the so-called antioxidant nutrients like vitamins C and E, beta-carotene, and selenium, may be much higher than their current RDA. The RDAs focus only on the prevention of nutritional deficiencies in population groups; they do not define "optimal" intake for an individual.

Another factor the RDAs do not adequately take into consideration are environmental and life-style factors, which can destroy vitamins and bind minerals. For example, even the Food and Nutrition Board acknowledges that smokers require at least twice as much vitamin C compared with nonsmokers.[3] But what about other nutrients and smoking? And what about the effects of alcohol consumption, food additives, heavy metals (lead, mercury, etc.), carbon monoxide, and other chemicals associated with our modern society that are known to interfere with nutrient function? Dealing with hazards of modern living may be another reason why many people take supplements.

While the RDAs have done a good job at defining nutrient intake levels to prevent nutritional deficiencies, there is still much to be learned regarding the optimum intake of nutrients.

Take a Multiple Vitamin-Mineral Formula

In an effort to increase their intake of essential nutrients, many Americans look to multiple vitamin-mineral supplements. In 1991 alone, over four hundred million dollars was spent on such products. Do these products provide any benefit? To highlight the potential benefit of taking a multivitamin-mineral supplement for improved health, vitality, and function, the results of two important clinical studies are discussed below.

A MULTIPLE VITAMIN-MINERAL SUPPLEMENT IMPROVES INTELLIGENCE IN CHILDREN

A study published in the medical journal *The Lancet* demonstrated that supplementing the diet with a multiple vitamin-mineral formula can increase nonverbal intelligence in children.[4] This study demonstrates the essential role of many vitamins and minerals in brain function. Nutrients especially important to brain and nervous-system function include thiamine, niacin, vitamin B_6, vitamin B_{12}, copper, iodine, iron, magnesium, manganese, potassium, and zinc. A deficiency of any of these essential nutrients will result in impaired brain and nervous-system function.

The study was performed on ninety children between the ages of twelve and thirteen. The children were divided into three groups: One group took no tablet; one group took a typical multiple vitamin-mineral tablet; and the last group took a tablet that looked and tasted just like the multiple yet contained no vitamins or minerals.

The results of this well-controlled study demonstrated that the group taking the supplement, but not the placebo group or the remaining thirty who took no tablet, had a significant increase in nonverbal intelligence. It is a well-accepted fact that a deficiency of a number of vitamins and minerals will result in impaired mental performance. Apparently, many of the children were suffering from "subclinical" vitamin and mineral deficiencies to an extent that hampered nerve-cell function and impaired mental performance. In other words, low levels of nutrients in the diet will not allow the brain to function properly. By providing the brain the nutrients it needs (through either diet or supplementation) to function at its optimal level, these nutritional deficiencies can be reversed and/or prevented.

MULTIPLE VITAMIN-MINERAL SUPPLEMENT IMPROVES IMMUNE FUNCTION IN THE ELDERLY

Aging is associated with decreased immune-system function. Recent evidence supports the hypothesis that many of the age-related defects in immune function are due to nutrient deficiency. The elderly are at the highest risk of nutritional deficiency. Nutrient deficiency is still the major cause of impaired immune function throughout the world.

The effect of a multiple vitamin-mineral supplement on immune function in the elderly was examined in a clinical study also published in *The Lancet*.[5] The study was double-blind and lasted for twelve months. The results of the study indicated that the elderly subjects receiving the nutritional supplement demonstrated improvements in many immune system parameters, and had significantly fewer infections compared with the placebo group.

This study highlights the essential role nutrition plays in maintaining a healthy immune system. Nutrients especially important to proper immune function include vitamin B_6, vitamin C, and zinc. These are required for the manufacture of antibodies, thymus gland hormones, and other important immune-system components. A deficiency of these or virtually any other nutrient will result in impaired immune-system function.

As the immune system is responsible for protecting against infection as well as against cancer and other diseases, the first step in enhancing immune function is proper nutrition. The closer an individual's essential nutrient intake is to optimal, the better chance he or she has that the immune system will function optimally—another good reason to take a multiple vitamin-mineral formula.

A Quick Guide to Vitamins and Minerals

Vitamins are classified into two groups: fat-soluble (A, D, E, and K) and water-soluble (the B vitamins and vitamin C). Vitamins function along with enzymes in chemical reactions necessary for human bodily function, including energy production. Vitamins and enzymes also work together to act as catalysts in speeding up the making or breaking of chemical bonds that join molecules together.

Minerals function, along with vitamins, as components of body enzymes. Minerals are also needed for proper composition of bone and blood and for the maintenance of normal cell function.

Throughout this book there are examples of certain health conditions that can be improved through diet supplementation with a specific vitamin or mineral. However, since this section is geared toward basic foundations for good health, the following recommendations for daily intake levels of vitamins and minerals are designed to provide an optimum intake range for maintaining good health. These recommended levels are most easily attained by taking a good multiple vitamin-mineral formula and then adding specific nutrients like vitamin C and calcium as needed.

Table 24.1   Daily Optimal Vitamin-Mineral Supplementation

Vitamin	Range for Adults in International Units (IU), micrograms (mcg), or milligrams (mg)
Vitamin A (retinol)	5,000–10,000 IU
Vitamin A (from beta-carotene)	10,000–75,000 IU
Vitamin D	100–400 IU
Vitamin E (d-alpha tocopherol)	400–1,200 IU
Vitamin K (phytonadione)	60–900 mcg
Vitamin C (ascorbic acid)	500–9,000 mg
Vitamin B_1 (thiamine)	10–90 mg
Vitamin B_2 (riboflavin)	10–90 mg
Niacin	10–90 mg
Niacinamide	10–30 mg
Vitamin B_6 (pyridoxine)	25–100 mg
Biotin	100–300 mcg
Pantothenic acid	25–100 mg
Folic acid	400–1,000 mcg
Vitamin B_{12}	400–1,000 mcg
Choline	150–500 mg
Inositol	150–500 mg
Minerals	*Range*
Boron	1–2 mg
Calcium	250–750 mg
Chromium	200–400 mcg
Copper	1–2 mg
Iodine	50–150 mcg
Iron	15–30 mg
Magnesium	250–750 mg
Manganese (citrate)	10–15 mg
Molybdenum (sodium molybdate)	10–25 mcg
Potassium	200–500 mg

Minerals (cont.)	Range (cont.)
Selenium (selenomethionine)	100–200 mcg
Silica (sodium metasilicate)	200–1,000 mcg
Vanadium (sulfate)	50–100 mcg
Zinc (picolinate)	15–30 mg

Final Comments

With the information available at this time, it appears that enhancing the diet with vitamin and mineral supplements may be of great benefit to a wide number of individuals. In addition to vitamins and minerals, there are many other nutritional supplements that provide exceptional health benefits, including bioflavonoids; coenzyme Q_{10}; carnitine; glucosamine sulfate; chondroitin sulfate; glandular products such as liver, thymus, spleen, and pancreatic extracts; bee byproducts (pollen, royal jelly, and propolis); chlorophyll; spirulina, chlorella, and other algae products; wheat and barley grass juice; wheat germ products; and lecithin.

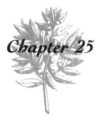

Chapter 25

A QUICK GUIDE TO
MEDICINAL HERBS

The World Health Organization has estimated that as much as 80 percent of the world's population relies on herbal medicines. This widespread use of natural medicinals is not restricted to Third World countries. Findings suggest that 30 to 50 percent of all medical doctors in France and Germany rely on herbal preparations as their primary medicines. So why aren't herbs more appreciated in the United States?

Because a natural product cannot be patented, drug companies prefer to develop synthetic substances as medicines. Nonetheless, it is a generally unknown fact that, for the past thirty years, about 25 percent of all prescription drugs in the United States have contained active ingredients obtained from plants.

One of the great fallacies promoted by the United States medical establishment has been that there is no firm scientific evidence for the use of many natural therapies, including herbal medicine. This assertion is simply not true. In fact, during the last ten to twenty years, there has been an explosion of scientific information concerning plants, crude plant extracts, and nutritional substances from plants as medicinal agents.

Throughout this book there are numerous examples of herbs that offer a more effective and safer alternative to drugs. Herbs will certainly play a major role in the medicine of the future, as there is an increasing amount of scientific evidence documenting their effectiveness. There is also a growing appreciation of the harmonious healing properties herbs possess.

It is often asked, What advantages do herbal medicines have over synthetic drugs? As a general rule, herbs are less toxic than their synthetic counterparts and offer less risk of side effects. Obviously, there are exceptions to this rule. In addition, the mechanism of action of an herb is often to correct the underlying cause of an illness. In contrast, a synthetic drug is often designed to alleviate the symptom (effect) without addressing the underlying cause. It has also been demonstrated with many plants that the whole plant or crude extract is much more effective than its isolated constituents or synthetic drugs.

Herbal Preparations

Herbal products come in many forms. Herbal teas are quite popular beverages that can have some medicinal effects. Most physicians and practitioners who use herbs for treatment tend to use stronger preparations, known as extracts. In most instances, there is no real comparison between an extract and the dried herb used in teas. An extract is more effective and has a higher concentration of active ingredients, a longer shelf life, and a greater degree of standardization.

Examples of extracts include tinctures, fluid extracts, and solid extracts. Tinctures are made using an alcohol and water mixture as the solvent. The herb is soaked in an alcoholic solution for a specified amount of time, depending on the herb. This soaking usually is from several hours to days; however, some herbs may be soaked for much longer periods of time. The solution is then pressed, yielding the tincture.

Fluid extracts are more concentrated than tinctures. They are made by distilling off some of the alcohol, typically by using methods that do not require elevated temperatures, such as vacuum distillation and filtration techniques. Tinctures are often formed from fluid extracts by adding alcohol.

A solid extract is produced by further concentration of the extract by the mechanisms described above for fluid extracts. The solvent is completely removed and then the extract is usually ground into coarse granules or a fine powder. A solid extract can also be diluted with alcohol and water to form a fluid extract or tincture.

STRENGTHS OF EXTRACTS

The potencies or strengths of herbal extracts are generally expressed in two ways. If they contain known active compounds, their strengths are commonly expressed in terms of the content of these active compounds. Otherwise, the strength is expressed in terms of their concentration. A 4:1 concentration means that one unit of measure of the extract is equivalent to, or derived from, four units of the crude herb. One gram of a 4:1 extract is concentrated from four grams of crude herb.

A tincture is typically a 1:10 or 1:5 concentration (10 or 5 units of extract come from 1 unit of herbs), while a fluid extract is usually 1:1. Hence, a solid extract is typically at least four times as potent as an equal amount of fluid extract, and forty times as potent as a tincture, if they are produced from the same quality of herb.

Typically, one gram of a 4:1 solid extract is equivalent to 4 milliliters of a fluid extract (one seventh of an ounce), and 40 milliliters of a tincture (almost one and a half ounces).

Stating the content of active constituents is the best method, as it allows for dosage to be based on activity. This method produces a more consistent clinical response. An analogy would be stating the level of caffeine in a cup of coffee. More companies in the United States are adopting this preferred method.

Most Important Herbal Medicines

Here is a concise guide to twenty-eight of the most important herbal medicines in the United States. It is beyond the scope of this chapter to extensively review the major herbs in current use. Therefore, only a concise guide to twenty-eight of the most important herbal medicines is provided. Although all the herbs discussed can be used safely for prolonged periods of time when taken at the recommended levels, it is best to utilize herbs, as you would most medicines, only when their use is indicated. While some herbs are suited for long-term use, others are not. For a more detailed discussion, consult my book *The Healing Power of Herbs*.

Aloe vera

Bilberry or European blueberry

Bromelain

Dandelion

Dong quai

Echinacea or purple coneflower

Feverfew

Garlic

Ginger

Ginkgo biloba

Ginseng, Chinese or Korean

Ginseng, Siberian

Goldenseal

Gotu kola

Gugulipid

Hawthorn

Lapacho

Licorice

Lobelia or Indian tobacco

Mahuang

Milk thistle

Sarsaparilla

Saw palmetto berry

St. John's wort

Tea tree oil

Turmeric

Uva ursi or bearberry

Valerian

Aloe vera

Aloe vera products, both for internal and external use, are widely used in
the United States. Despite widespread use, there are very few controlled

studies on aloe vera. From the information currently available, it can be concluded that aloe vera can be used topically in the treatment of minor burns, cuts, and abrasions.[1-4] The use of aloe orally, other than for its well-documented laxative effect, has not been fully studied. Preliminary and anecdotal studies indicate that aloe vera juice may offer some "tonic" and antiulcer effects on the gastrointestinal tract. The polysaccharide component of aloe vera, acemannan, possesses significant immune-enhancing and antiviral activity. Preliminary studies indicate it may be useful as an adjunct to current AIDS therapy.[5]

Aloe vera gel can be applied liberally for topical use. A wide range of products are available on the market; however, pure aloe vera gel is sufficient.

Commercially prepared aloe vera juice can be consumed as a beverage or tonic. As detailed information is currently lacking as to the optimal dose for these types of products, it is recommended that no more than one quart be consumed in any one day.

The dose of acemannan being used in HIV/AIDS patients is 800 to 1,600 milligrams per day. This would correspond to a dose of approximately ½ to 1 liter per day for most aloe vera juice products. There may be great variation in the amount of acemannan from one manufacturer to the next.

Bilberry or European blueberry (Vaccinium myrtillus)

KEY USES OF BILBERRY

Diabetic retinopathy

Macular degeneration

Cataract

Glaucoma

Varicose veins

Vaccinium myrtillus, or bilberry, is a shrubby perennial plant that grows in the woods and forest meadows of Europe. The fruit is a blueblack berry that differs from an American blueberry in that its meat is also blue-black.

The active components of bilberries are its flavonoids, specifically its anthocyanosides. Bilberry extracts have been widely used in Europe in the treatment of various vascular disorders and several eye diseases. Clinical studies have demonstrated a positive effect in the treatment of capillary fragility, various disturbances of blood flow to the brain (similar to the effect of *Ginkgo biloba*), varicose veins, and blood in the urine not caused by infection.[6,7,8]

Perhaps the most significant therapeutic application for bilberry extracts is in the field of ophthalmology. Interest in bilberry anthocyanosides first began when it was observed during World War II that British Royal Air Force pilots reported improved nighttime vision on bombing raids after consuming bilberries. Subsequent studies showed that the administration of bilberry extracts to healthy subjects resulted in improved nighttime visual acuity, quicker adjustment to darkness, and faster restoration of visual acuity after exposure to glare.

It appears that, in addition to their effect on blood vessels, anthocyanosides have an affinity for the part of the retina responsible for vision. This affinity is consistent with several of the clinical effects observed, including positive results in degeneration of the macular portion of the retina, cataracts, retinitis pigmentosa, diabetic retinopathy, and nightblindness.[9,10]

The standard dose of bilberry extract is based on its anthocyanoside content, as calculated by its anthocyanidin percentage. Widely used pharmaceutical preparations in Europe are standardized for anthocyanidin content (typically, 25 percent). These extracts are also available in the United States. The standard dose is 80 to 160 milligrams three times daily. Extensive studies in humans and animals have shown bilberry extracts are without toxic effects even when given at huge levels for long periods of time.

Bromelain

KEY USES OF BROMELAIN

Inflammation

Sports injuries

Respiratory tract infections

Menstrual cramps

Bromelains are sulfur-containing, protein-digesting enzymes (proteolytic enzymes, or proteases) obtained from the pineapple plant. Bromelain use as an anti-inflammatory agent is discussed in detail on page 80. Briefly, bromelain has been shown to be useful in a number of health conditions including angina, arthritis, indigestion, upper respiratory tract infections, athletic injuries, and trauma.[11]

The activity of bromelain is expressed in a variety of enzyme units. The use of milk clotting units (m.c.u.) is the officially recognized method. For most indications, the recommended m.c.u. range is 1,200 to 1,800. Unless bromelain is being used as a digestive aid, administration should be on an empty stomach (before or between meals). As a digestive aid, take bromelain with meals. The typical dosage is 250 to 750 milligrams three times per day. Bromelain is extremely safe to use. In human studies, very large doses of bromelain (nearly 2.0 grams) have been given without side effects.

Dandelion (Taraxacum officinale)

KEY USES OF DANDELION ROOT

Liver disorders

Water retention

Obesity

The dandelion is a perennial plant found almost everywhere on the planet. The root is the portion of the plant used most extensively, although the leaves probably possess a greater diuretic effect. Generally regarded as a liver remedy, dandelion has a long folk use throughout the world. Studies in humans and laboratory animals have shown that dandelion enhances the flow of bile, improving such conditions as liver congestion (cholestasis), bile duct inflammation, hepatitis, gallstones, and jaundice.[12] As a general tonic for the liver, dandelion root can be given at the following dosages three times daily:

Dried root (or as tea), 4 grams

Tincture—alcohol-based tinctures of dandelion are not recommended, due to the extremely high dosage required

Fluid extract (1:1), 4 to 8 milliliters (1 to 2 teaspoons)

Powdered solid extract (4:1), 250 to 500 milligrams

Dong quai (Angelica sinensis)

KEY USES OF DONG QUAI

Menopausal symptoms

Premenstrual syndrome

In Asia, dong quai's reputation is perhaps second only to ginseng. Predominantly regarded as a "female" remedy, dong quai has been used to treat such conditions as menstrual cramps, menopausal symptoms, and to assure a healthy pregnancy and easy childbirth.[13] Scientific investigation has shown that dong quai produces a balancing effect on estrogen activity and a tonic effect on the uterus.[14,15] Dong quai is often referred to as a tonic for the female glandular system. Long-term use is appropriate at recommended levels. Three-times-a-day dosages are as follows:

Dried root (or as tea), 1 to 2 grams

Tincture (1:5), 4 to 6 milliliters (1 to 1½ teaspoons)

Fluid extract (1:1), 0.5 to 2 milliliters (¼ to ½ teaspoon)

Solid extract (4:1), 125 to 500 milligrams

Echinacea or purple coneflower (Echinacea angustifolia)

KEY USES OF ECHINACEA ROOT

Viral infections

Impaired immune function

Wound healing

Echinacea is a North American herb used extensively by Native Americans. They employed it to combat illness more than they used any other plant. The root was used most often: externally, for the healing of wounds, burns, abscesses, and insect bites; internally, for infections, joint pains, and as an antidote for rattlesnake bites.[16]

Today, echinacea is still one of the most widely used herbs. Its primary clinical applications have been in cases of infections or when immune-system enhancement is desired. Clinical and experimental studies have confirmed these applications.[16,17] Although much of the clinical data are based on injectable products, oral administration is thought to yield similar results over time. In fact, there is some evidence indicating that oral administration may have a more profound effect on enhancing immunological activity.

As a general immunological stimulant during infection, echinacea can be administered in any of the forms and dosages given below three times daily:

Dried root (or as tea), 0.5 to 1 gram

Freeze-dried plant, 325 to 650 milligrams

Juice of aerial portion of E. *purpurea* stabilized in 22 percent ethanol, 1 to 2 milliliters

Tincture (1:5), 2 to 4 milliliters (½ to 1 teaspoon)

Fluid extract (1:1), 1 to 2 milliliters (¼ to ½ teaspoon)

Solid (dry powdered) extract (6.5:1 or 3.5 percent echinacoside), 100 to 250 milligrams

Feverfew (Tanacetum parthenium)

KEY USES OF FEVERFEW

Migraine headaches

Arthritis

Fever

Inflammation

Feverfew is cultivated throughout Europe and the United States as a decorative plant. The flowers are small and daisylike, with yellow disks and from ten to twenty white, toothed rays. Feverfew has been used for centuries for the treatment of migraines, fever, and arthritis. The modern use of feverfew has focused on its help for migraine headaches. This is discussed in detail on page 193.

Although a double-blind, placebo-controlled study demonstrated no apparent benefit from oral feverfew in rheumatoid arthritis, the dosage used was extremely small (76 milligrams dried, powdered feverfew leaf corresponding to two medium-size leaves). Patients also continued to take aspirin and other NSAIDs, a practice that has been suggested to reduce the efficacy of feverfew.[18]

The effectiveness of feverfew is dependent upon adequate levels of parthenolide, the active ingredient. While low dosages (50 milligrams per day) appeared useful in preventing migraines, higher dosages may be necessary for treating an acute migraine, and in treating rheumatoid arthritis. The standard dosages are as follows three times a day:

Dried leaves or by infusion (tea), 1 to 2 grams

Tincture (1:5), 4 to 6 milliliters (1 to 1½ teaspoons)

Fluid extract (1:1), 1 to 2.0 milliliters (¼ to ½ teaspoon)

Powdered solid extract (4:1), 250 to 500 milligrams

Garlic (Allium sativum)

KEY USES OF GARLIC

Infections

Elevated cholesterol levels

High blood pressure

Diabetes

Garlic's effect in lowering blood cholesterol levels and blood pressure has been discussed fully on page 138. Garlic has been used throughout history all over the world for the treatment of a wide variety of conditions, especially infections. Its antibiotic activity was noted by Louis Pasteur in 1858, and garlic was used by Albert Schweitzer in Africa for the treatment of amoebic dysentery.

Recent research has shown garlic to have antimicrobial activity against many types of bacteria, virus, worms, and fungi.[19] Garlic is especially active against *Candida albicans*, being more potent than nystatin, gentian violet, and six other reputed antifungal agents. In addition to its antibiotic activity, garlic has also been shown to enhance various aspects of the immune system, which supports its historical use in the treatment of a variety of infectious conditions.

Garlic possesses important anticancer properties. The famous Greek physician Hippocrates prescribed eating garlic as treatment for cancers. Based on animal research and some human studies, this recommendation may have been extremely wise. Several garlic components have displayed significant immune-enhancing as well as anticancer effects.[20] Human studies showing garlic's immune-enhancing and anticancer effects are largely based on population studies. From these studies it appears that there is an inverse relationship between cancer rates and garlic consumption; that is, cancer rates are lowest where garlic consumption is greatest. For example, in China, a study comparing populations in different regions found that death from gastric cancers in regions where garlic consumption was high was significantly less that in regions with lower garlic consumption.

Perhaps the best (and most economical) way to get the benefits of garlic is to consume it regularly in the diet. A variety of commercial preparations exist on the market that may also be of benefit. Simply follow the manufacturers' instructions.

Ginger (Zingiber officinale)

KEY USES OF GINGER

Nausea and vomiting with pregnancy

Motion sickness and vertigo

Arthritis

Historically, the majority of complaints for which ginger was used concerned the gastrointestinal system. Ginger is an excellent carminative (a substance that promotes the elimination of intestinal gas) and intestinal spasmolytic (a substance that relaxes and soothes the intestinal tract).

A clue to ginger's success in eliminating gastrointestinal distress is offered by recent double-blind studies that demonstrated ginger to be very effective in preventing the symptoms of motion sickness, especially seasickness. Several studies have shown ginger to be superior to Dramamine, a commonly used over-the-counter and prescription drug for motion sickness.[21,22,23] Ginger reduces all symptoms associated with motion sickness including dizziness, nausea, vomiting, and cold sweating.

Ginger has also been used to treat the nausea and vomiting associated with pregnancy. Recently, the benefit of ginger was confirmed in hyperemesis gravidarum, the most severe form of pregnancy-related nausea and vomiting.[24] This condition usually requires hospitalization. Ginger root powder at a dose of 250 milligrams four times a day brought about a significant reduction in both the severity of the nausea and the number of attacks of vomiting.

Ginger has also been shown to have anti-inflammatory properties. In one clinical study, seven patients with rheumatoid arthritis, in whom conventional drugs had provided only temporary or partial relief, were treated with ginger.[25] One patient took 50 grams per day of lightly cooked ginger, while the remaining six took either 5 grams of fresh or 0.1 to 1 gram of powdered ginger daily. All patients reported substantial improvement, including pain relief, joint mobility, and decrease in swelling and morning stiffness.

Most clinical studies have used powdered ginger root at a dose of 1 gram per day. Fresh ginger root may yield even better results. An equivalent dose would be approximately 10 grams or one third of an ounce of fresh ginger root—roughly a quarter-inch slice. Fresh ginger root is available at most grocery stores. If you have a juice extractor, fresh ginger is a fantastic addition to fresh fruit and vegetable juices, especially pineapple, carrot, and apple.

Ginkgo biloba

KEY USES OF *GINKGO BILOBA*

Decreased blood supply to the brain

Senility, ringing in the ears, dizziness

Impotence

Varicose veins

Alzheimer's disease

Ginkgo biloba may be the most important plant-derived medicine available. An extract of the *Ginkgo biloba* leaves offers great benefit to many elderly people with impaired blood flow to the brain (cerebral insufficiency). The symptoms of cerebral insufficiency include short-term memory loss, vertigo, headache, ringing in the ears, depression, and impotence (in males). These symptoms are often referred to as "symptoms of aging."

In a recent review, an analysis was made on the quality of research of more than forty clinical studies of a standardized extract of *Ginkgo biloba* leaves in the treatment of cerebral insufficiency.[26] The results of the analysis indicate that the quality of the research reviewed was on a par with the research methods used in investigating the drug Hydergine (ergoloid mesylates), an approved drug in the treatment of dementia, including Alzheimer's disease. The analysis further substantiated that ginkgo is effective in reducing all symptoms of cerebral insufficiency, including impaired mental function (senility). *Ginkgo biloba* extract has been extensively studied and appears to work by increasing blood flow to the brain, resulting in an increase in oxygen and glucose utilization.

Ginkgo biloba extract is one of the most popular medicines in France and Germany. In Germany, more than five million prescriptions are written each year for ginkgo. Unfortunately, most American physicians have never heard of it. There are so many people in the United States who could benefit from ginkgo extract, which is available in health-food stores, if they only knew about it.

In order to take advantage of ginkgo's effect on improving brain function, be sure that the product is the same quality as that used in the clinical studies. The product should be standardized to contain 24 percent ginkgo flavoglycosides. The standard dosage of this extract is 40 milligrams three times a day. Ginkgo is extremely safe to use, as there have been no reports of significant adverse reactions at the prescribed dose. Gingko is well suited for long-term use. In fact, the longer gingko is used, the more obvious the benefits become.

Ginseng, Chinese or Korean (Panax ginseng)

KEY USES OF *PANAX GINSENG*

Recovery from illness

Stress and fatigue

Diabetes

Improvement of mental and physical performance

Enhancement of sexual function

Protection against radiation

Korean or Chinese ginseng is a small perennial plant that originally grew wild in the damp woodlands of northern China, Manchuria, and Korea. Ginseng is, without question, the most famous medicinal plant of China, where it has been generally used alone or in combination with other herbs for its revitalizing properties, especially for people recovering from a long illness. It is regarded as being more potent than Siberian ginseng (see below).

The mental and physical revitalizing effects of ginseng have been demonstrated in both animal studies and double-blind clinical trials in humans.[27] In one double-blind clinical study, nurses who had switched from day to night duty rated themselves for competence, mood, and general well-being, and were given a test for mental and physical performance along with blood-cell counts and blood chemistry evaluation.[28] The group administered ginseng demonstrated higher scores in competence, well-being, and mental and physical performance when compared with those receiving a placebo. In another double-blind study that was performed on university students in Italy, ginseng extract was compared with placebo in various tests of mental performance.[29] A favorable effect of ginseng was observed in attention, mental arithmetic, logical deduction, integrated brain-body function, and reaction time to sounds. It is interesting to note that in the course of the trial, the students taking ginseng also reported a greater sensation of well-being.

From a practical standpoint, ginseng's antifatigue properties may be useful whenever fatigue or lack of energy is apparent. Athletes, in particular, may derive some benefit from ginseng use. The dosage of ginseng is related to the ginsenoside content of ginseng. The use of standardized ginseng preparations is recommended to ensure sufficient ginsenoside content, consistent therapeutic results, and reduced risk of toxicity. The typical dose of these extracts (taken one to three times daily) for general tonic effects should contain a saponin content of at least 25 milligrams of ginsenoside Rg1 with a ratio of ginsenoside Rg1 to Rb1 of 2:1. Check the label carefully to determine the levels of ginsenoside in proper ratio. The standard dose for high-quality ginseng root is in the range of 4 to 6 grams daily.

As each individual's response to ginseng is unique, care must be taken to observe possible ginseng toxicity. It is best to begin at lower doses and increase gradually. The most common side effects of taking too much ginseng are anxiety, irritability, nervousness, insomnia, hypertension, breast pain, and menstrual changes. Upon the appearance of any of these side effects, dosage should be reduced or the product should be discontinued.

Ginseng, Siberian (Eleutherococcus senticosus)

KEY USES OF SIBERIAN GINSENG

Stress and fatigue

Atherosclerosis

Improvement of mental and physical performance

Impaired kidney function

Eleutherococcus senticosus, or Siberian ginseng, is a shrub that grows abundantly in parts of Siberia, Korea, China, and Japan. Siberian ginseng root extract has been administered to more than twenty-one hundred healthy human subjects in clinical trials.[30] These studies indicated Siberian ginseng: (1) increased the ability of humans to withstand many adverse physical conditions (heat, noise, motion, work-load increase, exercise, and decompression); (2) increased mental alertness and work output; (3) improved the quality of work under stressful conditions: and (4) enhanced athletic performance.

The standard dosage of the fluid extract used in the majority of studies ranged from 2.0 to 4.0 milliliters (up to 16.0 milliliters), one to three times a day, for periods up to sixty consecutive days. In multiple dosing regimens, there is usually a two- to three-week interval between courses. Siberian ginseng is regarded as being less potent than *Panax ginseng.* Nonetheless, the same side effects may occur. Upon the appearance of any side effect, use should be discontinued. Three-times-daily dosages for various forms of Siberian ginseng are as follows:

Dried root, 2 to 4 grams

Tincture (1:5), 10 to 20 milliliters (2½ to 5 teaspoons)

Fluid extract (1:1), 2.0 to 4.0 milliliters

Solid (dry powdered) extract (20:1 containing greater than 1 percent eleutheroside E), 100 to 200 milligrams

Goldenseal (Hydrastis canadensis)

KEY USES OF GOLDENSEAL ROOT

Parasitic infections of the gastrointestinal tract

Infections of mucous membranes

Inflammation of the gallbladder

Cirrhosis of the liver

Goldenseal was used extensively by Native Americans as an herbal medication and clothing dye. Its medicinal application centered around its ability to soothe the mucous membranes that line the respiratory, digestive, and urinary tracts in inflammatory conditions induced by allergy or infection.

The medicinal value of goldenseal (as well as barberry and Oregon grape root) is thought to be due to its high content of alkaloids, of which berberine has been the most widely studied.[31,32,33] The broad antibiotic effects of berberine, combined with its anti-infective and immune-stimulating actions, supports the historical use of berberine-containing plants in infections of the mucous membranes: the linings of the oral cavity, throat, sinuses, bronchi, urinary tract, and gastrointestinal tract. Goldenseal's historical use is also supported by several clinical studies that have shown berberine has much success in the treatment of acute diarrhea.[34,35,36] Berberine has been found effective against diarrheas caused by *E. coli* (traveler's diarrhea), *Shigella dysenteriae* (shigellosis), *Salmonella paratyphi* (food poisoning), *Giardia lamblia* (giardiasis), and *Vibrio cholerae* (cholera). Presumably, goldenseal would have similar effects.

For best results, goldenseal extracts standardized for berberine content are preferred. Here are the dosages for various forms of goldenseal to be taken up to three times per day:

Dried root or as infusion (tea), 2 to 4 grams

Tincture (1:5), 6 to 12 milliliters (1½ to 3 teaspoons)

Fluid extract (1:1), 1 to 2 milliliters (¼ to ½ teaspoon)

Solid (powdered dry) extract (4:1 or 8 to 12 percent alkaloid content), 250 to 500 milligrams

Gotu kola (Centella asiatica)

KEY USES OF GOTU KOLA

Cellulite

Wound healing

Varicose veins

Scleroderma

Gotu kola has been utilized as a medicine in India and Indonesia since prehistoric times with use centered around its ability to heal wounds and relieve leprosy. Modern research has substantiated its effectiveness in both of these applications.[37]

Regarding healing wounds, the outcome of gotu kola's complex actions is a balancing effect on participating cells and tissues, particularly connective tissues. This makes gotu kola useful in a wide range of conditions in which enhancing wound healing is required, such as after surgery or trauma. In the United States, the most popular use of gotu kola has been in the treatment of cellulite and varicose veins. Both of these uses are supported by clinical studies showing positive effects.[37,38]

For maximum benefit, use gotu kola extracts standardized to contain 70 percent triterpenic acids at a dose of 60 to 120 milligrams per day.

Gugulipid (Commiphora mukul)

KEY USES OF GUGULIPID

Elevated cholesterol and triglyceride levels

Atherosclerosis

Hypothyroidism

Gugulipid is the standardized extract of the oleoresin of *Commiphora mukul* (mukul myrrh tree), an Indian medicinal tree. It was discussed fully on page 136. Gugulipid lowers both cholesterol and triglyceride levels. The dosage is based on its guggulsterone content. The standard dosage is 25 milligrams of guggulsterone three times per day.

Hawthorn (Crataegus oxyacantha)

KEY USES OF HAWTHORN

Atherosclerosis

High blood pressure

Congestive heart failure

Angina

As discussed on page 117, hawthorn extracts are effective in reducing blood pressure, angina attacks, and serum cholesterol levels, and in preventing the depositing of cholesterol in arterial walls. The dosage depends on the type of preparation and source material. Here are the three-times-daily dosages for various hawthorn preparations.

Crataegus berries or flowers (dried), 3 to 5 grams, or as an infusion

Crataegus fluid extract (1:1), 1 to 2 milliliters (½ to 1 teaspoon)

Crataegus freeze-dried berries, 1 to 1.5 grams

Crataegus flower extract (standardized to contain 1.8 percent vitexin-4'-rhamnoside, or 10 percent procyanidins), 100 to 250 milligrams

Lapacho (Tabebuia avellanedae)

KEY USES OF LAPACHO

Infections

Candida albicans

Lapacho is a tree that is native to Brazil. The Indians there also refer to the tree as pau d'arco or ipe roxo. The inner bark has been used for medicinal purposes for centuries as a folk remedy for a wide variety of afflictions including infections, cancers, ulcers, respiratory problems, poor circulation, and constipation.[39]

Lapacho was extensively studied by the National Cancer Institute (NCI). After initial positive results with crude extracts, it was felt that the compound lapachol was the most active anticancer agent. Lapachol entered phase I clinical trials at NCI in 1968, but after finding it difficult to obtain therapeutic blood levels of lapachol without some mild toxic side effects such as nausea, vomiting, and anti–vitamin-K activity, the NCI abandoned further research.[39]

The usual form of administration of lapacho is as a decoction (tea produced by boiling, rather than steeping) with the standard dose being 1 cup of decocted bark two to eight times per day. The decoction is made by boiling 1 teaspoon of lapacho for each cup of water for five to fifteen minutes.

Licorice *(Glycyrrhiza glabra)*

KEY USES OF LICORICE

Peptic ulcer

Premenstrual tension syndrome

Low adrenal function

Viral infections

Licorice root is one of the most extensively investigated botanical medicines. In addition to its use in peptic ulcers (see page 208), licorice can be used to balance estrogen levels in the premenstrual syndrome and during menopause; to improve adrenal function; and to enhance the immune system during viral infections.[40,41,42] It is important to follow a high-potassium, low-sodium diet when taking licorice. Taking too much licorice can lead to the loss of potassium and retention of sodium in the body. Licorice should not be used in patients with a history of high blood pressure, kidney failure, or current use of medicines for the heart. Three-times-daily dosages are:

Powdered root, 1 to 4 grams

Fluid extract (1:1), 4 to 6 milliliters (1 to 1½ teaspoons)

Solid (dry powdered) extract (4:1), 250 to 500 milligrams

Lobelia or Indian tobacco *(Lobelia inflata)*

KEY USES OF LOBELIA

Smoking deterrent

Expectorant in asthma, bronchitis, and pneumonia

Lobelia or Indian tobacco is an annual or biennial plant native to North America. The therapeutic actions of lobelia center around its lobeline content. Lobelia is a very effective expectorant in such conditions as pneumonia, asthma, and bronchitis.[43] Because lobeline has many of the same pharmacological actions as nicotine, it is often used orally as a smoking deterrent and to lessen nicotine withdrawal. Lobelia is safe at the prescribed levels. However, too much lobelia can produce severe nausea and vomiting as well as other signs of toxicity. Three-times-daily dosages are as follows:

Dried herb or as infusion (tea), 0.5 to 1 gram

Tincture (1:5), 4 to 6 milliliters (1 to 1½ teaspoons)

Fluid extract (1:1), 0.5 to 1 milliliter (⅛ to ¼ teaspoon)

Solid (dried powdered) extract (1 percent lobeline content), 200 milligrams

Mahuang (Ephedra sinica)

KEY USES OF MAHUANG

Asthma

Hay fever

Common cold

Weight-loss aid

Mahuang's medicinal use in China dates from approximately 2800 B.C. It was used primarily in the treatment of the common cold, asthma, hay fever, bronchitis, edema, arthritis, fever, hypotension, and hives. Western medicine's interest in mahuang began in 1923 with the demonstration that the isolated alkaloid ephedrine possessed a number of pharmacological effects. Ephedrine was synthesized in 1927, and since that time, both ephedrine and pseudoephedrine have been used extensively in over-the-counter cold and allergy medications.

The dosage of mahuang is dependent on the alkaloid content. The average total alkaloid content of *Ephedra sinica* is 1 to 3 percent. For asthma and as a weight-loss aid, the dose of ephedra should have an ephedrine content of 12.5 to 25.0 milligrams, and be taken two to three times daily. For the crude herb this would require a dose of 500 to 1,000 milligrams three times daily. Standardized preparations are preferred, as they are more dependable for therapeutic activity. For example, *Ephedra sinica* extracts are available with a standardized alkaloid content of 10 percent. The dosage of a 10-percent alkaloid-content extract would be 125 to 250 milligrams three times daily.

Too much ephedra can lead to increased blood pressure, increased heart rate, insomnia, and anxiety. Use should be discontinued upon the appearance of any of these symptoms. In addition, it is generally recommended that ephedra not be taken by patients with heart disease, high blood pressure, thyroid disease, diabetes, or difficulty in urination due to enlargement of the prostate gland; or by those on antidepressant drugs.

Milk thistle (Silybum marianum)

KEY USES OF MILK THISTLE

Liver disorders

Hepatitis

Cirrhosis of the liver

Psoriasis

Silybum marianum, or milk thistle, is a stout annual or biennial plant, found in dry rocky soils in southern and western Europe and some parts of the United States. The seeds, fruit, and leaves are used for medicinal purposes.

An extract of milk thistle known as silymarin is a remarkable medicine for the liver. In numerous clinical studies, silymarin has been shown to have positive effects in treating virtually every type of liver disease, including cirrhosis, hepatitis, and chemical- or alcohol-induced fatty liver.[44,45] The standard dose of milk thistle is based on its silymarin content (70 to 210 milligrams three times daily). For this reason, standardized extracts are preferred. Silymarin preparations are widely used in Europe, where a considerable body of evidence points to very low toxicity even when used for long periods of time.

Sarsaparilla (Smilax sarsaparilla)

KEY USES OF SARSAPARILLA

Psoriasis

Eczema

General tonic

Sarsaparilla species have been used all over the world in many different cultures for the same conditions, namely gout, arthritis, fevers, digestive disorders, and skin diseases. It contains saponins, or steroidlike
molecules, which bind to gut endotoxins. This effect may support the
plant's historical use as a "blood purifier" and tonic in human health
conditions associated with high endotoxin levels, most notably psoriasis,
eczema, arthritis, and ulcerative colitis.

In the United States, sarsaparilla has been widely touted as a "sexual
rejuvenator," with some commercial suppliers even claiming that it is a
rich source of human testosterone. The fact of the matter is that while
sarsaparilla may have good tonic effects, there is no actual testosterone
in the plant. It is unlikely that the steroidlike substances in sarsaparilla
are absorbed in any great degree. It is also unlikely that sarsaparilla has
any significant "anabolic" effects, as there is no clinical or experimental
evidence to support that it increases muscle mass.

The confusion arises because the sarsaparilla saponin, sarsapagenin,
can be synthetically transformed in the laboratory to testosterone. However, it is extremely unlikely that this reaction could take place in the
human body.

The three-times-daily dosage for sarsaparilla is as follows:

Dried root, 1 to 4 grams

Fluid extract (1:1), 8 to 16 milliliters (2 to 4 teaspoons)

Solid extract (4:1), 250 milligrams

Saw palmetto berry (Serenoa repens)

KEY USES OF SAW PALMETTO

Benign prostatic enlargement

Decreased function of testes

Serenoa repens (saw palmetto) is a small palm tree native to the
Atlantic coast of North America from South Carolina to Florida. The
berries of the plant are used for medicinal purposes, as discussed in

detail on page 215. For best results in the treatment of prostate enlargement, use the purified fat-soluble extract that contains not less than 85
percent and not more than 95 percent fatty acids and sterols. The dosage
is 160 milligrams twice daily.

St. John's wort (Hypericum perforatum)

KEY USES OF ST. JOHN'S WORT

Depression, anxiety

Sleep disturbances

AIDS (?)

St. John's wort, or hypericum, is a shrubby perennial plant native
to many parts of the world including Europe and the United States. A
tremendous amount of excitement about St. John's wort occurred after
researchers demonstrated in a preliminary study that the St. John's wort
components, hypericin and pseudohypericin, may inhibit a variety of
retroviruses including the retrovirus associated with AIDS (the human
immune-deficiency virus, or HIV).[46] More research is needed to determine if St. John's wort is an appropriate recommendation in AIDS
patients based on its antiviral activity.

Researchers have discovered that components in St. John's wort alter
brain chemistry in a way that improves mood, and there is clinical
research showing St. John's wort to be useful in relieving depression.
Clinical studies show a standardized extract of St. John's wort (0.125
percent hypericin) led to significant improvement in symptoms of anxiety, depression, and feelings of worthlessness.[47] In fact, the effectiveness
of the St. John's wort extract in relieving depression has been shown to
be greater than that produced by standard drugs used in depression,
including amitriptyline (Elavil) and imiprimine (Tofranil).[48] While these
drugs are associated with significant side effects (most often drowsiness,
dry mouth, constipation, and impaired urination), St. John's wort extract
is not associated with any significant side effect. In addition to improving
mood, the extract has been shown to greatly improve sleep quality, as
it was effective in relieving both insomnia and hypersomnia. No side
effects have been observed with the use of St. John's wort extract. The
dosage used in these studies has typically been 300 milligrams of the
extract (0.125 percent hypericin content) three times daily.

Tea tree oil (Melaleuca alternifolia)

KEY USES OF TEA TREE OIL

Topical antiseptic

Athlete's foot

Boils

Wound healing

Melaleuca alternifolia or "tea tree" is a small tree native to only one area of the world—the northeast coastal region of New South Wales, Australia. The leaves are the portion of the plant used medicinally; they are the source of a valuable therapeutic substance—tea tree oil. The medical world's first mention of tea tree appeared in the *Medical Journal of Australia* in 1930. A surgeon in Sydney reported some impressive results when a solution of tea tree oil was used for cleaning surgical wounds.[49]

Tea tree oil possesses significant antiseptic properties and is regarded by many as the ideal skin disinfectant. Reasons for this claim include its antimicrobial activity against a wide range of organisms; its good penetration of the skin; and its absence of irritating qualities. Tea tree oil has been used to treat the following conditions: acne, apthous stomatitis (canker sores), athlete's foot, boils, burns, carbuncles, corns, empyema, gingivitis, herpes, impetigo, infections of the nail bed, insect bites, lice, mouth ulcers, psoriasis, root canal soreness, skin and vaginal infections, ringworm and athlete's foot.[49]

A variety of products based on tea tree oil exist in the marketplace, including toothpastes, shampoos and conditioners, creams, hand and body lotions, soaps, gels, liniments, and nail polish removers. Apply as instructed on the product label.

Turmeric (Curcuma longa)

KEY USES OF TURMERIC AND CURCUMIN

Inflammation, arthritis

Liver and gallbladder disorders

The active component of turmeric is curcumin, a very powerful, yet safe, anti-inflammatory agent (see page 162). In addition to their use in inflammation, turmeric and curcumin have several other clinical applications. Most notable are atherosclerosis, liver disorders, gallstones, and the irritable bowel syndrome.

For medicinal effects, curcumin is recommended at a dose of 250 to 500 milligrams three times a day. Combining curcumin with bromelain may enhance its absorption and activity.

Uva ursi or bearberry (Arctostaphylos uva ursi)

KEY USES OF UVA URSI

Urinary tract infections

Water retention

Uva ursi is a small evergreen shrub found in the northern United States and in Europe. Uva ursi's most active ingredient is arbutin, which typically comprises 7 to 9 percent of the leaves.[50] At one time, arbutin was marketed as a urinary antiseptic and diuretic, despite the fact that the activity of arbutin is less than that of the total plant.[51] In order for arbutin to be active, it must be converted to another compound, hydroquinone, in the urinary tract. The arbutin molecule must be absorbed intact from the intestine. When arbutin is given alone, bacteria in the intestine break down much of the arbutin before it is absorbed. If the whole plant is given, the net effect is an increase in the amount of arbutin that is absorbed and converted to hydroquinone.

The activity of arbutin as an antibiotic in the urinary tract is dependent on an alkaline urine. The whole plant is of more value than isolated arbutin, as the other components of uva ursi serve to make the urine more alkaline. Three-times-daily dosages, during times of urinary-tract infection, are as follows:

Dried leaves or by infusion (tea), 1.5 to 4 grams

Tincture (1:5), 4 to 6 milliliters (1 to 1½ teaspoons)

Fluid extract (1:1), 0.5 to 2.0 milliliters (⅛ to ½ teaspoon)

Powdered solid extract (4:1), 250 to 500 milligrams

Valerian (Valeriana officinalis)

KEY USES OF VALERIAN

Insomnia

Anxiety

High blood pressure

Intestinal spasm

Valerian is a perennial plant native to North America and Europe. As discussed on page 226, valerian's prime use is as a sedative in the relief of insomnia, anxiety, and conditions associated with pain. Other conditions for which it has historically been used include migraine, hysteria, fatigue, intestinal cramps, and other nervous conditions. As a mild sedative, valerian may be taken in the following dosage thirty to forty-five minutes before retiring:

Dried root (or as tea), 1 to 2 grams

Tincture (1:5), 4 to 6 milliliters (1 to 1½ teaspoons)

Fluid extract (1:1), 1 to 2 milliliters (0.5 to 1 teaspoon)

Solid (dry powdered) extract (1.0 to 1.5 percent valtrate or 0.8 percent valeric acid), 150 to 300 milligrams

APPENDIX

Naturopathic Medical Schools, Physician Referral Organizations

Naturopathic Medical Schools

The Bastyr College of Natural Health Sciences in Seattle, Washington, is presently the only fully accredited school that trains naturopathic physicians, although the National College of Naturopathic Medicine in Portland, Oregon, is currently a candidate for accreditation. There is also a new school in Scottsdale, Arizona, the Southwest College of Naturopathic Medicine. All colleges offer a four-year doctoral program leading to the Doctor of Naturopathic Medicine (N.D.) degree. Pre-admission requirements at both schools are similar to those of conventional medical schools. For more information:

Bastyr College of Natural Health Sciences
144 N.E. 54th Street
Seattle, WA 98105
(206)523-9585

National College of Naturopathic Medicine
11231 S.E. Market Street
Portland, OR 97216
(503)255-4860

Southwest College of Naturopathic Medicine
6535 East Osborn Road
Scottsdale, AZ 85251
(602)998-0323

The American Association
of Naturopathic Physicians

The American Association of Naturopathic Physicians (AANP) is the professional organization of licensed naturopathic physicians. It is seeking to expand licensure of naturopaths in individual states and provinces. Although naturopaths practice in virtually every state and Canadian province, currently, only Alaska, Alberta, Arizona, British Columbia, Connecticut, District of Columbia, Hawaii, Manitoba, Montana, Ontario, Oregon, Saskatchewan, and Washington State offer licensure to naturopaths. The organization is also seeking to differentiate the professionally trained naturopath from unscrupulous individuals claiming to be naturopaths because they received a "mail order" degree. For more information and a referral service contact:

The American Association of Naturopathic Physicians
P.O. Box 20386
Seattle, WA 98102
(206)323-7610

American Holistic Medical Association

The American Holistic Medical Association is composed of medical doctors (M.D.s), osteopaths (D.O.s), and naturopaths (N.D.s) who share a common philosophy of encouraging personal responsibility for health and emphasizing the whole person.

American Holistic Medical Association
4101 Lake Boone Trail #201
Raleigh, NC 26707
(919)787-5146

GLOSSARY

Achlorhydria Absence of gastric acid

Acute Having a rapid onset, severe symptoms, and a short course; not chronic

Adrenaline A hormone that produces the "fight or flight" response; secreted by the adrenal gland. Also called epinephrine.

Aldosterone A hormone that causes the retention of sodium and water; secreted by the adrenal gland

Alkaloids A group of nitrogen-containing substances found in plants

Allopathy A term that describes the conventional method of medicine, which combats disease by using substances and techniques specifically against the disease or its symptoms

Amino acids A group of nitrogen-containing chemical compounds that form the basic structural units of proteins

Analgesic A substance that reduces the sensation of pain

Androgen A hormone that stimulates male characteristics

Anemia A condition in which the oxygen-carrying pigment (hemoglobin) in the blood is below normal limits

Anorexia The medical term for loss of appetite

Anthocyanidin A particular class of flavonoid that gives plants, fruits, and flowers colors ranging from red to blue

Antibody A protein manufactured by the body that binds to antigens to neutralize, inhibit, or destroy them

Antigen Any substance that, when introduced into the body, causes the formation of antibodies against it

Antihypertensive Blood pressure–lowering effect

Antioxidant A compound that prevents free-radical or oxidative damage

Artery A blood vessel that carries oxygen-rich blood away from the heart

Atherosclerosis A process in which fatty substances (cholesterol and triglycerides) are deposited in the walls of medium to large arteries, eventually leading to blockage of the artery

Autoimmune A process in which antibodies develop against the body's own tissues

Basal metabolic rate The rate of metabolism when the body is at rest

Basophil A type of white blood cell that is involved in allergic reactions

Benign Not serious. A mild disorder, usually not fatal.

Beta-carotene Pro-vitamin A. A plant carotene that can be converted to two vitamin A molecules.

Beta-cells The cells in the pancreas that manufacture insulin

Biofeedback A technique for developing conscious control of various involuntary functions like heart rate, intestinal motility, and body temperature

Bioflavonoid See **Flavonoid**.

Blood pressure The force exerted by blood as it presses against and attempts to stretch blood vessels

Bromelain The protein-digesting enzyme found in pineapple

Calorie A unit of heat. A nutritional calorie is the amount of heat necessary to raise 1 kilogram of water 1 degree Celsius.

Candida albicans A yeast common to the intestinal tract that can overgrow, leading to infection of the mouth, gastrointestinal tract, vagina, and other mucous membranes

Candidiasis A complex medical syndrome produced by a chronic overgrowth of the yeast *Candida albicans*

Carbohydrate Sugars and starches

Carcinogen Any agent or substance capable of causing cancer

Carcinogenesis The development of cancer caused by the actions of certain chemicals, viruses, and unknown factors on primarily normal cells

Cardiac output The volume of blood pumped from the heart in one minute

Cardiopulmonary Pertaining to the heart and lungs

Cardiotonic A compound that tones and strengthens the heart

Carotene A fat-soluble plant pigment, some of which can be converted into vitamin A by the body

Cartilage A type of connective tissue that acts as a shock absorber at joint interfaces

Cathartic A substance that stimulates the movement of the bowels, more powerful than a laxative

Cholagogue A compound that stimulates the contraction of the gallbladder

Choleretic A compound that promotes the flow of bile

Cholinergic Pertaining to the parasympathetic portion of the autonomic nervous system and the release of acetylcholine as a transmitter substance

Chronic Long-term or frequently recurring

Cirrhosis A severe disease of the liver characterized by the replacement of liver cells with scar tissue

Coenzyme A necessary nonprotein component of an enzyme, usually a vitamin or mineral

Colic Severe, spasmodic pain that occurs in waves of increasing intensity, reaches a peak, then abates for a short time before returning

Colitis Inflammation of the colon, usually accompanied by diarrhea with blood and mucus

Collagen The protein that is the main component of connective tissue

Congestive heart failure Chronic disease that results when the heart is not capable of supplying the oxygen demands of the body

Connective tissue The type of tissue that performs the function of providing support, structure, and cellular cement to the body

Coronary artery disease A condition that occurs when the heart receives an inadequate blood and oxygen supply due to atherosclerosis

Corticosteroid drugs A group of drugs similar to natural corticosteroid hormones, used predominately in the treatment of inflammation and to suppress the immune system

Corticosteroid hormones A group of hormones that control the body's use of nutrients and the excretion of salts and water in the urine; produced by the adrenal glands

Cushing's syndrome A condition caused by a hypersecretion of cortisone characterized by spindly legs, "moon face," "buffalo hump," abdominal obesity, flushed facial skin, and poor wound healing

Dehydration Excessive loss of water from the body

Demineralization   Loss of minerals from the bone

Dementia   Senility or loss of mental function

Dermatitis   Inflammation of the skin, sometimes due to allergy

Diastolic   The second number in a blood pressure reading, measuring pressure in arteries during the relaxation phase of the heartbeat

Disaccharide   A sugar composed of two monosaccharide units

Diuretic   A compound that causes increased urination

Diverticuli   Saclike outpouchings of the wall of the colon

Double-blind study   A way of controlling against experimental bias by insuring that neither the researcher nor the subject knows when an active agent or placebo is being used. If a placebo is used, the study is referred to as a double-blind placebo-controlled study.

Dysfunction   Abnormal function

Edema   Accumulation of fluid in tissues (swelling)

Eicosapentaenoic acid (EPA)   An omega-3 fatty acid found primarily in cold-water fish

Electroencephalogram   A machine that measures and records brain waves

Elimination diet   A diet that eliminates allergenic foods

Emulsify   The dispersement of large fat globules into smaller, uniformly distributed particles

Enteric-coated   A special way of coating a tablet or capsule to ensure that it does not dissolve in the stomach before it can reach the intestinal tract

Enzyme   An organic catalyst that speeds chemical reactions

Epidemiology   Study of the occurrence and distribution of diseases in human populations

Epinephrine   See **Adrenaline**.

Epithelium   The cells that cover the entire surface of the body and line most of the internal organs

Essential fatty acids   Fatty acids that the body cannot manufacture; linoleic and linolenic acids

Estrogens   Hormones that stimulate female sex characteristics

Excretion   The process of elimination of waste products from a cell, tissue, or the entire body

Extracellular   The fluid space outside a cell

Fibrin   A white, insoluble protein formed by the clotting of blood. It serves as the starting point for wound repair and scar formation.

Fibrinolysis The dissolution of fibrin or a blood clot by the action of enzymes that convert insoluble fibrin into soluble particles

Flavonoids Plant pigments responsible for the color of many fruits and flowers. They exert a wide variety of physiological effects on the human body.

Free radicals Highly reactive molecules, characterized by an unpaired electron, that can bind to and destroy cellular compounds

Gerontology The study of aging

Glucose A monosaccharide found in the blood; one of the body's primary energy sources

Goblet cell A goblet-shaped cell that secretes mucus

Ground substance The thick, gellike material in which the cells' fibers, and blood capillaries of cartilage, bone, and connective tissue are embedded

Helper T cell Lymphocytes that help in the immune response

Hematocrit An expression of the percentage of blood occupied by blood cells

Holistic medicine A form of therapy aimed at treating the whole person, not just the part or parts in which symptoms occur

Hormone A secretion of an endocrine gland that controls and regulates body functions

Hyperglycemia High blood sugar

Hypersecretion Excessive secretion

Hypertension High blood pressure

Hypochlorhydria Insufficient gastric acid output

Hypoglycemia Low blood sugar

Hypolipidemic Characterized by elevations of cholesterol and triglycerides in the blood

Hypotension Low blood pressure

Immunoglobulins Antibodies

Incidence The number of new cases of a disease that occur during a given period (usually years) in a defined population

Infarction Death to a localized area of tissue due to lack of oxygen supply

Insulin A hormone that lowers blood sugar levels; secreted by the pancreas

Interferon A potent immune-enhancing substance that is produced by the body's cells to fight off viral infection and cancer

Jaundice   A condition caused by elevation of bilirubin in the body and characterized by yellowing of the skin

Keratin   An insoluble protein found in hair, skin, and nails

Lesion   Any localized, abnormal change in tissue formation

Lethargy   A feeling of tiredness, drowsiness, or lack of energy

Leukocyte   White blood cell

Leukotrienes   Inflammatory compounds produced when oxygen interacts with polyunsaturated fatty acids

Lipids   Fats, phospholipids, steroids, and prostaglandins

Lipotropic   Promoting the flow of lipids to and from the liver

Lymph   Fluid that flows through the lymphatic system to be returned to the blood; contained in lymphatic vessels

Lymphocyte   A type of white blood cell found primarily in lymph nodes

Macular degeneration   A degenerative condition of the portion of the retina responsible for vision

Malabsorption   Impaired absorption of nutrients, most often due to diarrhea

Malaise   A vague feeling of being sick or of physical or mental discomfort

Malignant   A term used to describe a condition that tends to worsen and eventually cause death

Mast cell   A cell found in many tissues of the body that contributes greatly to allergic and inflammatory processes by secreting histamine and other inflammatory particles

Metabolism   A collective term for all the chemical processes that take place in the body

Metabolite   A product of a chemical reaction

Metalloenzyme   An enzyme containing a metal at its active site

Microbe   A popular term for microorganism

Molecule   The smallest complete unit of a substance that can exist independently and still retain the characteristic properties of the substance

Monosaccharide   A simple, one-unit, sugar like fructose and glucose

Mortality rate   The number of deaths per one hundred thousand of a given population per year

Mucosa   Another term for mucous membrane

Mucous membrane   The soft, pink tissue that lines most of the cavities and tubes in the body, including the respiratory tract, gastrointestinal tract, genitourinary tract, and eyelids. Mucous membrane secretes mucus.

Mucus   The slick, slimy fluid that is secreted by and acts as a lubricant and mechanical protector of the mucous membranes

Myelin sheath   A white fatty substance that surrounds nerve cells to aid in nerve-impulse transmission

Neoplasia   Medical term for a tumor formation, characterized by a progressive, abnormal replication of cells

Neurofibrillary tangles   Clusters of degenerated nerves

Neurotransmitters   Substances that modify or transmit nerve impulses

Night blindness   The inability to see well in dim light or at night

Nocturia   The disturbance of a person's sleep at night by the need to pass urine

Oligoantigenic diet   See **Elimination diet**

Otitis media   Acute infection of the middle ear

Pancreatin   A product that contains a potent concentration of digestive enzymes; obtained from the pancreas of a pig

Papain   The protein-digesting enzyme of papaya

Parkinson's disease   A slowly progressive, degenerating nervous-system disease characterized by resting tremor, pill rolling of the fingers, a masklike facial expression, shuffling gait, and muscle rigidity and weakness

Pathogen   Any agent, particularly a microorganism, that causes disease

Pathogenesis   The process by which a disease originates and develops, particularly the cellular and physiologic processes

Peristalsis   Successive muscular contractions of the intestines as they move food through the intestinal tract

Physiology   Study of the functioning of the body, including the physical and chemical processes of cells, tissues, organs, and systems

Physostigmine   A drug that blocks the breakdown of acetylcholine

Phytoestrogen   A plant compound that exerts estrogen effects

Piles   A common name for hemorrhoids

Placebo   An inert or inactive substance used for comparison to test the efficacy of another substance

Polysaccharide   A molecule composed of many sugar molecules linked together

Prostaglandin   A hormonelike compound manufactured from essential fatty acids

Psychosomatic   Pertaining to the relationship of the mind and body.

Commonly used to refer to those physiological disorders thought to be caused entirely or partly by psychological factors.

Putrefaction The process of breaking down protein compounds by rotting

Recommended Dietary Allowance (RDA) Recommended dietary allowance of vitamins and minerals needed daily to maintain a healthy body

Saccharide A sugar molecule

Satiety A feeling of fullness or gratification

Saturated fat A fat whose carbon atoms are bonded to the maximum number of hydrogen atoms; found in animal products like meat, milk, milk products, and eggs

Sclerosis The process of hardening or scarring

Senile dementia Mental deterioration associated with aging

Submucosa The tissue just below the mucous membrane

Suppressor T cell Lymphocytes controlled by the thymus gland that suppress the immune response

Syndrome A group of signs and symptoms that occur together in a pattern characteristic of a particular disease or abnormal condition

T cell A lymphocyte that is under the control of the thymus gland

Tonic A substance that exerts a gentle strengthening effect on the body

Trans-fatty acid The type of fat found in margarine

Uremia The retention of urine by the body and the presence of high levels of urine components in the blood

Urinalysis The analysis of urine

Urticaria Hives

Vasoconstriction The constriction of blood vessels

Vitamin An essential compound necessary to act as a catalyst in normal processes of the body

Western diet A diet characteristic of Western societies; that is, a diet high in fat, refined carbohydrates, and processed foods, and low in dietary fiber

Wheal The characteristic lesion in hives; a small welt

SOURCE NOTES

Chapter 1 — Making Medicine or Making Money?

1. Administrative Prices: Hearing Before the Subcommittee on Antitrust and Monopoly of the Committee of the Judiciary, U.S. Senate. U.S. Government Printing Office. Washington, DC, 1960
2. Dickson M: The pricing of pharamceuticals: An international comparison. Clin Therap 14:604–610, 1992
3. Safavi K T and Hayward R A: Choosing between apples and apples: Physicians' choices of prescription drugs that have similar side effects and efficacies. J Gen Int Med 7:32–37, 1992
4. Goldfinger S E: Physicians and the pharmaceutical industry. Ann Int Med 112:624–626, 1990
5. Council on Ethical and Judicial Affairs of the American Medical Association: Gifts to physicians from industry. JAMA 265:501, 1991
6. Waud D R: Pharmaceutical promotions—A free lunch? New Eng J Med 327:351–353, 1992
7. Wilkes M S, Doblin B H, and Shapiro M F: Pharmaceutical advertisements in leading medical journals: Experts' assessments. Ann Int Med 116:912–919, 1992
8. Avorn J, Chen M, and Hartley R: Scientific versus commercial sources of influence on the prescribing behavior of physicians. Am J Med 73:4–8, 1982
9. Leigh J P: International comparisons of physicians' salaries. Int J Health Serv 22:217–220, 1992

10. Curzer H J: Do physicians make too much money? Theoretical Med 13:45–65, 1992

11. Salive M E: The practice and earnings of preventive-medicine physicians. Am J Prev Med 8:257–262, 1992

12. Wortis J and Stone A: The addiction to drug companies. Biol Psychiatry 32:847–849, 1992

Chapter 2 — Natural Medicine:
A Rational Alternative

1. White L B, Tursky B, and Schwartz G (eds.): Placebos: Theory, Research and Mechanisms. Guilford, New York, NY, 1985

2. Ader R (ed.): Psychoneuroimmunology. Academic Press, New York, NY, 1981

3. Justiani F R: Iatrogenic disease: An overview. M Sinai J Med 51:210–214, 1984

4. Amundson L H: Iatrogenesis: A review. Continuing Ed June: 411–424, 1985

5. Steel K, Gertman P M, Crescenzi C, and Anderson J: Iatrogenic illness on a general medical service at a university hospital. New Eng J Med 304:638–642, 1981

6. National Research Council: Nutrition Education in U.S. Medical Schools. National Academy Press, Washington, DC, 1985

Chapter 3 — Acne Medications

1. Michaelsson G, Vahlquist A, and Juhlin L: Serum zinc and retinol-binding protein in acne. Br J Dermatol 96:283–286, 1977

2. Michaelsson G, Juhlin L, and Ljunghall K: A double-blind study of the effect of zinc and oxytetracycline in acne vulgaris. Br J Dermatol 97:561–565, 1977

3. Cunliffe W J, Burke B, Dodman B, and Gould D J: A double-blind

trial of a zinc sulphate/citrate complex and tetracycline in the treatment of acne. Br J Dermatol 101:321–325, 1979

4. Dreno B, Amblard P, Agache P, et al.: Low doses of zinc gluconate for inflammatory acne. Acta Derm Venereol 69:541–543, 1989

5. Weimar V, Puhl S, Smith W, and Broeke J: Zinc sulphate in acne vulgaris. Arch Dermatol 114:1776–1778, 1978

6. Kugman A, Mills O, Leyden J, et al.: Oral vitamin A in acne vulgaris. Int J Dermatol 20:278–285, 1981

7. Semon H and Herrmann F: Some observations on the sugar metabolism in acne vulgaris, and its treatment by insulin. Br J Dermatol 52:123–128, 1940

8. Grover R and Arikan N: The effect of intralesional insulin and glucagon in acne vulgaris. L Invest Dermatol 40:259–261, 1963

9. Abdel K M, El Mofty A, Ismail A, and Bassili F: Glucose tolerance in blood and skin of patients with acne vulgaris. Ind J Dermatol 22:139–149, 1977

10. Offenbach E and Pistunyer F: Beneficial effect of chromium-rich yeast on glucose tolerance and blood lipids in elderly patients. Diabetes 29:919–925, 1980

11. McCarthy M: High-chromium yeast for acne? Med Hypoth 14:307–310, 1984

12. Michaelsson G and Edqvist L: Erythrocyte glutathione peroxidase activity in acne vulgaris and the effect of selenium and vitamin E treatment. Acta Dermatol Venereol (StockH) 64:9–14, 1984

13. Snider B and Dieteman D: Pyridoxine therapy for premenstrual acne flare. Arch Dermatol 110:103–111, 1974

14. Bassett I B, Pannowitz D L and Barnetson RSC: A comparative study of tea-tree oil versus benzoyl peroxide in the treatment of acne. Med J Australia 153:455–458, 1990

Chapter 4 — Angina Medications

1. Cherchi A, Lai C, Angelino F, et al.: Effects of L-carnitine on exercise tolerance in chronic stable angina: a multicenter, double-blind, randomized, placebo-controlled crossover study. Int J Clin Pharm Ther Toxicol 23:569–572, 1985

Orlando G and Rusconi C: Oral L-carnitine in the treatment of chronic cardiac ischaemia in elderly patients. Clin Trials J 23:338–344, 1986

Kamikawa T, Suzuki Y, Kobayashi A, et al.: Effects of L-carnitine on exercise tolerance in patients with stable angina pectoris. Jap Heart J 25:587–597, 1984

Pola P, Savi L, Serrichio M, et al.: Use of physiological substance, acetyl-carnitine, in the treatment of angiospastic syndromes. Drugs Exptl Clin Res X:213–217, 1984

2. Opie L H: Role of carnitine in fatty acid metabolism of normal and ischemic myocardium. Am Heart J 97:373–378, 1979

3. Rebuzzi A G, Schiavoni G, Amico C M, et al.: Beneficial effects of L-carnitine in the reduction of the necrotic area in acute myocardial infarction. Drugs Exptl Clin Res 10:219–223, 1984

4. Folkers K and Yamamura Y (eds.): Biomedical and Clinical Aspects of Coenzyme Q_{10}, volumes 1–4. Elsevier Science Publ, Amsterdam, vol. 1:1977, vol. 2:1980, vol. 3:1982, vol. 4:1984

Folkers K, Vadhanavikit S, and Mortensen S A: Biochemical rationale and myocardial tissue data on the effective therapy of cardiomyopathy with coenzyme Q_{10}. Proc Natl Acad Sci 82:901–904, 1985

Mortensen S A, Vadhanavikit S, and Folkers K: Deficiency of coenzyme Q_{10} in myocardial failure. Drugs Exptl Clin Res 10:487–502, 1984

5. Kitamura N, Yamaguchi A, Otaki M, Sawatani O, et al.: Myocardial tissue level of coenzyme Q_{10} in patients with cardiac failure. In: Folkers K, Yamamura Y (eds): Biomedical and Clinical Aspects of Coenzyme Q_{10}, vol. 4: 243–252. Elsevier Science Publ, Amsterdam, 1984

Littarru G P, Ho L, and Folkers K: Deficiency of coenzyme Q_{10} in human heart disease, Part II. Int J Vit Nutr Res 42:413, 1972

Folkers K, Littarru G P, Ho L, et al.: Evidence for a deficiency of coenzyme Q_{10} in human heart disease. Int J Vit Nutr Res 40:380, 1970

Folkers K, Vadhanavikit S, and Mortensen S A: Biochemical rationale and myocardial tissue data on the effective therapy of cardiomyopathy with coenzyme Q_{10}. Proc Natl Acad Sci 82:901, 1985

6. Kamikawa T, Kobayashi A, Yamashita T, et al.: Effects of coenzyme Q_{10} on exercise tolerance in chronic stable angina pectoris. Am J Cardiol 56:247, 1985

7. Turlapaty PDMV and Altura B M: Magnesium deficiency produces spasms of coronary arteries: Relationship to etiology of sudden-death ischemic heart disease. Sci 208:199–200, 1980

Altura B M: Ischemic heart disease and magnesium. Magnesium 7:57–67, 1988

8. Lindberg J S, Zobitz M M, Poindexter J R, and Pak CYC: Magnesium bioavailability from magnesium citrate and magnesium oxide. J Am Coll Nutr 9:48–55, 1990

9. Petkov V: Plants with hypotensive, antiatheromatous and coronarodilating action. Am J Chin Med 7:197–236, 1979

Ammon HPT and Handel M: Crataegus, toxicology and pharmacology. Planta Medica 43:101–120, 318–322, 1981

O'Conolly V M, Jansen W, Bernhoft G, and Bartsch G: Treatment of cardiac performance (NYHA stages I to II) in advanced age with standardized crataegus extract. Fortschr Med 104:805–808, 1986

10. Mavers VWH and Hensel H: Changes in local myocardial blood flow following oral administration of a crataegus extract to non-anesthetized dogs. Arzneim Forsch 24:783–785, 1974

Roddewig V C and Hensel H: Reaction of local myocardial blood flow in non-anesthetized dogs and anesthetized cats to oral and parenteral application of a crataegus fraction (oligomere procyanidins). Arzneim Forsch 27:1407–1410, 1977

Rewerski V W, Piechocki T, Tyalski M, and Lewak S: Some pharmacological properties of oligomeric procyanidin isolated from hawthorn (Crataegus oxyacantha). Arzneim Forsch 17:490–491, 1967

11. Osher H L, Katz K H, and Wagner D J: Khellin in the treatment of angina pectoris. New Eng J Med 244:315–321, 1951

12. Anrep G V, Kenawy M R, and Barsoum G S: Coronary vasodilator action of khellin. Am Heart J 37:531–542, 1949

Conn J J, Kisane R W, Koons R A, and Clark T E: Treatment of angina pectoris with khellin. Ann Int Med 36:1173–1178, 1952

Chapter 5 — Antacids

1. Graham D Y, Smith J L, and Patterson D J: Why do apparently healthy people use antacid tablets? Am J Gastroenterol 78:257–260, 1983

2. Bolla K I, Briefel G, Spector D, et al.: Neurocognitive effects of aluminum. Arch Neurol 49:1021–1026, 1992

Flaten T P: Geographical associations between aluminum in drinking water and death rates with dementia (including Alzheimer's disease), Parkinson's disease, and amyotrophic sclerosis in Norway. Environ Geochem Health 12:152–157, 1990

Perl D P, Gajdusek D C, Garruto R M, et al.: Intraneuronal aluminum accumulation in amyotrophic lateral sclerosis and Parkinsonism-dementia of Guam. Science 217:1053–1055, 1982

3. Weberg R and Berstad A: Gastrointestinal absorption of aluminum from single doses of aluminum-containing antacids in man. Eur J Clin Invest 16:428–432, 1986

Weberg R, Berstad A, Aaseth J, and Falch J A: Mineral-metabolic side effects of low-dose antacids. Scand J Gastroenterol 20:741–746, 1985

Taylor G A, Ferrier I N, McLoughlin I J, et al.: Gastrointestinal absorption of aluminum in Alzheimer's disease: Response to aluminum citrate. Age Ageing 21:81–90, 1992

4. Grossman M, Kirsner J, and Gillespie I: Basal and histalog-stimulated gastric secretion in control subjects and in patients with peptic ulcer or gastric cancer. Gastroenterol 45:15–26, 1963

5. Recker R: Calcium absorption and achlorhydria. New Eng J Med 313:70–73, 1985

6. Nicar M J and Pak CYC: Calcium bioavailability from calcium carbonate and calcium citrate. J Clin Endocrin Metab 61:391–393, 1985

7. Editorial: Citrate for calcium nephrolithiasis. Lancet i:955, 1986

8. Cushner H M, Copley J B, and Foulks C J: Calcium citrate, a new phosphate-binding and alkalinizing agent for patients with renal failure. Curr Ther Res 40:998–1004, 1986

9. Barrie S A: Heidelberg pH capsule gastric analysis. In: Pizzorno J E and Murray M T: A Textbook of Natural Medicine. JBC Publ, Seattle, WA, 1985

Bray G W: The hypochlorhydria of asthma in childhood. Br Med J i:181–197, 1930

Rabinowitch I M: Achlorhydria and its clinical significance in diabetes mellitus. Am J Dig Dis 18:322–333, 1949

Carper W M, Butler T J, Kilby J O, and Gibson M J: Gallstones, gastric secretion and flatulent dyspepsia. Lancet i:413–415, 1967

Rawls W B and Ancona V C: Chronic urticaria associated with hypochlorhydria or achlorhydria. Rev Gastroent Oct:267–271, 1950

Gianella R A, Broitman S A, and Zamcheck N: Influence of gastric acidity on bacterial and parasitic enteric infections. Ann Int Med 78:271–276, 1973

De Witte T J, Geerdink P J, and Lamers C B: Hypochlorhydria and hypergastrinaemia in rheumatoid arthritis. Ann Rheum Dis 38:14–17, 1979

Ryle J A and Barber H W: Gastric analysis in acne rosacea. Lancet ii:1195–1196, 1920

Ayres S: Gastric secretion in psoriasis, eczema and dermatitis herpetiformis. Arch Derm July:854–859, 1929

Dotevall G and Walan A: Gastric secretion of acid and intrinsic factor in patients with hyper and hypothyroidism. Acta Med Scand 186:529–533, 1969

Howitz J and Schwartz M: Vitiligo, achlorhydria, and pernicious anemia. Lancet i:1331–1334, 1971

10. Rafsky H A and Weingarten M: A study of the gastric secretory response in the aged. Gastroenterol May:348–352, 1946

Davies D and James T G: An investigation into the gastric secretion of a hundred normal persons over the age of sixty. Brit J Med i:1–14, 1930

11. Mojaverian P, et al.: Estimation of gastric residence time of the Heidelberg capsule in humans. Gastroenterol 89:392–397, 1985

12. Wright J: A proposal for standardized challenge testing of gastric acid secretory capacity using the Heidelberg capsule radiotelemetry system. J John Bastyr Coll Nat Med 1:3–11, 1979

Chapter 6 — Arthritis Medications

1. Murray M T and Pizzorno J E: Encyclopedia of Natural Medicine. Prima Publ, Rocklin, CA, 1990

2. Petersdorf R et al. (eds.): Harrison's Principles of Internal Medicine. McGraw-Hill, New York, NY, 1983, pp. 517–524

3. Bland J H and Cooper S M: Osteoarthritis: A review of the cell biology involved and evidence for reversibility. Management rationally related to known genesis and pathophysiology. Seminars Arthr Rheum 14:106–133, 1984

4. Sokoloff L (ed.): Osteoarthritis. Clinics in Rheum Dis 11:(2), 1985

5. Brooks P M, Potter S R, and Buchanan W W: NSAID and osteoarthritis—help or hindrance? J Rheumatol 9:3–5, 1982

6. Perry G H, Smith MJG, and Whiteside C G: Spontaneous recovery of the hip joint space in degenerative hip disease. Ann Rheum Dis 31:440–448, 1972

7. Newman NM and Ling RSM: Acetabular bone destruction related to non-steroidal anti-inflammatory drugs. Lancet: ii; 11–13, 1985

8. Solomon L: Drug-induced arthropathy and necrosis of the femoral head. J Bone Joint Surg 55B:246–251, 1973

9. Ronningen H and Langeland N: Indomethacin treatment in osteoarthritis of the hip joint. Acta Orthop Scand 50:169–174, 1979

10. Smith M D, Gibson R A, and Brooks P M: Abnormal bowel permeability in ankylosing spondylitis and rheumatoid arthritis. J Rheumatol 12:299–305, 1985

Zaphiropoulos G C: Rheumatoid arthritis and the gut. Br J Rheumatol 25:138–140, 1986

Segal A W, Isenberg D A, Hajirousou V, et al.: Preliminary evidence for gut involvement in the pathogenesis of rheumatoid arthritis. B J Rheumatol 25:162–166, 1986

11. Bjarnason I, So A, Levi A J, et al.: Intestinal permeability and inflammation in rheumatoid arthritis: Effects of nonsteroidal anti-inflammatory drugs. Lancet ii:1171–1174, 1984

12. Sullivan M X and Hess W C: Cystine content of fingernails in arthritis. J Bone Joint Surg 16:185–188, 1935

13. Senturia B D: Results of treatment of chronic arthritis and rheumatoid conditions with colloidal sulphur. J Bone Joint Surg 16:119–125, 1934

14. Childers N F: A Diet to Stop Arthritis. Somerset Press, Somerville, NJ, 1981

15. Darlington L G, Ramsey N W, and Mansfield J R: Placebo-controlled blind study of dietary manipulation therapy in rheumatoid arthritis. Lancet i:236–238, 1986

Hicklin J A, McEwen L M, and Morgan J E: The effect of diet in rheumatoid arthritis. Clin Allergy 10:463–467, 1980

Panush R S: Delayed reactions to foods: Food allergy and rheumatic disease. Ann Allergy 56:500–503, 1986

16. Skoldstam L, Larsson L, and Lindstrom F D: Effects of fasting and lactovegetarian diet on rheumatoid arthritis. Scandinav J Rheumatol 8:249–255, 1979

Kroker G P, Stroud R M, Marshall R T, et al.: Fasting and rheumatoid arthritis: A multicenter study. Clin Ecology 2:137–144, 1984

17. Kjeldsen-Kragh J, Haugen M, Borchgrevink C F, et al.: Controlled trial of fasting and one-year vegetarian diet in rheumatoid arthritis. Lancet 338:899–902, 1991

18. Kremer J, Michaelek A V, Lininger L, et al.: Effects of manipulation of dietary fatty acids on clinical manifestation of rheumatoid arthritis. Lancet i:184–187, 1985

Nielsen G L, Faarvang K L, Thomsen B S, et al.: The effects of dietary supplementation with n-3 polyunsaturated fatty acids in patients with rheumatoid arthritis: a randomized, double-blind trial. Eur J Clin Invest 22:687–691, 1992

19. Darlington L G: Do diets rich in polyunsaturated fatty acids affect disease activity in rheumatoid arthritis? Ann Rheum Dis 47:169–172, 1988

Jantti J, Nikkari T, Solakivi T, et al.: Evening primrose oil in rheumatoid arthritis: Changes in serum lipids and fatty acids. Ann Rheum Dis 48:124–127, 1989

20. Cody V, Middleton E, and Harborne J B: Plant Flavonoids in Biology and Medicine—Biochemical, Pharmacological, and Structure-activity Relationships. Alan R Liss, New York, NY, 1986

Cody V, Middleton E, Harborne J B, and Beretz A: Plant Flavonoids in Biology and Medicine II—Biochemical, Pharmacological, and Structure-activity Relationships. Alan R Liss, New York, NY, 1988

21. Srivastava K C and Mustafa T: Ginger (Zingiber officinale) and rheumatic disorders. Med Hypoth 29:25–28, 1989

22. Setnikar I, Pacini A, and Revel L: Antiarthritic effects of glucosamine sulfate studied in animal models. Arzneim Forsch 41:542–545, 1991

23. Vaz A L: Double-blind clinical evaluation of the relative efficacy of ibuprofen and glucosamine sulfate in the management of osteoarthrosis of the knee in out-patients. Curr Med Res Opin 8:145–149, 1982

Crolle G and D'este E: Glucosamine sulfate for the management of arthrosis: a controlled clinical investigation. Curr Med Res Opin 7:104–114, 1981

Tapadinhas M J, Rivera I C, and Bignamini A A: Oral glucosamine sulfate in the management of arthrosis: report on a multi-centre open investigation in Portugal. Pharmatherapeutica 3:157–168, 1982

D'Ambrosia E D, Casa B, Bompani R, Scali G, and Scali M: Glucosamine sulfate: a controlled clinical investigation in arthrosis. Pharma-therapeutica 2:504–508, 1982

24. Vaz A L: Double-blind clinical evaluation of the relative efficacy of ibuprofen and glucosamine sulfate in the management of osteoarthrosis of the knee in out-patients. Curr Med Res Opin 8:145–149, 1982

25. Schwartz E R: The modulation of osteoarthritic development by vitamins C and E. Int J Vit Nutr Res supplement 26:141–146, 1984

      Bates C J: Proline and hydroxyproline excretion and vitamin C status in elderly human subjects. Clin Sci Molec Med 52:535–543, 1977

      Krystal G, Morris G M, and Sokoloff L: Stimulation of DNA synthesis by ascorbate in cultures of articular chondrocytes. Arth Rheum 25:318–325, 1982

26. Mullen A and Wilson CWM: The metabolism of ascorbic acid in rheumatoid arthritis. Proc Nutr Sci 35:8A–9A, 1976

27. Subramanian N: Histamine degradation potential of ascorbic acid. Agents and Actions 8:484–487, 1978

      Levine M: New concepts in the biology and biochemistry of ascorbic acid. New Eng J Med 314:892–902, 1986

28. Machtey, I. and Ouaknine: L. Tocopherol in osteoarthritis: A controlled pilot study. J Am Geriat Soc. 1978: 26; 328–330

29. Schwartz E R: The modulation of osteoarthritic development by vitamins C and E. Int J Vit Nutr Res supplement 26:141–146, 1984

30. Munthe E and Aseth J: Treatment of rheumatoid arthritis with selenium and vitamin E. Scand J Rheumatol 53(suppl.):103, 1984

31. Tarp U, Overvad K, Hansen J C, and Thorling E B: Low selenium level in severe rheumatoid arhtritis. Scand J Rheumatol 14:97–101, 1985

      Tarp U, Overvad K, Thorling E B, Hansen J C, and Graudal H: Selenium treatment in rheumatoid arhtritis. Scand J Rheumatol 14:364–368, 1985

32. Pandley S P, Bhattacharya S K, and Sundar S: Zinc in rheumatoid arthritis. Indian J Med Res 81:618–620, 1985

      Simkin P A: Treatment of rheumatoid arthritis with oral zinc sulfate. Agents and Actions (supplement) 8:587–595, 1981

      Mattingly P C and Mowat A G: Zinc sulphate in rheumatoid arthritis. Ann Rheum Dis 41:456–457, 1982

33. Pasquier C, Mach P S, Raichvarg D, et al.: Manganese-containing superoxide-dismutase deficiency in polymorphonuclear leukocytes of adults with rheumatoid arthritis. Inflammation 8:27–32, 1984

34. Barton-Wright E C and Elliott W A: The pantothenic acid metabolism of rheumatoid arthritis. Lancet ii:862–863, 1963

35. General Practitioner Research Group: Calcium pantothenate in arthritis conditions (report). Practitioner 224:208–211, 1980

36. Anand J C: Osteoarthritis and pantothenic acid. J Coll Gen Pract 5:136–137, 1963

Anand J C: Osteoarthritis and pantothenic acid. Lancet ii:1168, 1963

37. Kaufman, W. The Common Form of Joint Dysfunction: Its Incidence and Treatment. E. L. Hildreth Company, Brattleboro, VT, 1949

Hoffer, A: Treatment of arthritis by nicotinic acid and nicotinamide. Canad Med Ass J 81:235–239, 1959

38. Marcolongo R, Giordano N, Colombo B, et al.: Double-blind multicentre study of the activity of S-adenosyl-methionine in hip osteoarthritis. Curr Therap Res 37:82–94, 1985

39. Di Padova C: S-Adenosylmethionine in the treatment of osteoarthritis: Review of clinical studies. Am J Med 83:Supplement 5A:60–65, 1987

40. Taussig S and Batkin S: Bromelain, the enzyme complex of pineapple (Ananas comosus), and its clinical application: An update. J Ethnopharmacol 22:191–203, 1988

Murray M T: Healing Power of Herbs. Prima Publishing, Rocklin, CA, 1991

41. Srimal R and Dhawan B: Pharmacology of diferuloyl methane (curcumin), a non-steroidal anti-inflammatory agent. J Pharm Pharmac 25:447–452, 1973

42. Deodhar S D, Sethi R, and Srimal R C: Preliminary studies on antirheumatic activity of curcumin (diferuloyl methane). Ind J Med Res 71:632–4, 1980

43. Wright V: Treatment of osteo-arthritis of the knees. Ann Rheum Dis 23:389–391, 1964

Clarke G R, Willis L A, Stenner L, and Nichols P J R: Evaluation of physiotherapy in the treatment of osteoarthrosis of the knee. Rheumatol Rehab 13:190–197, 1974

Vanharantha H: Effect of shortwave diathermy on mobility and radiological stage of the knee in the development of experimental osteoarthritis. Am J Phys Med 61:59–65, 1982

Chapter 7 — Asthma, Hayfever, and Antihistamine Medications

1. Kaliner M and Lemanske R: Rhinitis and asthma. JAMA 268:2807–2829, 1992

2. Sly R M: Asthma mortality, East and West. Ann Allergy 69:81–84, 1992

3. Irving A and Jones W: Methods for testing impairment of driving due to drugs. Eur J Clin Pharm 43:61–66, 1992

4. Kemp J P: Antihistamines—is there anything safe to prescribe? Ann Allergy 69:276–280, 1992

5. Shirakawa T and Morimoto K: Lifestyle effect on total IgE. Allergy 46:561–569, 1991

6. Brostoff J and Challacombe S J (eds.): Food Allergy and Intolerance. W B Saunders, Philadelphia, PA, 1987

7. Heiner D C: Respiratory diseases and food allergy. Ann Allergy 53:657–664, 1984

8. Pelikan Z: Nasal response to food ingestion challenge. Arch Otolaryngol Head Neck Surg 114:525–530, 1988

9. Warrington R J, Sauder P J, and McPhillips S: Cell-mediated immune responses to artificial food additives in chronic urticaria 16:527–533, 1986

10. Freedman B J: A diet free from additives in the management of allergic disease. Clin Allergy 7:417–421, 1977

11. Lindahl O, Lindwall L, Spangberg A, et al.: Vegan diet regimen with reduced medication in the treatment of bronchial asthma. J Asthma 22:45–55, 1985

12. Dorsch W and Weber J: Prevention of allergen-induced bronchial constriction in sensitized guinea pigs by crude alcohol-onion extract. Agents Actions 14:626–630, 1984

13. Olusi S O, Ojutiku O O, Jessop WJE, and Iboko M I: Plasma and white blood cell ascorbic-acid concentrations in patients with bronchial asthma. Clinica Chimica Acta 92:161–166, 1979

14. Anderson R, Hay I, Van Wyk H A, and Theron A: Ascorbic acid in bronchial asthma. S A Med J 63:649–652, 1983

15. Spannhake E W and Menkes H A: Vitamin C—New tricks for an old dog. Am Rev Resp Dis 127:139–141, 1983

16. Johnston C S, Retrum K R, and Srilakshmi J C: Antihistamine effects and complications of supplemental vitamin C. J Am Diet Assoc 92:988–989, 1992

17. Foreman J C: Mast cells and the actions of flavonoids. J Allergy Clin Immunol 127:546–550, 1984

18. Cody V, Middleton E, Harborne J B, and Beretz A: Plant Flavonoids in Biology and Medicine II—Biochemical, Pharmacological, and Structure-activity Relationships. Alan R Liss, New York, NY, 1988

19. Petrakis P L, Kallianos A G, Wender S H, et al.: Metabolic studies of quercetin labelled with C_{14}. Arch Biochem and Biophys 85:264–271, 1959

20. Taussig S: The mechanism of the physiological action of bromelain. Med Hypoth 6:99–104, 1980

21. Personal communication with Jonathan Wright, M.D., Kent, Washington, June 1985

22. Simon S W: Vitamin B_{12} therapy in allergy and chronic dermatoses. J Allergy 2:183–185, 1951

23. Garrison R and Somer E: The Nutrition Desk Reference, Chapter 5—Vitamin Research: Selected Topics, pp 93–94. Keats Publ, New Canaan, CT, 1985

24. Collip P J, Goldzier S III, Weiss N, et al.: Pyridoxine treatment of childhood asthma. Ann Allergy 35:93–97, 1975

25. Reynolds R D and Natta C L: Depressed plasma pyridoxal phosphate concentrations in adult asthmatics. Am J Clin Nutr 41:684–688, 1985

26. Duke J A and Ayensu E S: Medicinal Plants of China. Reference Publications, Algonac, MI, 1985

27. Kasahara Y, Hikino H, Tsurufuji S, et al.: Anti-inflammatory actions of ephedrines in acute inflammations. Planta Medica 54:325–331, 1985

28. American Pharmaceutical Association: Handbook of Nonprescription Drugs, 8th ed. American Pharmaceutical Association, Washington, DC, 1986

29. Tinkelman D G and Avner S E: Ephedrine therapy in asthmatic children. JAMA 237:553–557, 1977

Chapter 8 — Blood Pressure–Lowering Medications

1. Medical Research Council Working Party on Mild Hypertension: MRC trial of treatment of mild hypertension: principal results. Br Med J 291:97–104, 1980

2. Report by the management committee: The Australian therapeutic trial in mild hypertension. Lancet. i:1261–1267, 1980

3. Veterans Administration Cooperative Study Group on Antihypertensive Agents: Effects of treatment on morbidity in hypertension: II, Results of patients with diastolic blood pressure averaging 90 through 114 mm Hg. JAMA 213:1143–1151, 1970

4. U.S. Public Health Service Hospitals Cooperative Study Group: Treatment of mild hypertension: Results of a ten-year intervention trial. Circ Res 40 (supplement I):I98–I105, 1977

5. Helgeland A: Treatment of mild hypertension: a five-year controlled drug trial, the Oslo study. Am J Med 69:725–732, 1980

6. Multiple Risk Factor Intervention Trial Research Group: Baseline rest electrocardiographic abnormalities, antihypertensive treatment, and mortality in the Multiple Risk Factor Intervention Trial. Am J Cardiol 55:1–15, 1985

7. Miettinen T A: Multifactorial primary prevention of cardiovascular diseases in middle-aged men—risk factor changes, incidence, and mortality. JAMA 254:2097–2102, 1985

8. Amery A, Birkenhager W, Brixko P, et al.: Mortality and morbidity results from European Working Party on High Blood Pressure in the Elderly Trial. Lancet i:1349–1354, 1985

9. Hypertension Detection and Follow-up Program Cooperative Group: Five-year findings of the Hypertension Detection and Follow-up Program, I. Reduction in mortality in persons with high blood pressure, including mild hypertension. JAMA 242:2562–2571, 1979

10. Freis E D: Rationale against the drug treatment of marginal diastolic systemic hypertension. Am J Cardiol 66:368–371, 1990

11. Alderman M H: Which antihypertensive drugs first—and why! JAMA 267:2786–2787, 1992

12. Rouse I L, Beilin L J, Mahoney D P, et al.: Vegetarian diet and blood pressure. Lancet ii:742–743, 1983

13. Lang T, Degoulet P, Aime F, et al.: Relationship between coffee

drinking and blood pressure: Analysis of 6,321 subjects in the Paris region. Am J Cardiol 52:1238–1242, 1983

14. Gruchow H W, Sobocinski M S, and Barboriak J J: Alcohol, nutrient intake, and hypertension in US adults. JAMA 253:1567–1570, 1985

15. Pierkle J L, Schwartz J, Landis J R, and Harlan W R: The relationship between blood lead levels and blood pressure and its cardiovascular risk implications. Am J Epidemiol 121:246–258, 1985

16. Glauser S, Bello C, and Gauser E: Blood-cadmium levels in normotensive and untreated hypertensive humans. Lancet i:717–718, 1976

17. Kaplan N M: Non-drug treatment of hypertension. Ann Int Med 102:359–373, 1985

18. Trowell H, Burkitt D, and Heaton K: Dietary Fibre, Fibre-depleted Foods and Disease. Academic Press, New York, NY, 1985

19. Iimura O, Kijima T, Kikuchi K, et al.: Studies on the hypotensive effect of high potassium intake in patients with essential hypertension. Clin Sci 61(Supplement 7):77s–80s, 1981

20. Khaw K T and Barrett-Connor: Dietary potassium and blood pressure in a population. Am J Clin Nutr. 39:963–968, 1984

21. Skrabal F, Aubock J, and Hortnagl H: Low sodium/high potassium diet for prevention of hypertension: Probable mechanisms of action. Lancet ii:895–900, 1981

22. Meneely G and Battarbee H: High sodium–low potassium environment and hypertension. Am J Cardiol 38:768–781, 1976

23. Singer P: Alpha-linolenic acid vs. long-chain n-3 fatty acids in hypertension and hyperlipidemia. Nutr 8:133–135, 1992

24. Knapp H R: Omega-3 fatty acids, endogenous prostaglandins, and blood pressure regulation in humans. Nutr Rev 47:301–313, 1989

25. Kendler B S: Garlic (Allium sativum) and onion (Allium cepa): A review of their relationship to cardiovascular disease. Prev Med 16:670–685, 1987

26. Foushee D, Ruffin J, and Banerjee U: Garlic as a natural agent for the treatment of hypertension: A preliminary report. Cytobios 34:145–152, 1982

27. Yoshioka M, Matsushita T, and Chuman Y: Inverse association of serum ascorbic acid level and blood pressure or rate of hypertension in male adults aged 30–39 years. Int J Vit Nutr Res 54:343–347, 1984

28. McCarron D A and Morris C D: Epidemiological evidence associating dietary calcium and calcium metabolism with blood pressure. Am J Nephrol 6(Supplement 1):3–9, 1986

29. Whelton P K and Klag J: Magnesium and blood pressure: Review of the epidemiologic and clinical trial experience. Am J Cardiol 63:26G–30G, 1989

30. Sowers J R, Zemel M B, Standley P R, and Zemel P C: Calcium and hypertension. J Lab Clin Med 114:338–348, 1989

31. Motoyama T, Sano H, and Fukuzaki H: Oral magnesium supplementation in patients with essential hypertension. Hypertension 13:227–232, 1989

32. Ammon HPT and Handel M: Crataegus, toxicology and pharmacology. Planta Medica 43:101–120, 318–322, 1981

33. Murray M T: The Healing Power of Herbs. Prima Publishing. Rocklin, CA, 1991

Chapter 9 — Cholesterol-Lowering Medications

1. National Research Council: Diet and Health, Implications for Reducing Chronic Disease Risk. National Academy Press, Washington, DC, 1989

2. Wilson PWF: High-density lipoprotein, low-density lipoprotein and coronary artery disease. Am J Cardiol 66:7A–10A, 1990

3. Stamler J and Shekelle R: Dietary cholesterol and human coronary artery disease. Arch Pathol Lab Med 112:1032–1040, 1988

4. The Expert Panel: Report of the National Cholesterol Education Program Expert Panel on detection, evaluation, and treatment of high cholesterol in adults. Arch Int Med 148:136–169, 1988

5. Committee of Principal Investigators: World Health Organization Clofibrate Trial: A co-operative trial in the primary prevention of ischemic heart disease using clofibrate. Br Heart J 40:1069–1118, 1978

6. Schauss A: Dietary Fish Oil Consumption and Fish Oil Supplementation. In: A Textbook of Natural Medicine. Pizzorno J E and Murray M T (eds), V:Fish Oils:1–7. Bastyr College Publications, Seattle, WA, 1991

7. Von Schacky C: Prophylaxis of atherosclerosis with marine omega-3 fatty acids, a comprehensive strategy. Ann Int Med 107:890–899, 1987

8. Cobias L, Clifton P S, Abbey M, et al.: Lipid, lipoprotein, and hemostatic effects of fish vs. fish oil w-3 fatty acids in mildly hyperlipidemic males. Am J Clin Nutr 53:1210–1216, 1991

9. Fraser G E, Sabate J, Beeson W L, and Strahan T M: A possible protective effect of nut consumption on risk of coronary heart disease. Arch Int Med 152:1416–1424, 1992

10. Mensink R P and Katan M B: Effect of dietary trans-fatty acids on high-density and low-density lipoprotein cholesterol levels in health subjects. New Eng J Med 323:439–445, 1990

11. Robertson J, Brydon W G, Tadesse K, et al.: The effect of raw carrot on serum lipids and colon function. Am J Clin Nutr 32:1889–1892, 1979

12. Stanto J L and Keast D R: Serum cholesterol, fat intake, and breakfast consumption in the United States adult population. J Am Coll Nutr 8:567–572, 1989

13. Ripsin C M, Keenan J M, Jacobs D R, et al.: Oat products and lipid lowering, a meta-analysis. JAMA 267:3317–3325, 1992

14. Cerda J, Robbins F L, Burgin C W, et al.: The effects of grapefruit pectin on patients at risk for coronary heart disease without altering diet or lifestyle. Clin Cardiol 11:589–594, 1988

15. Ornish D, Brown S E, Scherwitz L W, et al.: Can lifestyle changes reverse coronary heart disease. Lancet 336:129–133, 1990

16. Resnicow K, Barone J, Engle A, et al.: Diet and serum lipids in vegan vegetarians: A model for risk reduction. J Am Diet Assoc 91:447–453, 1991

17. The Coronary Drug Project Group: Clofibrate and niacin in coronary heart disease. JAMA 231:360–381, 1975

18. Canner P L and the Coronary Drug Project Group: Mortality in Coronary Drug Project patients during a nine-year post-treatment period. J Am Coll Cardiol 8:1245–1255, 1986

19. Henkin Y, Johnson K C, and Segrest J P: Rechallenge with crystalline niacin after drug-induced hepatitis from sustained-release niacin. JAMA 264:241–243, 1990

20. Welsh A L and Ede M: Inositol hexanicotinate for improved nicotinic acid therapy. Int Record Med 174:9–15, 1961

21. El-Enein AMA, Hafez Y S, Salem H, and Abdel M: The role of nicotinic acid and inositol hexaniacinate as anticholesterolemic and antilipemic agents. Nutr Rep Intl 28:899–911, 1983

22. Sunderland G T, Belch JJF, Sturrock R D, et al.: A double-blind randomised placebo-controlled trial of hexopal in primary Raynaud's disease. Clin Rheumatol 7:46–49, 1988

23. Satyavati G V: Gum guggul (Commiphora mukul)—The success

story of an ancient insight leading to a modern discovery. Ind J Med Res 87:327–335, 1988

24. Nityanand S, Srivastava J S, and Asthana O P: Clinical trials with gugulipid, a new hypolipidaemic agent. J Assoc Phys India 37:321–328, 1989

25. Lau B H, Adetumbi M A, and Sanchez A: Allium sativum (garlic) and atherosclerosis: a review. Nutr Res 3:119–128, 1983

26. Arsenio L, Bodria P, Magnati G, et al.: Effectiveness of long-term treatment with pantethine in patients with dyslipidemias. Clin Ther 8:537–545, 1986

27. Gaddi A, Descovich G, Noseda G, et al.: Controlled evaluation of pantethine, a natural hypolipidemic compound, in patients with different forms of hyperlipoproteinemia. Atheroscl 50:73–83, 1984

28. Kelley M D: Hypercholesterolemia: The cost of treatment in perspective. Sout Med J 83:1421–1425, 1991

Chapter 10 — Common-Cold Medications

1. Hutton N, Wilson M H, Mellits E D, et al.: Effectiveness of an antihistamine-decongestant combination for young children with the common cold: A randomized, controlled clinical trial. J Pediatr 118:125–130, 1991

2. Gaffey M J, Kaiser D L, and Hayden F G: Ineffectiveness of oral terfenadine in antural colds: evidence against histamine as a mediator of common cold symptoms. Pediatr Infect Dis J 7:223–228, 1988

3. Graham NMH, Burrell C J, Douglas R M, et al.: Adverse effects of aspirin, acetaminophen, and ibuprofen on immune function, viral shedding, and clinical status in rhinovirus-infected volunteers. J Infect Dis 162:1277–1282, 1990

4. Sanchez A, Reeser J, Lau H, et al.: Role of sugars in human neutrophilic phagocytosis. Am J Clin Nutr 26:1180–1184, 1973

5. Pauling L: Vitamin C and the Common Cold. Freeman, San Francisco, CA, 1970

6. Hemila H: Vitamin C and the common cold. Br J Nutr 67:3–16, 1992

7. Baird I, Hughes R, Wilson H, et al.: The effects of ascorbic acid and

flavonoids on the occurrence of symptoms normally associated with the common cold. Am J Clin Nutr 32:1686–1690, 1979

8. Eby G A, Davis D R, and Halcomb W W: Reduction in duration of common colds by zinc gluconate lozenges in a double-blind study. Antimicrob Agents Chemother 25:20–24, 1984

9. Murray M T: The Healing Power of Herbs. Prima Publishing, Rocklin, CA, 1991

10. Abe N, Ebina T, and Ishida N: Interferon induction by glycyrrhizin and glycyrrhetinic acid in mice. Microbiol Immunol 26:535–539, 1982

11. Chang H M and But PPH: Pharmacology and Applications of Chinese Materia Medica, Volume 2, pp 1041–1046. World Scientific Publishing, Teaneck, NJ, 1987

Chapter 11 — Corticosteroids

1. Kershner P and Wang-Cheng R: Psychiatric side effects of steroid therapy. Psychosomatics 30:135–139, 1989

2. Brostoff J and Challacombe S J (eds.): Food Allergy and Intolerance. W B Saunders, Philadelphia, PA, 1987

3. Workman E M, Jones A, Wilson A J, and Hunter J O: Diet in the management of Crohn's disease. Human Nutr: Applied Nutr 38A:469–473, 1984

4. Jones V A, Workman E, Freeman A H, et al.: Crohn's disease: maintenance of remission by diet. Lancet ii:177–180, 1985

5. Schauss A: Dietary fish oil consumption and fish oil supplementation, In: A Textbook of Natural Medicine. Pizzorno J E and Murray M T (eds.). V:Fish Oils:1–7 Bastyr College Publications, Seattle, WA, 1991

6. Simopoulos A P: Summary of the NATO Advanced Research Workshop on Dietary w₃ and 26 Fatty Acids: Biological effects and nutritional essentiality. J Nutr 119:521–528, 1989

7. Kendler B S: Gamma-linolenic acid: physiological effects and potential medical applications. J Appl Nutr 39:79–93, 1987

8. Swank R L and Pullen M H: The Multiple Sclerosis Diet Book. Doubleday, Garden City, NY, 1977

9. Swank R L: Multiple sclerosis: Fat-oil relationship. Nutr 7:368–376, 1991

10. Ransberger K: Enzyme treatment of immune complex diseases. Arthr Rheum 8:16–19, 1986

11. Ransberger K and van Schaik W: Enzyme therapy in multiple sclerosis. Der Kassenarzt 41:42–45, 1986

12. Taussig S and Batkin S: Bromelain: The enzyme complex of pineapple (Ananas comosus) and its clinical application, an update. J Ethnopharm 22:191–203, 1988

13. Murray M T: Healing Power of Herbs. Prima Publishing, Rocklin, CA, 1991

14. Ammon HPT and Wahl M A: Pharmacology of Curcuma longa. Planta Medica 57:1–7, 1991

Chapter 12 — Cortisone Creams, Lotions, and Ointments

1. Sloper K S, Wadsworth J, and Brostoff J: Children with atopic eczema, I: Clinical response to food elimination and subsequent double-blind food challenge. Quart J Med 80:677–693, 1991

2. Biagi P L, Bordini A, Masi M, et al.: A long-term study on the use of evening primrose oil (Efamol) in atopic children. Drugs Exptl Clin Res 4:285–290, 1988

3. Proctor M, Wilkenson D, Orenberg E, et al.: Lowered cutaneous and urinary levels of polyamines with clinical improvement in treated psoriasis. Arch Dermatol 115:945–949, 1979

4. Rosenberg E and Belew P: Microbial factors in psoriasis. Arch Dermatol 118:1434–1444, 1982

5. Lithell H, Bruce A, Gustafsson B, et al.: A fasting and vegetarian diet treatment trial on chronic inflammatory disorders. Acta Derm Vener (StockH) 63:397–403, 1983

6. Maurice PDL, Allen B R, Barkley ASJ, et al.: The effects of dietary supplementation with fish oil in patients with psoriasis. Br J Dermatol 1117:599–606, 1987

7. Bittiner S B, Tucker WFG, Cartwright I, and Bleehen S S: A double-blind, randomized, placebo-controlled trial of fish oil in psoriasis. Lancet i:378–380, 1988

8. Monk B E and Neill S M: Alcohol consumption and psoriasis. Dermatologica 173:57–60, 1986

9. Evans F Q: The rational use of glycyrrhetinic acid in dermatology. Br J Clin Practice 12:269–79, 1958

10. Kumagai A, Nanaboshi M, Asanuma Y, et al.: Effects of glycyrrhizin on thymolytic and immunosuppressive action of cortisone. Endocrinol Japon 14:39–42, 1967

11. Okimasa E, Moromizato Y, Watanabe S, et al.: Inhibition of phospholipase A_2 by glycyrrhizin, an anti-inflammatory drug. Acta Med Okayama 37:385–391, 1983

12. Mann C and Staba E J: The chemistry, pharmacology, and commercial formulations of chamomile. Herbs, Spices, and Medicinal Plants 1:235–280, 1984

13. Weber G and Galle K: The liver, a therapeutic target in dermatoses. Med Welt 34:108–111, 1983

Chapter 13 — Diabetes Medications

1. University Group Diabetes Program: A story of the effectiveness of hypoglycemic agents on vascular complications in patients with adult-onset diabetes: II, Mortality results. Diabetes 19:789–830, 1970

2. Burkitt D and Trowell H: Western Diseases: Their Emergence and Prevention. Harvard Univ Press, Cambridge, MA, 1981

3. National Research Council: Diet and Health, Implications for Reducing Chronic Disease Risk. National Academy Press, Washington, DC, 1989

4. Anderson J: Diabetes. A Practical Approach to Daily Living. Arco Press, New York, NY, 1981

5. Anderson J W and Ward K: High-carbohydrate, high-fiber diets for insulin-treated men with diabetes mellitus. Am J Clin Nutr 32:2312–2321, 1979

6. Simpson HCR, Simpson R W, Lousley S, et al.: A high-carbohydrate leguminous-fiber diet improves all aspects of diabetic control. Lancet 1:1–5, 1981

7. Hughes T, Gwynne J, Switzer B, et al.: Effects of caloric restriction

and weight loss on glycemic control, insulin release and resistance and atherosclerotic risk in obese patients with type II diabetes mellitus. Am J Med 77:7–17, 1984

8. Mooradian A D and Morley J E: Micronutrient status in diabetes mellitus. Am J Clin Nutr 45:877–895, 1987

9. Murray M T and Pizzorno J E: Encyclopedia of Natural Medicine. Prima Publishing, Rocklin, CA, 1990

10. Anderson R A: Chromium, glucose tolerance, and diabetes. Biol Trace Element Res 32:19–24, 1992

11. Urberg M and Zemel M B: Evidence for synergism between chromium and nicotinic acid in the control of glucose tolerance in elderly humans. Metabolism 36:896–899, 1987

12. Vallerand A L, Cuerrier J P, Shapcott D, et al.: Influence of exercise training on tissue chromium concentrations in the rat. Am J Clin Nutr 39:402–409, 1984

13. Ceriello A, Giugliano D, Russo P D, and Passariello N: Hypomagnesemia in relation to diabetic retinopathy. Diabetes Care 5:558–559, 1982

14. Coggeshall J C, Heggers J P, Robson M C, and Baker H: Biotin status and plasma glucose in diabetics. Ann NY Acad Sci 447:389–392, 1985

15. Bever B O and Zahnd G R: Plants with oral hypoglycemic action. Quart J Crude Drug Res 17:139–196, 1979

16. Murray M T: Healing Power of Herbs. Prima Publishing, Rocklin, CA, 1991

17. Welihinda J, Arvidson G, Gylfe E, et al.: The insulin-releasing activity of the tropical plant Momordica charantia. Acta Biol Med Germ 41:1229–1240, 1982

18. Sharma K K, Gupta R K, Gupta S, and Samuel K C: Antihyperglycemic effect of onion: effect on fasting blood sugar and induced hyperglycemia in man. Ind J Med Res 65:422–429, 1977

19. Shanmugasundaram ERB, Rajeswari G, Baskaran K, et al.: Use of Gymnema sylvestre leaf extract in the control of blood glucose in insulin-dependent diabetes mellitus. J Ethnopharm 30:281–294, 1990

20. Baskaran K, Ahamath B K, Shanmugasundaram K R, and Shanmugasundaram ERB: Antidiabetic effect of a leaf extract from Gymnema sylvestre in non-insulin-dependent diabetes mellitus patients. J Ethnopharm 30:295–305, 1990

Chapter 14 — Gout Medications

1. Faller J and Fox I H: Ethanol-induced hyperuricemia. New Eng J Med 307:1598–1602, 1982
2. Blau L W: Cherry diet control for gout and arthritis. Tex Report Biol Med 8:309–311, 1950
3. Bindoli A, Valente M, and Cavallini L: Inhibitory action of quercetin on xanthine oxidase and xanthine dehydrogenase activity. Pharmacol Res Comm 17:831–839, 1985
4. Busse W W, Kopp D E and Middleton E: Flavonoid modulation of human neutrophil function. J Allergy Clin Immunol 73:801–809, 1984
5. Lewis A S, Murphy L, McCalla C, et al.: Inhibition of mammalian xanthine oxidase by folate compounds and amethopterin. J Biol Chem 259:12–15, 1984
6. Oster K A: Xanthine oxidase and folic acid. Ann Int Med 87:252, 1977
7. Ball G V and Sorensen L B: Pathogenesis of hyperuricemia in saturnine gout. New Eng J Med 280:1199–1202, 1969

Chapter 15 — Headache Medications

1. Brostoff J and Challacombe S J (eds.): Food Allergy and Intolerance. W B Saunders, Philadelphia, PA, 1987
2. Mansfield L E, Vaughan T R, Waller S T, et al.: Food allergy and adult migraine: Double-blind and mediator confirmation of an allergic etiology. Ann Allergy 55:126–129, 1985
3. Carter C M, Egger J, and Soothill J F: A dietary management of severe childhood migraine. Hum Nutr: Appl Nutr 39A:294–303, 1985
4. Hughes E C, Gott P S, Weinstein R C, and Binggeli R: Migraine: A diagnostic test for etiology of food sensitivity by a nutritionally supported fast and confirmed by long-term report. Ann Allergy 55:28–32, 1985
5. Egger J, Carter C M, Wilson J, et al.: Is migraine food allergy? Lancet ii:865–869, 1983
6. Monro J, Brostoff J, Carini C, and Zilkha K: Food allergy in migraine. Lancet ii:1–4, 1980

7. Littlewood J T, Glover V, and Sandler M: Red wine contains a potent inhibitor of phenolsulphotransferase. Br J Clin Pharm 19:275–278, 1985
8. Swanson D R: Migraine and magnesium: Eleven neglected connections. Perspect Biol Med 31:526–557, 1988
9. Ramadan N M, Halvorson H, Vande-Linde A, et al.: Low brain magnesium in migraine. Headache 29:590–593, 1989
10. Galland L D, Baker S M, and McLellan R K: Magnesium deficiency in the pathogenesis of mitral valve prolapse. Magnesium 5:165–174, 1986
11. Fernandes J S, Pereira T, Carvalho J, et al.: Therapeutic effect of a magnesium salt in patients suffering from mitral valvular prolapse and latent tetany. Magnesium 4:283–289, 1985
12. Johnson E S, Kadam N P, Hylands D M, and Hylands P J: Efficacy of feverfew as prophylactic treatment of migraine. Br Med J 291:569–573, 1985
13. Murphy J J, Heptinstall S, and Mitchell JRA: Randomized double-blind placebo-controlled trial of feverfew in migraine prevention. Lancet ii:189–192, 1988
14. Murray M T: The Healing Power of Herbs. Prima Publishing, Rocklin, CA, 1991

Chapter 16 — Laxatives

1. Sonnenberg A and Koch T R: Epidemiology of constipation in the United States. Dis Colon Rectum 32:1–8, 1989
2. Leicester R and Hunt R: Peppermint oil to reduce colonic spasm during endoscopy. Lancet ii:989, 1982
3. Somerville K, Richmond C, and Bell G: Delayed-release peppermint oil capsules (Colpermin) for the spastic colon syndrome: a pharmacokinetic study. Br J Clin Pharmacol 18:638–640, 1984
4. Rees W, Evans B, and Rhodes J: Treating irritable bowel syndrome with peppermint oil. Br Med J ii:835–836, 1979

Chapter 17–Peptic Ulcer Medications

1. Ateshkadi A, Lam N P, and Johnson C A: Helicobacter pylori and peptic ulcer disease. Clin Pharm 12:34–48, 1993

2. Rydning A, Berstad A, Aadland E, and Odegaard B: Prophylactic effects of dietary fiber in duodenal ulcer disease. Lancet 2:736–739, 1982

3. Kang J Y, Tay H H, Guan R, et al.: Dietary supplementation with pectin in the maintenance treatment of duodenal ulcer. Scand J Gastroenterol 23:95–99, 1988

4. Harju E and Larme T K: Effect of guar gum added to the diet of patients with duodenal ulcers. J Parenteral Enteral Nutr 9:496–500, 1985

5. Andre C, Moulinier B, Andre F, and Daniere S: Evidence for anaphylactic reactions in peptic ulcer and varioliform gastritis. Ann Allergy 51:325–328, 1983

6. Siegel J: Immunologic approach to the treatment and prevention of gastrointestinal ulcers. Ann Allergy 38:27–29, 1977

7. Kumar N, Kumar A, Broor S L, et al.: Effect of milk on patients with duodenal ulcers. Brit Med J 293:666, 1986

8. Werbach M R: Nutritional Influences on Illness. Third Line Press, Tarzana, CA, 1987

9. Cheney G: Rapid healing of peptic ulcers in patients receiving fresh cabbage juice. Cal Med 70:10–14, 1949

10. Cheney G: Anti-peptic ulcer dietary factor. J Am Diet Assoc 26:668–672, 1950

11. Glick L: Deglycrrhizinated liquorice in peptic ulcer. Lancet ii:817, 1982

12. Tewari S N and Wilson A K: Deglycyrrhizinated liquorice in duodenal ulcer. Practitioner 210:820–825, 1972

13. Morgan A G, McAdam WAF, Pacsoo C, and Darnborough A: Comparison between cimetidine and Caved-S in the treatment of gastric ulceration, and subsequent maintenance therapy. Gut 23:545–551, 1982

14. Kassir Z A: Endoscopic controlled trial of four drug regimens in the treatment of chronic duodenal ulceration. Irish Med J 78:153–156, 1985

15. Turpie A G, Runcie J, and Thomson T J: Clinical trial of deglycyrrhizinated liquorice in gastric ulcer. Gut 10:299–303, 1969

16. Rees WDW, Rhodes J, Wright J E, et al.: Effect of deglycyrrhizinated

liquorice on gastric mucosal damage by aspirin. Scand J Gastroenterol
14:605–607, 1979

Chapter 18 — Prostate Medications

1. Hinman F: Benign Prostatic Hyperplasia. Springer-Verlag, New
York, 1983
2. Fahim M, Fahim Z, Der R, and Harman J: Zinc treatment for the
reduction of hyperplasia of the prostate. Fed Proc 35:361, 1976
3. Hart J P and Cooper W L: Vitamin F in the treatment of prostatic
hyperplasia. Report Number 1, Lee Foundation for Nutritional Research, Milwaukee, WI, 1941
4. Scott W W: The lipids of the prostatic fluid, seminal plasma and
enlarged prostate gland of man. J Urol 53:712–718, 1945
5. Horton R: Benign prostatic hyperplasia: A disorder of androgen
metabolism in the male. J Am Geri Soc 32:380–385, 1984
6. DeRosa G, Corsello S M, Ruffilli M P, et al.: Prolactin secretion after
beer. Lancet 2:934, 1981
7. Judd A M, MacLeod R M, and Login I S: Zinc acutely, selectively and
reversibly inhibits pituitary prolactin secretion. Brain Res 294:190–192, 1984
8. Vescovi P P, Gerra G, Rastelli G, et al.: Pyridoxine (vit. B6) decreases
opiods-induced hyperprolactinemia. Horm Metabol Res 17:46–47, 1985
9. Dufour B, Choquenet C, Revol M, et al.: A clinical study of the effects
of an extract of Pygeum africanum on the functional symptoms of benign
prostatic hypertrophy. Ann Urol 18:193–195, 1984
10. Ranno S, Minaldi G, and Viscusi G: Efficacy and tolerability in the
treatment of prostatic adenoma with Tadenan 50. Progr Med
42:165–169, 1986
11. Ask-Upmark E: Prostatitis and its treatment. Acta Medica Scand
181:355–357, 1967
12. Ohkoshi M, Kawamura N, and Nagakubo I: Clinical evaluation of
Cernilton in chronic prostatitis. Jap J Clin Urol 21:73–85, 1967
13. Boccafoschi and Annoscia S: Comparison of Serenoa repens extract
with placebo by controlled clinical trial in patients with prostatic adeno-
matosis. Urologia 50:1257–1268, 1983
14. Cirillo-Marucco E, Pagliarulo A, Tritto G, et al.: Extract of Serenoa

repens (PermixonR) in the early treatment of prostatic hypertrophy. Urologia 5:1269–1277, 1983

15. Tripodi V, Giancaspro M, Pascarella M, et al.: Treatment of prostatic hypertrophy with Serenoa repens extract. Med Praxis 4:41–46, 1983

16. Emili E, Lo Cigno M, and Petrone U: Clinical trial of a new drug for treating hypertrophy of the prostate (Permixon). Urologia 50:1042–1048, 1983

17. Greca P and Volpi R: Experience with a new drug in the medical treatment of prostatic adenoma. Urologia 52:532–535, 1985

18. Duvia R, Radice G P, and Galdini R: Advances in the phytotherapy of prostatic hypertrophy. Med Praxis 4:143–148, 1983

19. Tasca A, Barulli M, Cavazzana A, et al.: Treatment of obstructive symptomatology caused by prostatic adenoma with an extract of Serenoa repens. Double-blind clinical study vs. placebo. Minerva Urol Nefrol 37:87–91, 1985

20. Cukier (Paris), Ducassou (Marseille), Le Guillou (Bordeaux), et al.: Permixon versus placebo. C R Ther Pharmacol Clin 4/25:15–21, 1985

21. Crimi A and Russo A: Extract of Serenoa repens for the treatment of the functional disturbances of prostate hypertrophy. Med Praxis 4:47–51, 1983

22. Champlault G, Patel J C, and Bonnard A M: A double-blind trial of an extract of the plant Serenoa repens in benign prostatic hyperplasia. Br J Clin Pharmacol 18:461–462, 1984

23. Champault G, Bonnard A M, Cauquil J, and Patel J C: Medical treatment of prostatic adenoma. Controlled trial: PA 109 vs placebo in 110 patients. Ann Urol 18:407–410, 1984

24. Mattei F M, Capone M, and Acconcia A.: Serenoa repens extract in the medical treatment of benign prostatic hypertrophy. Urologia 55:547–552, 1988

25. Bassi P, Artibani W, De Luca V, et al.: Standardized Pygeum africanum extract in the treatment of benign prostatic hypertrophy. Min Urol Nefrol 39:45–50, 1987

26. Buck A C, Rees RWM, and Ebeling L: Treatment of chronic prostatitis and prostadynia with pollen extract. Br J Urol 64:496–499, 1989

27. Dumrau F: Benign prostatic hyperplasia: Amino acid therapy for symptomatic relief. Am J Geriat 10:426–430, 1962

28. Feinblatt H M and Gant J C: Palliative treatment of benign prostatic hypertrophy: Value of glycine, alanine, glutamic acid combination. J Maine Med Assn 49:99–102, 1958

Chapter 19 — Sedative Medications

1. Kalow W: Variability of caffeine metabolism in humans. Arzneim Forsch 35:319–324, 1985

2. Leathwood P D, Chauffard F, Heck E, and Munoz-Box R: Aqueous extract of valerian root (valeriana officianalis L.) improves sleep quality in man. Pharmacol Biochem Behavior 17:65–71, 1982

3. Leathwood P D and Chauffard F: Aqueous extract of valerian reduces latency to fall asleep in man. Planta Medica 54:144–148, 1985

4. Lindahl O and Lindwall L: Double blind study of a valerian preparation. Pharmacol Biochem Behavior 32:1065–1066, 1989

5. Griffiths W, Lester B, Coulter J, and Williams H: Tryptophan and sleep in young adults. Psychophysiology 9:345–356, 1972

6. Wyatt R, Engelman K, Kupffer D, et al.: Effects of L-tryptophan (a natural sedative) on human sleep. Lancet ii:842–846, 1970

7. Hartman E: L-tryptophan: A rational hypnotic with clinical potential. Am J Psychiatry 134:366–370, 1977

8. Roufs J B: Review of L-tryptophan and eosinophilia-myalgia syndrome. J Am Diet Assn 92:844–850, 1992

9. Caston J C, Roufs J B, Forgarty C M, et al.: Treatment of refractory eosinophilia-myalgia syndrome associated with the ingestion of L-tryptophan–containing products. Adv Ther 7:206–228, 1990

10. Botez M, Cadotte M, Beaulieu R, and Pichette L: Neurologic disorders responsive to folic acid therapy. Can Med Assn J 115:217–223, 1976

Chapter 20 — Weight-Loss Aids

1. Anderson J W and Bryant C A: Dietary fiber: diabetes and obesity. Am J Gastroenterol 81:898–906, 1986

2. Hylander B and Rossner S: Effects of dietary fiber intake before meals on weight loss and hunger in a weight-reducing club. Acta Medica Scand 213:217–220, 1983

3. Rossner S, Zweigbergk D V, Ohlin A, and Ryttig K: Weight reduction

with dietary fibre supplements: Results of two double-blind studies. Acta Medica Scand 222:83–88, 1987

4. El-Shebini S M, Hanna L M, Topouzada S T, et al.: The role of pectin as a slimming agent. J Clin Biochem Nutr 4:255–262, 1988

5. Krotkiewski M: Effect of guar gum on body-weight, hunger ratings and metabolism in obese subjects. Br J Nutr 52:97–105, 1984

6. Halama W H and Maudlin J L: Distal esophageal obstruction due to a guar gum preparation. South Med J 85:642–646, 1992

7. Arch JRS, Ainsworth A T, and Cawthorne M A: Thermogenic and anorectic effects of ephedrine and congeners in mice and rats. Life Sci 30:1817–1826, 1982

8. Massoudi M and Miller D S: Ephedrine, a thermogenic and potential slimming drug. Proc Nutr Soc 36:135A, 1977

9. Dulloo A G and Miller D S: The thermogenic properties of ephedrine/methylxanthine mixtures: animal studies. Am J Clin Nutr 43:388–394, 1986

10. Dulloo A G and Miller D S: The thermogenic properties of ephedrine/methylxanthine mixtures: human studies. Int J Obesity 10:467–481, 1986

11. Astrup A, Breum L, Toubro S, et al.: The effect and safety of an ephedrine/caffeine compound compared to ephedrine, caffeine and placebo in obese subjects on an energy restricted diet, a double-blind trial. Int J Obesity 16:269–277, 1992

12. Kalow W: Variability of caffeine metabolism in humans. Arzneim Forsch 35:319–324, 1985

Chapter 21 — Building a Positive Mental Attitude

1. Peterson C: Explanatory style as a risk factor for illness. Cognitive Therap Res 12:117–130, 1988

2. Peterson C, Seligman M, and Valliant G: Pessimistic explanatory style as a risk factor for physical illness: A thirty-five year longitudinal study. J Person Soc Psych 55:23–27, 1988

3. Seligman M E: Learned Optimism. Alfred A. Knopf, New York, NY, 1990

Chapter 22 — Designing a Healthful Diet

1. Trowell H, Burkitt D, and Heaton K: Dietary Fibre, Fibre-depleted Foods and Disease. Academic Press, New York, NY, 1985
2. U.S. Dept. of Health and Human Services: The Surgeon General's Report on Nutrition and Health. Prima Press, Rocklin, CA, 1988
3. National Research Council: Diet and Health, Implications for Reducing Chronic Disease Risk. National Academy Press, Washington, DC, 1989
4. Murray M T and Pizzorno J E: Encyclopedia of Natural Medicine. Prima Press, Rocklin, CA, 1991
5. Brostoff J and Challacombe S J (eds.): Food Allergy and Intolerance. W B Saunders, Philadelphia, PA, 1987

Chapter 23 — The Importance of Exercise

1. Pollack M L, Wilmore J H and Fox S M: Exercise in Health and Disease. W B Saunders, Philadelphia, PA, 1984.
2. Farmer M E, Locke B Z, Mosciki E K, et al.: Physical activity and depressive symptomatology: The NHANES 1 epidemiologic follow-up study. Am J Epidemiol 1328:1340–1351, 1988
3. Wilmore J H: Alterations in strength, body composition and athropometric measurements consequent to a 10-week weight training program. Med Sci Sports 6:133–138, 1974
4. Ballor D L, Katch V L, Becque M D and Marks C R: Resistance weight training during calorie restriction enhances lean body weight maintenance. Am J Clin Nutr 47:19–25, 1988

Chapter 24 — A Quick Guide to Nutritional Supplements

1. Block G, Cox C, Madans J, et al.: Vitamin supplement use, by demographic characteristics. Am J Epidemiol 127:297–309, 1988

2. National Research Council: Diet and Health. Implications for Reducing Chronic Disease Risk. National Academy Press, Washington, DC, 1989

3. National Research Council: Recommended Dietary Allowances, 10th ed. National Academy Press, Washington, DC, 1989

4. Benton D and Roberts G: Effect of vitamin and mineral supplementation on intelligence of a sample of schoolchildren. Lancet 1:140–143, 1988

5. Chandra R K: Effect of vitamin and trace-element supplementation on immune responses and infection in elderly subjects. Lancet 340:1124–1127, 1992

Chapter 25 — A Quick Guide to Medicinal Herbs

1. Haller J S: A drug for all seasons, medical and pharmacological history of aloe. Bull NY Acad Sci 66:647–657, 1990

2. Klein A D and Penneys N S: Aloe vera. J Amer Acad Dermatol 18:714–719, 1988

3. Grindlay D and Reynolds T: The aloe vera leaf phenomena: A review of the properties and modern use of the leaf parenchyma gel. J Ethnopharmacol 16:117–151, 1986

4. Shelton R W: Aloe vera, its chemical and therapeutic properties. Int J Dermatol 30:679–683, 1991

5. McDaniel H R, Combs C, McDaniel R, et al.: An increase in circulating monocyte/macrophages (MM) is induced by oral acemannan (ACE-M) in HIV-1 patients. Am J Clin Pathol 94:516–517, 1990

6. Coget J M and Merlen J F: Anthocyanosides and microcirculation. J Mal Vasc 5:43–46, 1980

7. Amouretti M: Therapeutic value of Vaccinium myrtillus anthocyanosides in an internal medicine department. Therapeutique 48:579–581, 1972

8. Spinella G: Natural anthocyanosides in treatment of peripheral venous insufficiency. Arch Med Int 37:21–29, 1985

9. Scharrer A and Ober M: Anthocyanosides in the treatment of retinopathies. Klin Monatsbl Augenheilkd 178:386–389, 1981

10. Caselli L: Clinical and electroretinographic study on activity of anthocyanosides. Arch Med Int 37:29–35, 1985

11. Taussig S and Batkin S: Bromelain, the enzyme complex of pineapple (Ananas comosus) and its clinical application, an update. J Ethnopharmacol 22:191–203, 1988

12. Susnik F: Present state of knowledge of the medicinal plant Taraxacum officinale Weber. Med Razgledi 21:323–328, 1982

13. Duke J A and Ayensu E S: Medicinal Plants of China, pp 74–77. Reference Publications, Algonac, MI, 1985

14. Yoshiro K: The physiological actions of tang-kuei and cnidium. Bull Oriental Healing Arts Inst USA 10:269–278, 1985

15. Harada M, Suzuki M, and Ozaki Y: Effect of Japanese angelica root and peony root on uterine contraction in the rabbit in situ. J Pharm Dyn 7:304–311, 1984

16. Foster S: Echinacea, Nature's Immune Enhancer. Healing Arts Press, Rochester, VT, 1991

17. Bauer R and Wagner H: Echinacea species as potential immunostimulatory drugs. Economic and Med Plant Res 5:253–321, 1991

18. Pattrick M, Heptinstall S, and Doherty M: Feverfew in rheumatoid arthritis: A double blind, placebo controlled study. Ann Rheum Dis 48:547–549, 1989

19. Adetumbi M A and Lau B H: Allium sativum (garlic)—A natural antibiotic. Med Hypoth 12:227–237, 1983

20. Dausch J G and Nixon D W: Garlic: A review of its relationship to malignant disease. Prev Med 19:346–361, 1990

21. Mowrey D and Clayson D: Motion sickness, ginger, and psychophysics. Lancet i:655–657, 1982

22. Grontved A and Hentzer E: Vertigo-reducing effect of ginger root. ORL 48:282–286, 1986

23. Grontved A, Brask T, Kambskard J, and Hentzer E: Ginger root against seasickness: A controlled trial on the open sea. Acta Otolaryngol 105:45–49, 1988

24. Fischer-Rasmussen W, Kjaer S K, Dahl C, and Asping U: Ginger treatment of hyperemesis gravidarum. Eur J Ob Gyn Reproduct Biol 38:19–24, 1990

25. Srivastava K C and Mustafa T: Ginger (Zingiber officinale) and rheumatic disorders. Med Hypoth 29:25–28, 1989

26. Kleijnen J and Knipschild P: Ginkgo biloba for cerebral insufficiency. Br J Clin Pharamacol 34:352–358, 1992

27. Shibata S, Tanaka O, Shoji J, and Saito H: Chemistry and pharmacology of Panax. Economic Med Plant Res 1:217–284, 1985

28. Hallstrom C, Fulder S and Carruthers M: Effect of ginseng on the performance of nurses on night duty. Comp Med East & West 6:277–282, 1982

29. D'Angelo L, Grimaldi R, Caravaggi M, et al.: A double-blind, placebo-controlled clinical study on the effect of a standardized ginseng extract on psychomotor performance in healthy volunteers. J Ethnopharmacol 16:15–22, 1986

30. Farnsworth N R, Kinghorn A D, Soejarto D D, and Waller D P: Siberian ginseng (Eleutherococcus senticosus): current status as an adaptogen. Economic and Med Plant Res 1:156–215, 1985

31. Hahn F E and Ciak J: Berberine. Antibiotics 3:577–588, 1976

32. Amin A H, Subbaiah T V, and Abbasi K M: Berberine sulfate: Antimicrobial activity, bioassay, and mode of action. Can J Microbiol 15:1067–1076, 1969

33. Sun D, Courtney H S, and Beachey E H: Berberine sulfate blocks adherence of Streptococcus pyogenes to epithelial cells, fibronectin, and hexadecane. Antimicrob Agents and Chemother 32:1370–1374, 1988

34. Kamat S A: Clinical trial with berberine hydrochloride for the control of diarrhoea in acute gastroenteritis. J Assn Physicians India 15:525–529, 1967

35. Desai A B, Shah K M and Shah D M: Berberine in the treatment of diarrhoea. Ind Pediatr 8:462–465, 1971

36. Sharma R, Joshi C K, and Goyal R K: Berberine tannate in acute diarrhea. Ind Pediatr 7:496–501, 1970

37. Kartnig T: Clinical applications of Centella asiatica (L.) Urb Herbs Spices Medicinal Plants 3:146–173, 1988

38. Barletta S, Borgioli A and Corsi C: Results with Centella asiatica in chronic venous insufficiency. Gazz Med Ital 140:33–35, 1981

39. Willard T: Tabebuia Species. In: A Textbook of Natural Medicine, Chapter V:Tabebuia. Pizzorno J E and Murray M T (eds.), JBC Publications, Seattle, WA, 1987

40. Kumagai A, Nishino K, Shimomura A, Kin T, and Yamamura Y: Effect of glycyrrhizin on estrogen action. Endocrinol Japon 14:34–38, 1967

41. Armanini D, Karbowiak I, and Funder J: Affinity of liquorice derivatives for mineralocorticoid and glucocorticoid receptors. Clin Endocrinol 19:609–612, 1983

42. Abe N, Ebina T, and Ishida N: Interferon induction by glycyrrhizin and glycyrrhetinic acid in mice. Microbial Immunol 26:535–539, 1982

43. Cambar P, Shore S, and Aviado D: Bronchopulmonary and gastrointestinal effects of lobeline. Arch Int Pharmacodyn 177:1–27, 1969

44. Salmi H A and Sarna S: Effect of silymarin on chemical, functional, and morphological alteration of the liver. A double-blind controlled study. Scand J Gastroenterol 17:417–421, 1982

45. Scheiber V and Wohlzogen F X: Analysis of a certain type of 2 × 3 tables, exemplified by biopsy findings in a controlled clinical trial. Int J Clin Pharm 16:533–535, 1978

46. Meruelo D et al.: Therapeutic agents with dramatic antiretroviral activity and little toxicity at effective doses: Aromatic polycyclic diones hypericin and pseudohypericin. Proc Nat Acad Sci 85:5230–5234, 1988

47. Hobbs C: St. John's Wort, Hypericum perforatum L. HerbalGram 18/19:24–33, 1989

48. Proceedings from the 4th International Congress on Phytotherapy. Munich, Germany, September 10–13, 1992

49. Altman P M: Australian tea tree oil. Austral J Pharmacy 69:276–278, 1988

50. Merck Index, 10th ed., pp 796–797, p4721. Merck & Co, Rahway, NJ, 1983

51. Frohne V: Untersuchungen zur frage der harndesifizierenden wirkungen von barentraubenblatt-extracten. Planta Medica 18:1–25, 1970

INDEX